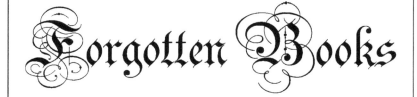

ISBN 978-1-397-30636-4
PIBN 11375359

1 MONTH OF
FREE
READING

at

www.ForgottenBooks.com

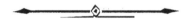

By purchasing this book you are eligible for one month membership to ForgottenBooks.com, giving you unlimited access to our entire collection of over 1,000,000 titles via our web site and mobile apps.

To claim your free month visit:
www.forgottenbooks.com/free1375359

THE

GLASGOW MEDICAL JOURNAL

EDITED BY

G. H. EDINGTON AND W. R. JACK

WITH THE ASSISTANCE OF

R. F. YOUNG (SUB-EDITOR OF "ABSTRACTS")

A. J. BALLANTYNE	L. FINDLAY
J. BROWNLEE	A. A. GRAY
R. M. BUCHANAN	R. MUIR
E. P. CATHCART	E. H. L. OLIPHANT
F. J. CHARTERIS	J. R. RIDDELL

FOR THE

Glasgow and West of Scotland Medical Association

JULY TO DECEMBER, 1914

VOL. LXXXII

GLASGOW:

ALEX. MACDOUGALL, 70 MITCHELL STREET

LONDON: H. K. LEWIS, 136 GOWER STREET

1914

THE

GLASGOW MEDICAL JOURNAL.

No. I. JULY, 1914.

ORIGINAL ARTICLES.

THE WORKING OF THE MIDWIVES ACT (ENGLAND, 1902).*

BY SIR FRANCIS HENRY CHAMPNEYS, BART., M.D., F.R.C.P.,
Honorary President of the Society ; Chairman of the Central Midwives Board.

LADIES AND GENTLEMEN,—In accordance with custom I am here to give, as your Honorary President, a discourse of some kind; and, in accordance with a suggestion from a leading member of your body, to talk to you to-night of the working of the Midwives Act in England.

The subject is a large one, and I would not consent to embark upon it did I not feel that I owe you something in return for the distinguished honour which you have done me.

No one except those who have actually done it can imagine the labour of setting in action the machinery expressed in a new Act of Parliament. Doing any new thing is laborious, but this has special difficulties of its own. Some of these will become apparent on consideration of the processes through which a Bill passes on its road to becoming an Act. It is, in the first place, drafted by a person of more or less skill.

In the first alternative possibilities of misreading and

* An Address delivered before the Obstetrical and Gynæcological Society of Glasgow, on Wednesday, 22nd April, 1914.

misunderstanding are reduced to a minimum. In this stage careful study will probably enable an intelligent person to realise in his imagination more or less completely the picture which existed in the mind of the draftsman. In the second alternative possibilities of misreading and misunderstanding are not anticipated, and the result is a picture which is blurred and which is capable of misreading and misunderstanding, to the detriment of the public and to the advantage of lawyers.

I remember an amusing experience of my own in illustration of this: Two distinguished gentlemen were dining with me, and, after the departure of the ladies, found themselves on either side of me. There had been a discusssion in the Courts on the meaning of an Act, and one of my guests, whom I will call A., remarked on 'the difficulty which had arisen, and on the obscurity of the Act. I (seeing difficulties ahead) said, "You can ask B., for I believe he drew it." "Do you draft these Bills," said A. "I do," said B. "Why do you make them so obscure," said A. "I make them as intelligible as is desirable," said B.

Well, to resume. When the Bill is presented to a Committee of its promoters it is "amended," as it is called. It may be improved, but is most likely to have its unity impaired; and, as this process goes on at every stage during its passage through Parliament, the picture is often so far distorted that those to whom it falls to set the Act in operation have to reconstruct the picture before they can do so; and this process of reconstruction is apt to be very difficult.

I hope, therefore, that those who eventually obtain a Bill for Scotland will have a kindly thought for those who have done their best to bring the Act into useful operation for England and Wales, and especially for my colleagues on the Central Midwives Board who have framed a code of rules in accordance with the Act, which has required very little revision since its first appearance, and is now of great value and utility.

Any help which I can give towards a Bill for Scotland will be willingly given.

What good has the Midwives Act done?—The answer to this question in the main lies in the statistics of the Registrar-General. It will be remembered that the appalling statistics of Matthews Duncan remained very little improved until the last few years.

In order to show the alteration which set in on the passing of the Midwives Act, I will quote from a statement by myself reported in the *Proceedings of the Royal Society of Medicine* (vol. iii, No. 9, July, 1910, pp. 231-2):—

"From Table A, giving the annual death-rates from puerperal sepsis per million of females living, it would be seen that the death-rate in 1902 was 118, and in 1907 it was 81. The census of 1901 showed that in England and Wales there were 16,800,000 women. The saving of life in 1907, as compared with 1902, was 37 per million. In other words, the lives of more than 621 women were saved in 1907, which would have been lost in 1902. Table B, calculated in the proportion of 1,000 births, showed the same thing, and these results were graphically set forth in diagrams A and B. Diagram C, showing the death-rates from puerperal sepsis and accidents of childbirth to 1,000 births, shows that this rate prior to 1903 was never below 4·41; in 1907 it was 3·83. Striking evidence was given before the Departmental Committee to the same effect. As regards infantile mortality, Dr. Robinson, of Rotherham, stated that while the death-rate in cases attended by midwives was 101 per 1,000 in 1907, the death-rate in cases not attended by midwives was 194; in 1908 the mortality in midwives cases was 92, in non-midwives cases 195."

I have been favoured by Dr. Stevenson, of the General Register Office, Somerset House, with a continuation of the figures up to and including 1911, and now give the calculation up to that date, which is arrived at by substituting the results of 1911 for those of 1907:—

"From Table A, giving the annual death-rates from puerperal sepsis per million of females living, it would be seen that the death-rate in 1902 was 118 and in 1911 it was 72. The census of 1911 showed that in England and Wales there were 18,672,986 women. The saving of life in 1911, as compared with 1902, was 46 per million. In other words, the lives of 859 women were saved in 1911 which would have been lost in 1902. Table C, showing the death-rates from puerperal sepsis and accidents of childbirth to 1,000 births, shows that this rate prior to 1903 was never below 4·41; in 1911 it was 3·67."

These figures show that the passing of the Midwives Act was followed by a sudden and considerable fall, and that the improvement since this has been gradual and comparatively slight.

It would seem that the great initial improvement in the puerperal mortality must have been due to improvement in the midwives; we may hope for still further improvement, not only in cases attended by midwives, but by medical practitioners, but can hardly expect so striking a change in the future.

Comments upon the Midwives Act (England and Wales), 1902, with references to the amending Bill of 1910 and the Bill for Scotland, 1912.

I shall not go through the whole Act, but shall only comment upon points of importance.

1. (2) England. Almost at the very outset a serious defect meets us in the qualifying words, "*habitually and for gain.*" By this clause a woman without education, training, or skill commits no offence in attending women in their confinements unless in can be proved that she does so (*a*) habitually, *and* (not "or") (*b*) for gain.

Both (*a*) and (*b*) have proved ambiguous, both have to be defined in any given case, and there is no authoritative definition of either. (*a*) "Habitually" may mean anything, and magistrates have declined to convict. (*b*) "For gain" is also indefinite. If payment is not demanded, and a money reward is given as a thank-offering, is that gain? Moreover, as above said, both (*a*) and (*b*) have to be proved before an offence is constituted.

I am glad to see that in the Bill for Scotland, 3 (2), these words are omitted. They are quite unnecessary, as the words at the end of the clause exempting "anyone rendering assistance in a case of emergency" completely cover all that is desirable.

1. (4) England. *Employment of uncertified substitute.*— This section has occasionally been invoked in order to interfere with *bonâ fide* training. The Board has always declined to endorse such a reading, which is manifestly absurd. On the other hand, the trainer is held fully responsible for the acts of her pupils.

3. *The constitution of the Board* (3. England, 5. Scotland).— I have little to say about this. It is obvious that midwives

and doctors should be represented; it is desirable that there should be a proportion of women; it is desirable that the great Government Departments concerned should be represented, including the Privy Council, which is the head of the whole machinery; and the Local Government Board, which is concerned in the administration of the Poor Law, and is in touch with the medical officers of health. Such representation is apt to prevent mutual misunderstanding, and to further the smooth working of the Act. But it is of the first importance that all who occupy seats on the Board should remember that the great aim of everyone concerned with the working of the Act should be, not the furtherance of the claims of constituents, but the guardianship of the lives and health of the poor mothers of our country. I am happy to say that I cannot remember an occasion when my Board has forgotten this primary duty.

I see that in the Bill for Scotland, as in the Amending Bill for England, 1910, a clause is inserted providing for the future revision of the constitution of the Board by a simple procedure not requiring the protracted machinery of an Act of Parliament. This should be helpful. (Scotland 6; Amending Bill, England 2.)

3 1. (*f*) England, prescribes among the duties of the Board that of deciding the conditions under which midwives may be suspended from practice.

8. (3) England, prescribes among the duties of the Local Supervising Authority that of "suspending any midwife from practice, in accordance with the rules under this Act, if such suspension appears necessary to prevent the spread of infection." Some difficulty is apt to arise under this head with the Local Supervising authority. Cases have occurred in which a midwife has been suspended indefinitely, which is not the intention of the Act, nor in the best interests of the community. A midwife who is infectious should be disinfected, and should then be allowed to resume her work. A midwife who has broken any rule of the Board regarding infection should be referred to the Board for penal proceedings.

In consequence of this the Central Midwives Board at the last revision of the rules framed an important Section F, which provides that all suspensions should be at once reported (with the grounds thereof) to the Board; and, also, that the period of suspension should not be longer that is required for adequate disinfection ; and that all suspensions longer than twenty-four hours should be at once reported, with reasons, to the Board, and should be subject to revision by the Board.

Both the Scottish Bill 8 (1) (*a*) and the English Amending Bill 8 (1) (*a*) provide powers for the Board to suspend a midwife in lieu of striking her name off the roll, and also to suspend her pending the decision of a penal case; also, (*b*) for the Local Supervising Authority which takes proceedings against a midwife, either before a Court of Justice or the Board, to suspend her from practice until the case had been decided. These rules should be very carefully considered in the light of our experience as above related. The proposal to compensate her for loss of practice (8 (2) in both) in suitable cases seems just.

Clause 9 (Scotland) and 9 (Amending Bill, England) provide power for the Board, if they think fit, to pay the expenses of any midwife summoned to appear before them. Such discretion would certainly be sometimes exercised in cases in which charges are proved to be frivolous or ill-founded.

Clause 10 (Scotland) and 10 (1) (England) enable the Board to prohibit any midwife removed from the roll from attending women in childbirth in any capacity (even as a monthly nurse). I highly approve of this power. No doubt the injunction would be used with discretion.

Clause 11 (Scotland) and 10 (2) Amending Bill (England) authorise a penalty of £5 for failing to surrender a certificate when called upon to do so. A very good and necessary regulation.

Clause 12 (Scotland) and 16 (England) provide for notification to local supervising authorities of the removal of names from the roll.

Clause 13 (Scotland) and 12 Amending Bill (England) provide for reciprocal treatment (a sort of *ad eundem* certification) of midwives certified in other parts of His Majesty's dominions, provided that the standard of training and examination is sufficient. This proviso is of great importance.

Clause 14 (Scotland) practically repeats Clause 9 (1) (Scotland) and 9 (1) Amending Bill (England) (see above), authorising the payment of the expenses of midwives summoned before the Board, at the discretion of the Board ; possibly an oversight.

Clause 15 (Scotland) corresponds with Section 4 (England, 1902), providing for appeal from the Board to the High Court.

The finance of the Board is provided for in Section 5 of the English Act, which calculates the amount to be paid by each district in proportion to *the number of midwives who have given notice of their intention to practise.*

In the Scottish Bill, Clause 16, the amount is in proportion to the *populations of the districts.* This is also the provision in the Amending Bill for England, 1910, Clause 3. It is a great improvement.

I do not know whether the Scottish Board will find a difficulty in getting in their money in the first instance. A new payment is always a grievance. If they do, they will find that quiet persistence will succeed, and that, after the first year or two, they will have no trouble.

The subsequent sections (English, 6-9 inclusive; Scottish, Clauses 17-19 inclusive) are practically identical, and require no comment.

Powers of entry (not in Midwives Act, 1902; present in Scottish Bill, Clause 20; and in Amending Bill (England), Clause 15).—The object of this clause is to exercise supervision over lying-in homes in the interest of mothers and children. It is very difficult to do good without doing harm, and the Central Midwives Board feared that this clause would tend to penalise the employment of a certified midwife in a lying-in home.

Notification of practice.—Clause 21 (1) (Scotland) corresponds with Clause 10 (England), except that the Scottish Bill contains two additional clauses (2 and 3) obliging a midwife who has not notified, and attends any woman in childbirth "in any capacity" (probably this means as a monthly nurse) in the absence of a doctor to notifiy the Local Supervisiug Authority within forty-eight hours; and similarly obliging a midwife to notify a change of address within three days (Scotland) or seven days (England). These new clauses appear in the English Amending Bill as 11 (1) and (2). I am afraid that trouble might arise out of this regulation.

Obtaining a certificate by false representation and wilful falsification of the roll are dealt with in identical clauses in the two Bills (11 and 12 England, and 22 and 23 Scotland).

Contribution towards training of midwives.—Clause 24 (Scotland) and Amending Bill of 1910 (England), Clause 13, authorise local supervising authorities to contribute towards the training of midwives. The training of midwives is becoming an increasingly difficult problem, and it may prove necessary in England to subsidise them in some such manner if they are to obtain the standard of excellence desired by all in the interests of the poorer mothers and babies.

Payment of fees of medical practitioners called in on advice of midwives.—The Act of 1902 contains no clause with this object. The Scottish Bill (25) authorises such payment by the Local Government Board, subject to a power to recover the same from the husband or guardian when either is able to repay it. The Amending Bill (England) (17) enables the medical practitioner to recover his fee from the Guardians of the Poor, who may recover it in their turn "from the patient or person liable to provide the patient with medical aid."

The payment of medical practitioners has been a great difficulty in working the Act; ghastly cases have occurred in which women have been allowed to die on account of the refusal of one medical practitioner after another to go to the help of a midwife. The promoters and administrators of the Act have been freely abused for the absence of any provision for the payment of doctors. The memory of the average person is notoriously short, but some are able to remember that, when the Bill was in the making, the practitioners and their representatives devoted their energies to attempting to prevent legislation rather than to the provision of payment of the doctor. The Insurance Act has considerably changed the situation, and should relieve the tension; it is too early at present to say to what extent.

Rules.—The Act (3, 1) says that the duties and powers of the Board shall be "to frame rules," which have to be approved by the Privy Council. This set of rules, inaugurated in 1903, and revised in 1907 and 1911, forms the code under which the Act is administered. They were the outcome of much hard and anxious work originally, and very little alteration became necessary at their subsequent revisions. I strongly advise those who are interested in framing a Bill for Scotland to consider them carefully. I think that they will find them useful, and, indeed, a great part of them might be studied with advantage by all practitioners of midwifery.

It will only be necessary to refer to certain points in the rules.

Section C, "regulating the course of training and the conduct of examinations, and the remuneration of the examiners" is the first section that we need consider to-day.

1. (1) prescribes attendance on not fewer than 20 labours, "making abdominal and vaginal examinations during the course of labour and personally delivering the patient." Twenty labours is none too many. The words which describe how they are to be attended have been very carefully selected, in order to prevent (*a*) mere looking on; (*b*) scamping of the experience by allowing several to count the same case.

Difficulty has been experienced at times in the matter of internal examinations. The Board insists on the exact fulfilment of its rule, on which the education of the touch of the midwife depends. Some training schools have found it difficult to provide sufficient cases for the pupils whom they accept; but the primary duty of the Board is to secure the proper training of the midwife. The granting of certificates by bodies or individuals other than the Board requires the careful supervision of the Board, and it is a common experience that signing of certificates is apt to become perfunctory. The training must occupy not less than three months. This time is confessedly very short, and is generally prolonged beyond the minimum. The question of increasing the duration of training is largely one of pecuniary means.

As a matter of fact a large proportion of successful candidates (about 58 per cent) never intend to practise as midwives, but desire the certificate of the Board as a qualification for appointments or as a superior nursing diploma. Some 42 per cent intend to practise as midwives. It also appears that the candidates who intend to practise as midwives, and those who intend to practise as monthly nurses, come for the most part from different institutions.

It is evident that the Act was not passed, with toil and strife, to add a gilt edge to monthly nurses, but to provide well-trained midwives for the poor. It is probable that the Board may

reconsider the duration of the training required, and that, in
so doing, the convenience and the pecuniary means of the real
midwife-candidate may principally be considered.

Rule C, 4, specifies the subjects on which candidates are liable
to be examined. At the next revision the Board may probably
add a clause referring to "serious skin eruptions," which are
mentioned in the Rule, E 19 (5), relating to the "conditions in
which medical help must be sent for."

Rule D concerns the "rules of procedure on the removal of
a name from the roll, and on the restoration to the roll of
a name removed." This rule is very precise, and the procedure
is minutely prescribed. Yet it has not infrequently happened
that a Local Supervising Authority has failed to understand it.
At the last revision of the rules, therefore, a note was prefixed
to the rule in order to guard against possible misapprehension.
This appears to have been of service in the way of preventing
misunderstanding.

The procedure is briefly as follows:—The Board receives a
complaint of some misconduct on the part of a midwife. The
Local Supervising Authority of her district finds or does not find
a "true bill." The solicitor of the Board formulates the charges.
The Penal Cases Committee of the Board decides whether to
cite the accused to appear before it. In a very few cases, where
the charges do not seem to warrant citation, a caution may be
administered, but a censure is never administered unless an
offence is either proved before the Board or admitted by the
accused.

The midwives who are cited are furnished with a copy of
their indictments in separate counts, to which alone they have
to answer, each count bearing a reference to the rule or section
in the Act concerned, where possible; this last proviso meaning,
in reality, such offences as are included in the phrases "mal-
practice, negligence, or misconduct" (Act, Section 8), where
these cannot be more specifically mentioned. The commonest
instance of this class is drunkenness, which naturally requires
no special rule to forbid it. Yet, on the principle that "what
is sauce for the goose is sauce for the gander," the Board's
practice is to require evidence of (*a*) drunkenness on duty, or
(*b*) repeated drunkenness, before it considers itself justified
in cancelling a certificate.

Here difficulty has sometimes occurred with the Local Supervising Authority. The Board, however, requires very definite evidence of intoxication, which is sometimes hard to get. In any case it is better to fail to convict a guilty person than to convict an innocent person; and, as a matter of experience, the lucky drunkard of to-day generally appears as the undoubted drunkard of to-morrow.

At the "Penal Board" the proceedings generally follow those of a Court of Law, except that no oath is administered, and witnesses cannot be compelled to attend. The accused may be defended by counsel or solicitor. Where no counsel or solicitor is retained, the Board, and especially the chairman, feels it to be its duty to see that the accused suffers no disadvantage thereby. In a large number, or even in the majority of cases, the accused does not appear in person, but sends in a defence, and statutory declarations of witnesses are accepted. The court is rather one of equity than of criminal law; but such an enquiry as is held has many advantages, and is as a matter of experience eminently fair.

In the only instance in which its decision has been appealed against to the High Court of Justice (Act, Section 4) it was strongly upheld, and its procedure favourably commented on by the judges concerned. In the course of the investigation, counts in the indictment are frequently expunged. At the end of the enquiry the Board deliberates in *camerâ*, and decides which counts it considers proved and which not proved, and strikes out the latter. Having settled its findings, it asks the Inspector of Midwives, or other similar official if present, concerning the general character of the accused, and the solicitor concerning any previous convictions. This is never done until the proof of the indictment is settled.

As regards sentence, the following are the sentences in use:—Removal from the roll; severe censure; censure; caution. The latter (caution to obey the rules) is the only pronouncement ever made without proof of the truth of the accusation.

There is another pronouncement not very long in force, which is found very convenient. In some cases, especially those in which no grave offence has been proved, and yet the Board is of opinion that the accused is a woman who may be very undesirable as a midwife, it decides that the counts of the indictment (as many as are proved) are proved, but suspends sentence and asks for a report from the Local Supervising Authority in 3 and 6 (or 3 or 6) months. If favourable, no further action is taken; if unfavourable, the name is erased from the roll.

This procedure answers well in the case of women who habitually break rules as to notifying the Local Supervising Authority, &c., and in whose case the gravity of the offence becomes cumulative by persistent repetition.

Copy of the wording used by the Board when judgment is postponed at the hearing of a penal case.—"The Board finds the charges proved, but suspends sentence until the next Penal Board after the expiration of six months from this date, and requests the Local Supervising Authority to furnish the Board with a report on your conduct and methods of practice at the end of three months and again at the end of six months."

A report in 3 and 6 months is often asked from the Local Supervising Authority also in cases where a censure is administered. But a censure is a sentence, and the midwife cannot be punished twice for the same offence; whereas postponement of sentence keeps the offence alive and suspends a Sword of Damocles over the midwife's head. This procedure, together with the reports, acts most beneficially, and works a real reform in many cases.

Rule E deals with the subjects of regulating, supervising and restricting, within due limits, the practice of midwives. The first point to be noted is the word "washable," as applied to the material of the midwife's dress. The word means exactly what it says. The sort of material is suggested in the phrase "such as linen, cotton, &c.," but otherwise the responsibility for the material being "washable material that can be boiled" is left to the midwife.

Rule 5 (disinfection) is one of special importance. It has been greatly improved at the last revision by bringing the woman, "whether acting as a midwife or as a nurse" or being "herself liable to be a source of infection," under the disability of being unable to practise until disinfected to the satisfaction of the Local Supervising Authority. The meshes of the net have been made smaller, and now catch the woman (1) who might have pleaded that she was not acting as a midwife;

(2) who, not having been in contact with an infected person, is herself infectious (as, for instance, from a foul ulcer of the leg); (3) and it is to be noted that it is not necessary to prove that a midwife has been *told* that a patient is septic—she is bound to suspect the condition herself, and to get disinfected.

Rule 6 obliges a midwife, "in cases where a doctor has been sent for, to await his arrival and faithfully carry out his instructions." Offences against this rule are not uncommon.

Rule 8 limits internal examinations to those absolutely necessary; but, as this rule was quoted in some quarters in opposition to Rule C 1 (1), obliging the pupil to watch the progress of her twenty labours by vaginal as well as by abdominal examinations, a footnote was appended to the effect that Rule E 8 was not to be taken as relieving a pupil from any of the obligations of Rule C 1 (1).

Rule 11 (puerperium) lays down the duration of responsibility of the midwife "in a normal case," and prescribes that duration as 10 days; and also obliges her, if she attends longer, to note the fact and its explanation in her register. It does not prescribe the number of visits, but leaves her the responsibility of paying as many as necessary. This rule is often important in penal proceedings.

Rule 13 obliges a midwife to take and record the pulse and temperature at each visit. It was inserted at the last revision. To have imposed it in 1903 would have meant that a very large number of *bonâ fide* midwives (*i.e.*, the untrained women in practice at the passing of the Act) might have been struck off as soon as they were on, which would have been contrary to the spirit of the Act. But it was felt in 1911 that the time had come to raise the standard, especially as it appeared from the penal experiences of the Board that a good many women either would not or could not learn to take the pulse and temperature, so important for the safety of their patients. Breaches of this rule have never, I think, been the *only* cause for removing a midwife from the roll. I may say that many local supervising authorities, by the help of their inspectors of midwives, have taken great pains to teach their old *bonâ fide* midwives these methods.

Rule 15 concerns the care of the child's eyes immediately the head is born, and gives a reference to page 42, where is to be found a leaflet on ophthalmia neonatorum drawn up by the chairman at the request of the Board.

Rule 17 deals with the difficult subject of laying out the dead. To forbid a woman to do this for a stillborn child which she had delivered, or for a woman on whom she had attended, would be absurd; any infection would already be incurred, and one disinfection would do. Again, no harm is done by her laying out a body in a case of non-infectious illness, if she is not attending a confinement at the time, and is disinfected afterwards. In the case, however, of her laying out a strange body, she is subject to the prohibition of the Local Supervising Authority. This rule was framed to meet the case of villages where there is only one woman to do nursing and midwifery. It sounds complicated, but represents real facts, and has not been complained against.

Rule 18 obliges the midwife to record any drug other than a simple aperient in her register. The Board deliberately refrained from scheduling approved drugs, or forbidden drugs, and placed the whole responsibility on the midwife.

Rule 19 prescribes the conditions in which medical help must be sent for. It is probably the most frequently broken of all the rules. The Board, in framing it, carefully avoided ordering the midwife to send for medical help, but obliged her to explain that the case is one in which a doctor is required, and to fill up the proper form, and hand it to the husband or the nearest relative or friend present. This is intended to prevent the doctor from saying that the midwife had sent for him and is responsible for his fee; but I am bound to say that it has not prevented this assertion in all cases, though unfounded. The choice of a medical practitioner rests with the patient or her representative. The rule then proceeds to give instances of cases in which medical help is required in cases of pregnancy, labour, lying-in, or where the child requires it. Finally, various forms of notification are appended.

Rule 27 (letters C.M.B.) forbids a midwife to append letters to her name. This became necessary on account of such appended letters as C.M.B., which gives a sort of impression that it is something more than merely " M.B.," and is probably as good as " C.M.G." This use of unauthorised capital letters after a name is not confined to midwives, nor even to women, and seems to be a relic of original sin.

Rule F, concerning suspension from practice, has already been commented on in connection with Section 8 (3) of the Midwives Act.

Forms of certificates and leaflets.—Appended to the rules are various certificates, also a leaflet on ophthalmia neonatorum, and one on cancer of the uterus, drawn up by the chairman at the request of the Board. The latter is an attempt to save lives which may sometimes be saved by prompt treatment, by making use of midwives as missionaries. They are given to all midwives on their certification, and are widely distributed by many local supervising authorities. Finally, there is a simple glossary.

Regulations governing training.—The course is prescribed in Rule C. It comprises, 1 (1), attendance on not fewer than twenty labours, including nursing of twenty lying-in women and their infants for ten days after labour, 1 (2). The certificates for the above are found in schedule, Forms III and IV. These can be signed by—C 1 (2)—(*a*) an approved medical practitioner; (*b*) a certified midwife, being the chief midwife or matron of an institution recognised by the Board; (*c*) a certified midwife, being the matron or superintendent nurse of a poor law institution; (*d*) a certified midwife approved by the Board. It will be seen that certificates can be signed either by (1) officials of an approved institution or (2) by approved doctors or midwives.

The approval of an institution carries with it the approval of its proper officers; but these are only approved so long as they remain attached to the institution. The approval of an individual doctor or midwife attaches to the individual as long as the approval lasts. These approved lists are revised yearly. The practice of the Board is to approve institutions when of a certain size and importance, such as the large lying-in hospitals, whose staffs can be trusted to be thoroughly competent; and to approve the individuals attached to smaller institutions.

In addition to this, in country districts especially, it is necessary sometimes to approve the best individual available, though unattached. This is particularly the case in Wales, where large mining populations exist apart from any large town. But in these cases the Board depends largely upon the Medical Officers of Health as to the desirability of approval.

In the earlier stages of the history of the Board great pressure was sometimes put upon the Board to add a small institution to the list of "approved institutions," which were inclined to look down upon smaller institutions in which individuals had to be approved. I remedied this by altering the title and putting all institutions, whether approved *en bloc* or individually, into one list, and the trouble instantly ceased.

The "course of instruction," by lectures, demonstrations, &c., is prescribed in Rule C 1 (3), and the subjects are scheduled in C 4. The course must extend over not less than three months, C 1 (3), and must consist of not less than fifteen lectures. (Schedule, Form V, p. 37.) The question of general education was carefully considered by the Board, and it was decided not to insist upon any standard higher than that mentioned in the schedule—"that she possesses sufficient elementary education to enable her to read and to take notes of cases." Any higher standard would undoubtedly deprive the country of some of the best women practising as midwives.

The Board believes that, so far as lectures are concerned, it is well to encourage large classes, and that for the following reasons :—

1. A large class means more adequate payment to the lecturer, and this makes it easier to secure one who is skilled in the difficult art of lecturing.

2. A large class certainly reacts upon the lecturer, stimulating him, while nothing is more depressing than to lecture to a very small class. This does not apply to practical instruction, in which moderate numbers are more satisfactory.

3. A large class probably reacts favourably upon its individual members.

For this reason the Board approached the lying-in hospitals of London, and some other large institutions, asking them whether they could not see their way to admit outside pupils for lectures only. All the lying-in hospitals, however, but one declined. The Board greatly regrets their decision. Their acquiescence might have given a real help towards the better training of the poorer midwives, who, it seems, are those who chiefly undertake the work of real midwives, and especially in rural districts.

A difficulty arises at times in connection with the distribution of the cases of midwifery and of the lectures. It is intended that these should be fairly distributed throughout the three months of training, and not be crowded into a very short time, the object being to secure that the candidate should live for a time in an obstetric atmosphere. As deviations from the desired course were known to occur, the Board has issued instructions that the dates of the twenty confinements shall be sent in with the schedule filled up before the examination.

The examination of midwives.—Examinations are held in London in February, April, June, August, October, and December; in provincial centres (Birmingham, Bristol, Leeds, Manchester, and Newcastle) in February, June, and October. The examination is both written and oral, the papers being set in London and sent down to the provinces. In some cases the papers are allowed to be written, under proper supervision, at other places, the candidates going to the authorised centre for the oral examination. As several days elapse between the written and oral examinations, this saves the expense of a double journey. The examiners consist of the rising obstetricians of the country, and of many who have already attained to eminence. I visit practically every oral examination in London, and listen at all or most of the tables, and I have been struck by the fairness and patience with which the examinations are conducted.

It occasionally happens that the number of examiners in a particular centre is short for an examination. In such cases an examiner is generally sent for from or to London, as the case may be. This brings the various centres into touch with each other, and also helps to keep the standard uniform. But it is interesting to record the fact that when the standard at a centre has appeared to differ from the average (as, for instance, by an unusually high or low percentage of rejections), the provincial examiners who have taken part in London examinations have always been able to assure me that the standard was practically identical. In some cases the Board has sent an expert to visit an examination and report. This has never revealed any serious discrepancy between standards, nor any serious defect.

In arriving at a conclusion no percentage of marks is recognised, but examiners are requested to weigh the whole examination, written and oral, and to decide on the one question, "Is the candidate safe to be allowed to practise as a midwife?"

Examiners are reminded that a candidate must never be asked where she was trained; each candidate appears as a number only. Each candidate has a card with her examination number. This she is obliged to produce or she is not allowed to enter the examination hall. The Board has felt obliged to enforce this rule strictly ever since two candidates, relying on their memory, gave wrong numbers, with the result that an erroneous announcement of the result was made, leading to confusion and very undesirable comment.

The length of training of midwives is certainly very short. Three months is a very short time to turn an ignorant untrained woman into a competent midwife, fit to deal with matters of life and death. It is certainly desirable that the duration of training should be prolonged, but the difficulty is the expense. As it is, a woman who is trained at an institution has to pay fees for her keep and instruction for at least three months, during which she is earning nothing, and this is often difficult.

The supply of midwives.—It early became likely that a large number of women who became candidates for the certificate of the Board had no intention of practising as midwives.

In 1907 I instituted an enquiry, with the approval of the Board, into this question, having slips given to all the candidates on which was written the question whether or not they intended to practise as midwives.

In 1910 the additional question was added, whether, if so, they intended to practise in rural districts.

From these enquiries it was found that the percentage of successful candidates intending to practise as midwives was 53 in 1907, and has sunk to 41·8 in 1913. The percentage of the total intending to practise in rural districts has fluctuated, but the percentage of the total successful candidates intending to practise in rural districts has sunk from 27·4 in 1910 to 20·7 in 1913, the decline being steady in each year.

It is plain from this that the number of women intending to

act as real midwives is steadily diminishing. Whether the supply will be equal to the demand remains to be seen, and I cannot at present make any sure statement on this point.

For the last two years I have had a table drawn out showing the destination of the successful candidates from various institutions.

From the tables it was found that, speaking generally, most of the great lying-in hospitals are principally engaged in training monthly nurses, while genuine midwives receive their training from other institutions. The one exception in London is the General Lying-in Hospital, which trains many who intend to practise as midwives; many of these, again, in rural districts.

Now, the Midwives Act was never intended merely to turn out gilt-edged monthly nurses, and it is plain that the work of the Board must be the training and supply of real midwives, especially for rural districts; and that institutions are valuable to the country in proportion as they subserve this purpose.

In 1912 the results were as follows:—*Medical schools* provided 99 successful candidates, of whom 16 intended to practise as midwives, or 16·1 per cent. *Lying-in institutions* provided 894 successful candidates, of whom 259 intended to practise as midwives, or 29 per cent. *Other institutions* (mostly rural, such as county nursing associations) provided 420 successful candidates, of whom 272 intended to practise, or 64·8 per cent.

In 1913 the results were as follows:—*Medical schools* provided 113 successful candidates, of whom 9 intended to practise as midwives, or 8 per cent. *Lying-in institutions* provided 828 successful candidates, of whom 211 intended to practise as midwives, or 25·5 per cent. *Other institutions* provided 434 successful candidates, of whom 294 intended to practise as midwives, or 67·7 per cent.

For the year 1912 the number from these three groups intending to practise as midwives was 547; in 1913 it was 514.

THE OPERATIVE TREATMENT OF FRACTURES, WITH SPECIAL REFERENCE TO PLATING.*

By GEO. H. EDINGTON, M.D., D.Sc., F.R.F.P.S.G.,

Surgeon, Western Infirmary; and Lecturer in Clinical Surgery, University of Glasgow.

THE accompanying skiagrams illustrate the immediate effect of operative treatment of fractures of the long bones, viz., the retention in good position of the fragments. Such an effect is so obvious that I would not have taken up the time of the meeting with the subject were it not that in connection with operative treatment there are certain drawbacks. These are important, and they are all the more worthy of consideration because they are liable to be overlooked or forgotten in the contemplation both of the excellent immediate and of the good late results of operative treatment.

Within the last nine months I have had under my care several cases, originally operated upon by other surgeons, which illustrate some of these drawbacks. In each of these cases the plate had been left *in situ*.

1. *Persistent sinus* may result, as in the case of a seaman, aged 47, in whom a fracture of the lower end of the right humerus had been plated. The wound had only partially closed, and a sinus was still present when I saw him nineteen months later. There was also considerable thickening of the bone in the neighbourhood of the plate. I removed the plate, the lower end of which was partly covered over by new bone, and the sinus healed.

2. In other two cases there was *persistent sinus, with cario-necrosis around the nail-holes*. The first of these was that of a man, aged 28. A fracture just below the middle of the tibia was plated in October, 1912. When I saw him in January, 1914, there was considerable thickening of the bone, which was

---

* Communication at the annual meeting of the Glasgow and West of Scotland Branch of the British Medical Association, held in the Western Infirmary, on 12th May, 1914.

very tender. I removed the plate, which was embedded in, but not completely covered over by, new bone; but the sinus did not close till some carious bone around one of the nail-holes had been scraped away. The other case was that shown in Fig. 8.

It is interesting to note that in all three cases the plate was partly covered over by new bone. This had to be opened up to allow of removal of the plate.

3. *Necrosis in compound fracture.*—In this case a woman, aged 37, had sustained a compound fracture of the right tibia at its lower end. Plating had been *immediately* performed, but violent sepsis, luckily localised, in its effects, had ensued; and when, two months later, the case came under my care I had to remove the plate and a considerable quantity of necrosed bone before healing set in.

That these are not by any means isolated cases must be patent to anyone who is familiar with recent surgical literature. At the meeting in Montreal, in 1912, of the American Surgical Association,[1] five papers dealing with the subject of fractures were submitted. It is quite evident to anyone studying these papers and the discussions following them that, quite apart from the risk of introduction of sepsis at the operation, plates and nails may be responsible for a good deal of trouble. Thus— " In many instances the apparatus produces so much 'irritation' long after union of the bone has occurred that it must be removed;"[2] and, "as a rule the presence of a plate, in place of stimulating osteogenesis between the broken bone ends, retards it."[3]

It must not be thought that the nails remain for an indefinite period firm in the bone. Undoubtedly in some cases they may be found firm months after insertion, but more usually they cause absorption of the bony walls of the nail-tracks to such an extent that the nails are quite loose and may be picked out with a dissecting forceps. This loosening of the nails may occur without obvious ill-effect (Fig. 7), or the nail may leave the plate and actually work its way towards the skin, as in Fig. 8. Another, and much more serious, effect is the weakening of the bone, so that fracture may occur at the site of one of the nail-tracts. This occurrence has actually been met with, and is mentioned in the volume already referred to. Lilienthal, who

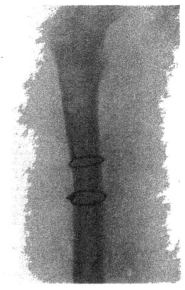

FIG. 1.   FIG. 2.

William J., aged 10 years. Spiral fracture of left femur, involving 3 inches of length of bone. Fragments held in position by circling loops of wire, which left *in situ.* Full use of limb three months after operation.

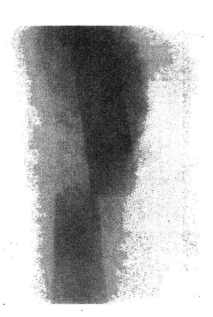

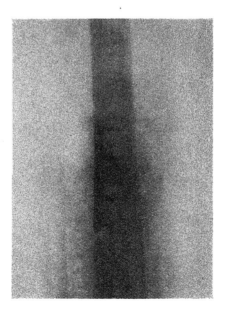

FIG. 3.   FIG. 4.

John L., aged 18 years, seaman. Transverse fracture of left femur, lower third. Fall of 30 feet into hold, striking limb on projecting ridge. Upper end of lower fragment displaced outwards and backwards into popliteal space. Perfect apposition by 4-nail plate applied outer side. Plate removed four weeks later ; pus-like fluid not examined. Union firm,

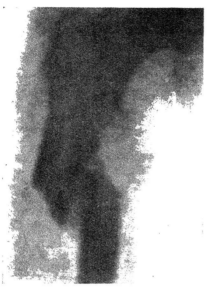

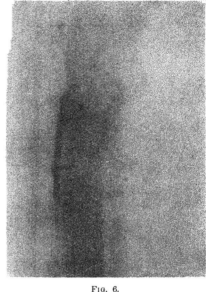

FIG. 5.

FIG. 6.

James H., aged 19 years. Fracture of left femur, upper third. Two and a half months after accident, firm union with angular deformity, riding, and 1½ inch shortening. Callus divided, ends of fragments rawed, and fixed in apposition by 4-nail plate on outer side.

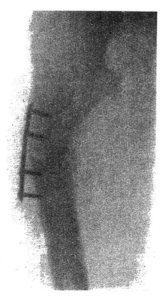

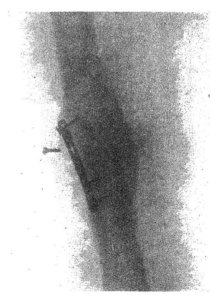

FIG. 7.

FIG. 8.

From same case as Figs. 6 and 7. Shows condition eight weeks later: some bowing of bone, and starting of lower nails. When seen twenty-six weeks later, good use of limb, with half an inch shortening. Eleven months after operation plate removed because of increasing pain and stiffness, of one month's duration.

Henry T., aged 46 years. Compound fracture, middle of right femur. Plated in February, 1913. Sinus persisted, and head of one nail projected from it shortly before admission in January, 1914. Plate and nails extracted. Six weeks later, carious bone scraped. Discharged 18th April, sinus still open.

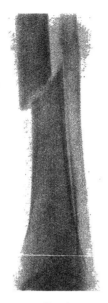
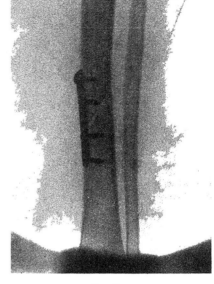

Fig. 9.   Fig. 10.

Thomas S., aged 15 years. Fracture of both bones of right leg caused by blow from heavy piece of metal. Transverse fracture of fibula at level of upper end of fracture of tibia. Approximation of tibial fragments by 4-nail plate, which removed one month later, when union almost firm. Yellow pus-like fluid from nail-holes, *sterile*.

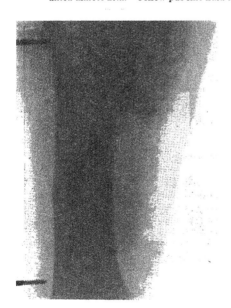

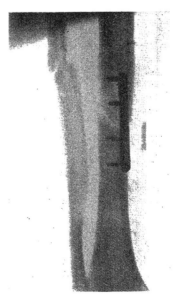

Fig. 11.   Fig. 12.

Thomas B., aged 35 years. Fell off loaded lorry, 10-12 feet, landing on feet. Compound fracture both bones of right leg, with some comminution of lower fragment of tibia, and with upper fragment projecting through wound. Tibia plated eight days later. Plate removed after four weeks, giving vent to a few drops of pus-like fluid, which *sterile*. Union not quite firm two weeks later, and plaster of Paris applied.

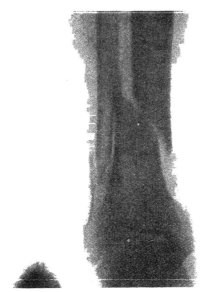

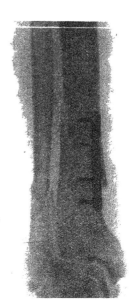

Fig. 13.   Fig. 14.

William G., aged 72 years. Fracture of both bones of right leg, which caught between two planks. Spiral oblique fracture lower third of tibia. Fibula broken at lower level. Approximately good position of tibia by plating. Two months later, good union. Discharged January, 1914, *retaining plate.*

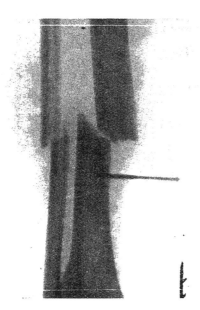
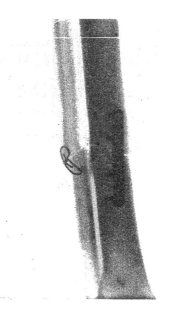

Fig. 15.   Fig. 16.

John M., aged 23 years. Transverse fracture of right leg, direct violence on football field. Fortnight later, wired fibula and plated tibia. Plate removed three weeks later, milky fluid escaping; *sterile.* Good union two months after operation, and two months later walking with slight limp, from restriction of movements at ankle.

mentions this case, says " it is self-evident that the mere presence of the screws in the shaft of a long bone must prove a source of weakness, because they mean the persistence of bony defects. With the screws removed, these defects would fill with new bone, and osseous homogeneity would be restored." [4]

The above notwithstanding, I think it may justly be claimed that the operative treatment of fractures of the long bones permits of their uniting with an avoidance of deformity to an extent which, in many cases, would not be attained by non-operative methods. It gives, on the whole, good results, but it is incumbent on the surgeon to attempt to obviate as far as possible the occurrence of such ill-results as are exemplified by the cases just narrated. I believe that, with this end in view, the plates should be removed before the case leaves the hands of the surgeon. While a considerable proportion of my own cases (*e.g.*, Figs. 1, 2, 5, 6, 7, 13, and 14) have gone home with the plates or wires *in situ,* and have remained well,* I have of late practised removal of the plate at the end of the fourth week. This necessitates re-opening the wound, but I think that the increased probability of a good *late* result is well worth it. I may add that this practice was instituted quite independently of, and was not suggested by, any signs of sepsis. In several cases, however, the removal of the plate was accompanied by the escape of pus-like fluid, which was *bacteriologically sterile.*

If it be intended to operate, simple fractures are usually plated within a few days of admission. In compound fractures, on the other hand, my practice is to wait for at least a week in order to be sure that the fracture is pursuing an aseptic course.

In no case is plating used as a substitute for splints, and I consider that careful immobilisation by the latter is a vital part of the treatment.

---

* Since the meeting at which this communication was read, the case illustrated by Figs. 5, 6, and 7 has required, eleven months after operation, removal of the plate on account of increasing pain and stiffness, of one month's duration, at the seat of fracture, thus confirming the experience of Estes (*vide supra*). The plate was covered over, except at its lower end, by thickened periosteum, and was slightly bent and lying in close apposition to the bone. The nails were loose in the nail-tracks.

There is not the same likelihood of late trouble when wire is used as a means of co-apting the fragments. This fact has long been known to surgeons in connection with fracture of the patella. Occasionally, however, the twisted ends of the wire may project, and may cause the formation of an adventitious bursa, or even of a sinus. In either case the wire may require to be removed.*

* Since writing the above, I have met with an example of adventitious bursa from this cause in a case where the clavicle had been wired ten months previously. The bursa was found after removal to have a very thick wall surrounding a small cavity in which lay the end of the wire.

REFERENCES.

[1] *Transactions*, vol. xxx, 1912.
[2] Estes, *loc. cit.*, p. 670.
[3] Martin and Barton, *loc. cit.*, p. 691.
[4] *Loc. cit.*, p. 683.

ACUTE SUPPURATIVE APPENDICITIS: SOME CONCLUSIONS FROM AN ANALYSIS OF A SERIES OF 100 CONSECUTIVE CASES.*

By ROBERT B. CARSLAW, M.A., M.B.,

Dispensary Surgeon, Western Infirmary ; and Assistant Surgeon, Victoria Infirmary, Glasgow.

ONE is apt to think that a series of 100 cases of acute suppurative appendicitis is much too short to give reliable data on which to found any conclusions. While this is undoubtedly true as regards any statistical results, there is at the same time, I think, a great deal to be learned from even a short series of consecutive cases seen and operated on by the same surgeon who, in collecting the details, has a definite personal recollection of almost every case. I, therefore, make no apology in presenting this series of cases, which have been operated on by me during the three years 1911, 1912, and 1913. They represent all the cases of acute suppurative appendicitis seen by me during these years, as in no case was operation refused by patient or surgeon. Sixty-eight of them were operated on in the Victoria Infirmary, Glasgow, in the wards of Mr. Maylard, Mr. Parry, and Mr. Grant Andrew (to whom I am indebted for permission to publish them); the remaining 33 occurred in my private practice.

Age and sex.—The age varied from 4 to 56 years, but 72 of the cases were between 10 and 30 years. The proportion of males to females, which was fairly constant in the various decades, was two to one.

Previous attacks.—Sixty-three had had no previous attack, 16 had had one previous attack, and 17 had had two or more previous attacks. In 5 cases there was no record. The percentage of those who submitted to operation during the first attack was 74 in 1913, whereas in 1911-12 it was only 60.

* Read at a meeting of the Glasgow Southern Medical Society held on 2nd April, 1914.

Duration of the symptoms.—The duration of the symptoms before the patient came to operation varied between two very wide limits, the shortest being that of one patient (a doctor) who was operated on within six hours of the onset of his illness, the longest being two months.

The appendix: 1. Its *situation.*—The appendix was removed at the operation in 94 cases; its situation was *iliac* in 48, *retro-cæcal* in 26, and *pelvic* in 20. The pelvic position was relatively much more common in females (30 per cent) than in males (17 per cent).

2. *Concretions.*—One or more concretions were found in 20 of the cases. The concretion, whether lying inside a non-perforated appendix (in 5 cases) or inside a perforated gangrenous appendix (in 14 cases), was always situated just beyond a stenosis of the lumen. This stenosis was usually found at the base (in 13 cases), but sometimes at the middle of the appendix (in 6 cases).

3. *Perforation.*—In 61 of the 94 appendices removed a perforation was found. Like the concretions, it was very often situated just beyond a stenosis, its position being determined by the presence of the concretion. Thus it occurred at the *base* in 11 cases (in 9 of which a concretion was present), and in the *middle* in 12 cases (in 6 of which a concretion was present). In 1 case there were two stenoses, and just distal to each there were a gangrenous patch, a perforation, and a concretion. In several cases where there was no gross perforation, a deep gangrenous ulcer was found opposite the concretion. In 30 cases where the perforation was at the tip of the appendix no concretion was present, the position of the perforation being determined by the distribution of the blood supply.

Types of cases.—I have found it impossible to arrange my cases in accordance with the usual classification of gangrenous appendix, localised abscess, and general peritonitis, as so many of the cases presented conditions common to more than one of these types. Taking, for example, a case of localised abscess of four days' duration, which has come to operation because the abscess has for the last twelve or twenty-four hours been leaking into the general peritoneal cavity; the peritonitis caused by this leakage, at first local, soon becomes general. Again, we often find a somewhat similar case coming to operation because an abscess has suddenly ruptured into the general peritoneal cavity, which is thus flooded with pus. The peritonitis met with in these two cases differs both in its origin and character from the acute free spreading peritonitis which may be present in a case of acute gangrenous perforative appendicitis of one or two days' duration.

The term "general peritonitis" is, I think, an unfortunate one under which to classify cases, as we may have in some which are not very acute a large quantity of purulent fluid in the general peritoneal cavity (this fluid, being more defensive than offensive in character); whereas the truly acute general peritonitis is rarely met with except in the late stages of the disease. I have therefore used the term "free spreading peritonitis," meaning by this an acute peritonitis which is not localised in any way by adhesions, and which, although in different cases varying in character and extent, would, if left alone, rapidly become truly general, and involve the whole peritoneal cavity.

Although reluctant to employ a complicated classification, I have found it necessary to divide my cases into the following six types:—

Type I.—Appendix distended with pus (19 cases).

The *appendix* wall is thickened, the lumen is stenosed (at the base in 15, at the middle in 4 cases), the mucous membrane is inflamed, ulcerated, or gangrenous (6 cases). There is no perforation, and no gangrene of the outer wall of the appendix. In 13 cases bacillus coli, in 2 cases staphylococcus, and in 1 pneumococcus were found; no record in 3 cases.

The situation of the appendix was iliac in 14 cases, retro-cæcal in 4, and pelvic in 1.

The *peritoneal cavity* presented various conditions, the only constant one being the absence of recent adhesions. Thus in 4 cases (3 retro-cæcal, 1 iliac) there was no free fluid; in 9 cases (8 iliac, 1 retro-cæcal) there was free serous fluid; in 5 cases (4 iliac, 1 pelvic) there was free sero-purulent fluid; and in 1 case (iliac) there was free purulent fluid in the general peritoneal cavity, from which a pure growth of staphylococcus was obtained.

The fluid was more turbid the nearer one approached the appendix, and, while being free in the general peritoneal cavity, was always more abundant in the pelvis.

As the condition of the appendix was the predominating feature in these cases, and as the peritonitis present was of a "defensive" or "protective" character, these cases are included under this type instead of under Type VI.

Symptoms.—With one exception these cases were in very good condition at the time of operation. The localised pain, tenderness, and rigidity were usually comparatively well marked, although in several cases so slight as to make the diagnosis doubtful. In 8 cases the pulse was not over 80. The exception referred to was a case in which the appendix was distended with pneumococcal pus and the general peritoneal cavity contained a large quantity of sero-purulent fluid. This patient, although seen within twelve hours of the onset of his symptoms, looked very ill and was very toxæmic (temperature 101°, pulse 132). There was general pain, tenderness, and rigidity over the whole of the abdomen.

Type II.—Gangrenous appendix (14 cases).

The *appendix* wall is gangrenous through all its coats, either in its whole length (9 cases) or in its distal half only (5 cases). In only 1 case was there a gross perforation, but in several there was a deep ulcer, opposite a concretion, almost through. In 7 cases bacillus coli was found, in 7 cases there was no record. The situation of the appendix was iliac in 10 cases, retro-cæcal in 1 case, and pelvic in 3 cases.

The *peritoneal cavity* presented various conditions, the only constant one being the absence of recent adhesions.

Thus, in 5 cases (all iliac) there was free serous fluid; in 7 cases (4 iliac, 1 retro-cæcal, 2 pelvic) there was free sero-purulent fluid, and in two cases (1 iliac, 1 pelvic) there was in the general peritoneal cavity free purulent fluid from which a growth of bacillus coli was obtained.

The fluid—as in Type I—while varying in character and extent was more abundant in the pelvis, and more turbid near the appendix.

Although in most of these cases there was a free peritonitis they are classed under Type II instead of under Type VI, as the predominating feature was the condition of the appendix, the peritonitis present being of a defensive or protective character.

Symptoms.—With the exception of 4 cases the general condition was good, the pulse being in one case only 60. The localised pain, tenderness, and rigidity were well marked in all except two.

The 4 cases referred to were toxæmic and had pain, tenderness, and rigidity over the whole of the abdomen.

Type III.—Localised abscess (28 cases).

The *appendix* was removed in 22 cases (8 iliac, 11 retro-cæcal, 3 pelvic); it was gangrenous in its whole length in 16 cases, in its distal half only in 6 cases. There was a perforation in 20 cases.

The *abscess* varied greatly in size, in several cases, especially those of long duration being very large. In 4 cases it was up to the umbilicus.

In 17 cases bacillus coli, in 3 cases bacillus coli and staphylococcus were found; in 8 cases there was no record.

The *peritoneal cavity* presented various conditions.

Thus, in 4 cases (1 iliac, 3 retro-cæcal) there was no free fluid; in 14 cases (4 iliac, 8 retro-cæcal, 2 pelvic) there was free serous fluid; in 1 case (iliac) there was sero-purulent fluid; in 7 cases the general peritoneal cavity was not seen; in 2 cases there was no record.

Symptoms.—The general conditions varied greatly—in 2 cases, both of short duration, it was very good; in the majority of the others it was fairly good, but in 8 cases, all of long duration, there was marked toxæmia. There was no general rigidity in any of the cases, but in those in which the abscess was very large there was distension.

Type IV.—Localised abscess leaking into the peritoneal cavity (16 cases).

In this type the adhesions which had been localising the abscess had given way at one place, and there had been a slight escape of the pus, usually downwards into the pelvis, or, in the case of a pelvic abscess, upwards into the general peritoneal cavity. Thus, in the immediate vicinity of the abscess there is a free spreading purulent peritonitis; the pelvis is usually full of pus; elsewhere there is serous or sero-purulent fluid in the general peritoneal cavity. In 1 case the abscess was very large, filling the whole pelvis and the lower half of the abdomen.

The *appendix* was removed in 15 cases (5 iliac, 5 retro-cæcal, 5 pelvic); it was gangrenous in its whole length in 11 cases, in its distal half only in 4 cases. There was a perforation in 14 cases.

In 11 cases bacillus coli, in 1 case bacillus coli and staphylococcus were found; in 4 cases there was no record.

Symptoms.—In none of these cases was the general condition at all good; the symptoms in all had become much worse when the leakage took place, usually from twelve to twenty-four hours before the patient was seen. In 6 of the cases there was marked toxæmia, 2 of these being deeply jaundiced. In about one-half of the cases the pain, tenderness, and rigidity which had been at first localised had become general and were accompanied by distension.

Type V.—Localised abscess ruptured into the general peritoneal cavity (7 cases).

In this type the adhesions, which had been localising the abscess, had suddenly given way, allowing a large quantity of pus into the general peritoneal cavity, and thus giving rise to an acute spreading general peritonitis.

In none of my cases was the abscess of less than five days' duration. In 1 case it was very large, filling the whole of the pelvis and the right side of the lower half of the abdomen.

The *appendix* was removed in all the cases (3 iliac, 2 retro-cæcal, 2 pelvic); it was gangrenous in its whole length in all but one; it was perforated in all.

In 5 cases bacillus coli, in 1 case bacillus coli and staphylococcus were found; in 1 case there was no record.

Symptoms.—The general condition was very bad in all, the symptoms in every case having been suddenly greatly exacerbated when the rupture took place, usually about six to twelve hours before the patient was seen. All the patients were very toxæmic, 1 was very deeply jaundiced, and 1 was moribund.

There was great distension in all, and generalised pain, tenderness, and rigidity in all except 2, both of whom died.

Type VI.—Free spreading peritonitis (17 cases).

In this type there are no adhesions and consequently no localisation of the pus. The acute spreading peritonitis varies in extent according to the duration of the symptoms and the virulence of the organisms. It is this spreading peritonitis, which has set in almost at the onset of the illness, which is the predominating feature of the case, and not the actual condition of the appendix.

The *appendix* was removed in all the cases (8 iliac, 3 retro-cæcal, 6 pelvic); it was gangrenous in its whole length in 8, in its distal half only in 8; it was perforated in 16.

There were no recent adhesions in the general *peritoneal cavity*; the peritonitis was absolutely general in 12 cases (in 6 of which there were *very* large quantities of pus); in 5 cases it was not absolutely general (3 of these being very early cases). In 12 cases bacillus coli, in 1 case bacillus coli and staphylococcus were found in the peritoneal pus; in 4 cases there was no record.

Symptoms.—The general condition was fairly good in 11 of the cases, but 6 of the cases were very toxæmic, three of them greatly distended. The pain, tenderness, and rigidity were generalised in all.

Bacteriological and histological examination.—In 74 of the cases a more or less thorough examination was made of the pus from the appendix and from the peritoneal cavity. In few of the private cases was a culture taken, but in most of the hospital cases the results got from stained films were verified by culture.

No histological record was kept, in the majority of the cases, of the cells of the fluids, but in my later cases a much more thorough examination has been made. Bacillus coli was found alone in 65 cases, in combination with staphylococcus in 6 cases; staphylococcus was found alone in 2 cases, and pneumococcus in 1 case. The peritoneal exudations which are found in the various types and stages of the disease vary very much in character. Within a few hours of the bacterial invasion of the peritoneum one finds a serous exudate which contains few cells. This fluid soon becomes sero-purulent in character, and the cells are found to be chiefly polymorphonuclear leucocytes. There are in addition, however, many mononuclear cells, some of which are undoubtedly the mononuclear leucocytes of the blood; others, which vary in size and in staining properties, are derived from the endothelial cells of the peritoneum and the lymphatics of the omentum. Both these varieties are actively phagocytic. As the cells become more numerous the fluid becomes frankly purulent. The cells, in colloquial language, are the defensive forces of the peritoneal cavity, which are called out at the first sign of danger. In the serous and sero-purulent fluids they are engaged in successful conflict with the bacteria, some of which are free in the fluid, but most of which have been ingested by the polymorphonuclear cells. At this stage we also find that some of the large mononuclear phagocytes have engulfed some polymorphonuclear cells. The cells have then the upper hand, and are not only destroying the bacteria, but are taking charge of them after death.

If the cells are able to take charge of the bacteria, this purulent fluid, which may be thick creamy pus, is "defensive" in character; but, on the other hand, if owing to the virulence of the bacteria or to their overwhelming number the bacteria are winning, then we find purulent fluid which might well be called "offensive." In it there are any number of bacteria free in the fluid, the polymorphonuclear cells are degenerated, there are few large mononuclear cells, and those present show little phagocytic activity. We find these various kinds of fluids in the various types of cases—for example, in Type I we find "offensive" pus inside the appendix, and "defensive" fluid, either serous, sero-purulent, or even purulent, in the general peritoneal cavity. The defensive forces of the peritoneal cavity are thus called out before there is any gross perforation of the wall of the appendix. It may be that this is due to the transudation of the bacterial products through the wall, but there is no doubt that the organisms themselves can migrate from the lumen of the appendix into the peritoneal cavity without producing necrosis, ulceration, or gangrene at the site of their invasion.

Again, in Type III we have a well localised abscess containing "offensive" pus, but there is usually at the same time a "defensive" exudate in the general peritoneal cavity; and in Type V we have a - peritoneal cavity containing "defensive" fluid, suddenly flooded with a quantity of "offensive" pus containing large numbers of active organisms and few, if any, living leucocytes.

Complications and sequelæ.—In almost one-third of the cases various complications and sequelæ arose which delayed convalescence.

A. Abdominal.—Re-collection of pus in the wound, 2 cases; secondary abdominal abscess, 1; pus from rectum, 3; septic thrombosis of appendix mesentery, 6; acute intestinal obstruction, 1; post-operative distension, 14; fæcal fistula, 9; ventral hernia, 6; hernia of portion of omentum, 1; gastro-intestinal hæmorrhage, 2; hæmaturia, 1; malposition of ascending colon, 1. *B. Pulmonary.*—Bronchitis, 3; bronchitis, pneumonia, 2; pneumonia, pleurisy, empyema, 1. *C.* Cardiac, 2. *D.* Femoral thrombosis, 2. *E.* Parotitis, 1. *F.* Jaundice, 9.

Mortality.—Reference has already been made to four deaths—

1. That of a boy, æt. 5, who was admitted in a moribund condition (his pulse being imperceptible), who died six hours after operation.

2. That of a young woman who developed a fresh spreading peritonitis after her gauze drain had been removed on the second day after operation, and who had a secondary abscess in the abdomen, a double pneumonia, and a left empyema—death taking place on the twenty-seventh day.

3. That of a young man with the cardiac complications.

4. That of a girl who died of acute intestinal obstruction on the twenty-first day, due to strangulation of a loop of ileum below an old tubercular adhesion.

Four additional deaths must be added to the above.

5. A boy, æt. 11, with a retro-cæcal localised abscess of five days' duration, whose condition before operation was fairly good (temperature 101° F., pulse 108), and whose appendix was removed without any difficulty. A gauze drain was inserted at the upper end of the wound, which was partially stitched. He was fairly well on the first day and on the morning of the second day after operation, his temperature being normal, and pulse about 100.

The gauze drain was removed on the second day after operation, and soon afterwards his pulse began to rise; by the next morning he was very ill, temperature 101° F., pulse 144, and by evening his temperature was 103° F., and the pulse uncountable. He died on the morning of the fourth day. The *post-mortem* showed that there was no peritonitis. There was passive congestion of both lungs. The pleura and pericardium were covered with petechial hæmorrhages. No bacteriological examination of the blood was made, but I am convinced that the early removal of the gauze drain had, by disturbing the thrombosed veins in its neighbourhood, indirectly given rise to a condition of acute septicæmia.

6. An unmarried woman, æt. 24 years, who had a leaking retro-cæcal abscess of 6 days' duration, who was deeply jaundiced, very toxæmic, and greatly distended. When the appendix was being removed it was noticed that there was septic thrombosis of the appendix mesentery. She was fairly well twenty-four hours after the operation; temperature, 100°; pulse, 100; and had passed flatus. She then had a very sudden collapse, and died in six hours from a very acute toxæmia apparently due to the separation of a septic thrombus in the mesentery of the appendix.

7. A girl, æt. 8 years, who had a very large abscess, filling the pelvis and the iliac and retro-cæcal fossæ, of seven days' duration, which had ruptured into the general peritoneal cavity twelve hours before operation. She was deeply jaundiced and very toxæmic; temperature, 100°; pulse, 132. There was neither pain nor tenderness, and no rigidity of the abdomen. At the operation it was noticed that the mesentery of the appendix, which was retro-cæcal in position, was in a condition of septic thrombosis.

There was absolutely no improvement after operation, the patient dying within thirty-six hours.

8. The last death, which occurred in August, 1912, occurred in a man of 26 years of age, who had an acute spreading peritonitis of two days' duration. He was not very ill before the operation, his temperature being 100° and pulse only 96, but there was marked distension. At the operation it was noticed that there was septic thrombosis of the appendix mesentery. His general condition improved greatly after the operation for five days, the only unfavourable symptom being the persistence of the distension, which was ,not relieved by a very satisfactory evacuation of his bowels on the fourth day. On the fifth day his gauze drain was removed, no anæsthetic being necessary, and there was no collection of pus behind it. Within four hours his pulse-rate had risen from 64 to 84, within eight hours it was 160, and he died within fourteen hours, with a temperature of 105·6°. During the last ten hours he was wildly delirious.

This man's death was a very great disappointment, as he was apparently so well—temperature 98°, pulse 64 on the morning of the fifth day—the only disturbing feature being the persistence of the distension. Curiously enough, the patient himself all along entertained not the slightest hope of recovery, although, when asked, he smilingly admitted that he felt perfectly well.

His death was due to a sudden acute toxæmia, the onset of which coincided with the removal of the gauze drain. Had this removal taken place on the second or third day after operation I would have had no doubt that the too early removal had determined the separation of a septic clot from the thrombosed mesentery, but it is more difficult to trace it to this when the removal was delayed till the fifth day. The gauze, which was saturated with pus, came out without the slightest difficulty.

In this series of 101 cases there have thus been 8 deaths, but as 1 of these, that due to acute obstruction, was in no way connected with the attack of appendicitis, it is permissible to leave it out in calculating the mortality percentage, which is therefore approximately 7 per cent.

It is rather striking that the deaths all occurred in the first half of the period over which this series of cases is spread; no death has occurred since August, 1912. In other words, I have had a series of 65 consecutive cases of acute suppurative appendicitis without a death.* One cannot, of course, draw any definite conclusions from so short a series, but I think that this is at least partly due to the operative treatment which I have employed during the last two years, the outstanding features of which are (1) short duration of the operation, (2) gentle handling of the inflamed tissues, and (3) efficient drainage when necessary.

Treatment. When to operate.—On the question of when to operate there has been, up till recently, great diversity of opinion. American surgeons were probably among the first to advocate early operation, and, with few exceptions, surgeons of all nationalities have now no hesitation in saying that every case should be operated on as soon as possible after the diagnosis has been made.

At a time when the specialists disagreed one could not blame the practitioner if he went in for the policy of "wait and see;" but now that this vexed question has once and for all been settled, it behoves the practitioner to see that the surgeon has the opportunity given him to carry out the policy of early operation. The advantages offered by early operation are so numerous and so evident that it is hard to understand how anyone can remain unconvinced.

In the first place, it must be admitted that the symptoms during the first twenty-four hours of an attack of acute appendicitis do not form a reliable index as to its subsequent course. The more experienced the observer the more readily does he confess his inability to say whether the inflammatory process is within the next twenty-four, thirty-six, or forty-eight hours to subside, or whether it is to increase in severity. One's ignorance at this early stage is even more profound, because, in any given case, it is impossible not only to predict

---

* To those 65 consecutive recoveries from acute suppurative appendicitis may be added 20 cases operated on since January, 1914, thus bringing the series (still unbroken) up to 88.

what is going to happen, but equally impossible to be *absolutely* certain as to the exact state of affairs at the moment. Thus, in 8 of my cases of Type I, in which the appendix was distended with pus, the pulse was not over 80 and the temperature not higher than 99° F.; in 3 of these cases the localised pain, tenderness, and rigidity were so very slight as to make the diagnosis of appendicitis doubtful, and yet in all these cases the appendix contained pus. Again, in 2 of my cases of Type II the localised pain, tenderness, and rigidity were very slight (in 1 the pulse was 60 and the temperature 98° F.), and yet in these 2 cases the appendix was completely gangrenous.

For these two reasons, then—one's inability to state the exact condition at the time, and one's ignorance as to the future progress—the plea for early operation is a strong one. The critic may retort that if every case of acute appendicitis is operated on in the early stages, then some have been submitted to operation which, if left alone and submitted to what is called the "expectant treatment" (a most speculative procedure), would have subsided, and which might then have been operated on in the interval stage. Quite apart from the fact that it is impossible to say what case will ever reach the interval stage, is it wrong to remove an appendix which is the seat of an acute catarrhal inflammation? It is done practically without risk, the patient makes a rapid recovery, and has a sound scar. Again, one knows how often a patient who would readily submit to operation when suffering pain, rebels when told that he must in cold blood in the interval stage have his appendix removed. Thus it happens that many mild cases are allowed to have attack after attack until the character of the attack suddenly changes, and operation becomes absolutely necessary. Unfortunately one cannot say that numerous antecedent attacks make the present one any safer.

It is no discredit to a surgeon, after recommending immediate operation, to find on opening the abdomen an appendix which is in a condition of acute catarrhal inflammation; it is, indeed, a matter for mutual congratulation on the part of practitioner and surgeon.

In the second place, coming to the type of case which at

the operation proves to have advanced past the catarrhal stage, what advantage does one gain by early operation? There can be no possible dubiety about this. It may be that, in certain cases, an appendix full of pus will remain quiescent for an indefinite period, but no one can deny that a patient going about with his appendix full of pus is in a very unsafe condition. In the vast majority of suppurative appendices the inflammatory process is progressive, and if left alone will extend until ulceration of all the coats of the appendix takes place and gangrene and perforation occur.

Again, taking Type VI (acute spreading peritonitis), we find that the severity and urgency of the symptoms forced the hand of the most determined believer in delay, and thus allowed most of these cases to be saved, whereas delay obviously meant death. The two deaths, in cases of this type, which occurred in my series, were in cases which were submitted to operation on the second day of the attack; every hour that was lost certainly reduced the chances of one of them who, partly because of a pre-existing cardiac condition, made no fight at all against the acute peritonitis which ultimately killed him on the fourth day after operation.

Coming now, in the third place, to the types of cases in which an *abscess* is present, one has to give well-founded reasons for immediate operation, for unfortunately it is believed, and preached, by not a few that if a localised abscess is found when the patient is first seen it is safe to delay. This is a most dangerous policy, for just as no one, however experienced, can tell what will take place within the first 24 or 48 hours of the acute attack, so no one can with certainty say that an abscess, no matter how well localised, will remain local. Out of 51 cases in which an abscess was present, the abscess was leaking into the general peritoneal cavity in 16, and had ruptured in 7. If it is admitted, then, that one cannot guarantee that a localised abscess will neither leak nor burst, it remains only to point out the very evident advantages to be gained by anticipating such an event.

The longer the delay in operating the greater the toxæmia, especially if the peritoneum has been flooded with "offensive" pus. The presence of an early spreading peritonitis, from a

leaking abscess, much more of an acute general peritonitis
from a ruptured abscess, not only causes a profound change
in the condition of the patient (thus making the prognosis
more grave), but practically ensures the occurrence of more
or less serious complications.

In this series there was one death out of 28 cases of localised
abscess, and this occurred in a patient who had been ill for
five days. *Post-mortem* examination showed that there was
no peritonitis, but the presence of petechial hæmorrhages on
the pleura and pericardium, in addition to the rapid exacerba-
tion of the symptoms, showed that death was due to an acute
toxæmia. Without a doubt this patient would have had a
better chance of recovery if operated on sooner.

Another strong plea for early operation in cases of localised
abscess is to be found in the fact that there were no complications in cases seen within four days of the onset of the
illness, whereas marked distension, fæcal fistula, and ventral
hernia occurred in the later cases. This is seen in the average
duration in bed, which was 26 days for cases operated on
before the fifth day, but as high as 38 for cases operated
on after the fifth day.

Contrasting the results of operation in the cases of localised
abscess with those of the cases which had been left until
leakage or *rupture* took place we find—(1) a mortality of
3½ per cent in Type III, 19 per cent in Type IV, and 29 per
cent in Type V; and (2) complications were neither so
frequent nor so varied in Type III as in Types IV and V.
This applied especially to post-operative distension and
pulmonary complications.

It is quite true that if every case of localised abscess could
safely be left until the abscess was adherent to the anterior
abdominal wall there would probably be no deaths at all, as
such an abscess can be easily and safely evacuated by a small
extra-peritoneal incision; but, as has been shown, this course
cannot *safely* be taken.

Thus, every case of acute appendicitis ought to be operated
on as soon as the diagnosis is made, and the surgeon who,
seeing cases in the more advanced stages, delays operation, is
courting failure, for not only does the general condition of
the patient become worse, but there is always the risk of

what is apparently a well-localised abscess changing its character, and either leaking or rupturing into the general peritoneal cavity.

In every case in this series the operation was performed as soon as the patient had been transferred either to a nursing home or to hospital. A large localised abscess adherent to the anterior abdominal wall can be safely opened in any circumstances, no matter how unfavourable, but it is advisable in all other cases to have good light and the other simple necessaries which are to be found in a modern operating theatre.

No preparatory treatment is necessary; a single application of a 4 per cent solution of iodine in rectified spirit, after dry shaving, being all that is required.

The incision.—For the great majority of cases the best incision is the *gridiron,* which gives in almost every case a perfect view of the field of operation, whether the appendix is retro-cæcal, iliac, or pelvic. This incision can be extended either upwards or downwards by cutting across the internal oblique and transversalis muscles. This extension may be necessitated by—(1) the retro-cæcal position of the appendix (extension upwards); (2) the pelvic position of the appendix (extension downwards); (3) the fixation of the cæcum; (4) incomplete relaxation owing to anæsthetic difficulties. There is no doubt that the gridiron incision is much less likely to be followed by ventral hernia than any other. I have not found that there is any tendency for a re-collection of pus to form behind it provided the gauze drain is left in for five days. In 72 of my cases the simple gridiron sufficed —in 13 of these the appendix was pelvic in position; a ventral hernia occurred in only 1. In 17 cases the simple gridiron incision was not sufficient, and an upward (in 8 cases) or a downward (in 9 cases) extension was made; a ventral hernia occurred in 2.

In very early cases in which the diagnosis may be doubtful, the *vertical incision through the right rectus muscle* is found to be very useful. This was employed in 6 of my cases, 3 of which were in 1911 before I had realised how much could be seen and done through a gridiron incision, even when the appendix was in the pelvis.   In 1 of these the partially stitched wound opened and a ventral hernia resulted.

For large abscess, adherent to the anterior abdominal wall, a small *extra-peritoneal* incision is often advisable.   In 4 of my cases this was done, the appendix not being looked for. In 2 cases the incision was a *subumbilical* one in the middle line—in one because the patient was moribund and great speed was essential, in the other to open a very large abscess reaching up to the umbilicus; in this case a ventral hernia resulted.

The peritoneum having been opened, rolls of gauze are introduced and the field of operation carefully walled off from the general peritoneal cavity.   This precaution is not of course taken in cases of acute spreading peritonitis.   While this is being done the character of the fluid, if any, in the general peritoneal cavity is noted.

The cæcum is then very gently displaced upwards and the base of the appendix looked for.   If the cæcum is fixed, as the result of old adhesions due to former attacks, no attempt is made to pull it up out of the abdomen.   The appendix is removed in the usual manner, the stump being ligated, carbolised, and invaginated by a purse-string suture when possible.

The appendix was removed at the time of operation in 94 of my cases; in 2 it was found impossible to ligate the stump (in 1 of these there was gangrene of the cæcum); in 12 it was impossible, or inadvisable, to turn in the stump after ligation owing either to the bad condition of the patient necessitating speed, or to fixation of the cæcum.

Should the tip of the appendix be inaccessible, especially if the appendix be distended with pus and likely to rupture, it is best to divide it at the base between two ligatures, and remove it base first.   This was found to be advisable in many cases of retro-cæcal and pelvic appendices.

Throughout the operation the cæcum should be handled very gently, not only on account of possible damage to the part actually touched, but also because of the danger of separating clots in the veins of the mesentery.   The retro-cæcal, retro-peritoneal tissues should be opened as little as possible, especially if there is a retro-cæcal abscess.   The operation should be performed quickly—it should *always* be completely finished within a quarter of an hour.

Drainage.—The question of drainage divides itself naturally into two parts—(1) Is drainage necessary? and (2) is drainage possible?

When discussing whether drainage is necessary one can very easily answer the question so far as the peritoneal fluids are concerned. If the peritoneal fluid is "defensive," reactionary, or protective in character, then it is not only unnecessary but inadvisable to remove it. On the other hand, the "offensive" fluid, in which the bacteria have gained the upper hand, must be removed if at all possible.

Again, if it is possible to remove the whole of the necrotic or gangrenous tissue involved, then no local drainage is necessary, as the whole of the active bacterial army, including the reserves, has been removed. On the other hand, if the gangrenous process, which originated in the appendix, has spread to the surrounding tissues, if the cæcum, the omentum, or the adjacent peritoneum has become necrotic or gangrenous, then it would be folly to leave this undrained. The bacterial army which we have been unable to remove, however diminished in numbers, may or may not be overwhelmed by the defensive forces of the peritoneum. In cases of doubt one may risk more if the doubtful area is situated in the pelvis (where it will be flooded with defensive fluid) than if it is in the retro-cæcal tissues.

Coming to the second question—Is drainage possible?—we find that in most cases it is not only possible, but very easily effected. In the case of the large localised abscess adherent to the anterior abdominal wall, all that is needed is the insertion of a large drainage-tube through a small extra-peritoneal incision. Again, in cases of abscess more deeply situated the best method of drainage is the insertion of gauze. The gauze soon becomes saturated, and after about twelve hours ceases to act as a drain, but by keeping the wound open and by inducing the formation of adhesions it isolates the local area of necrosis or gangrene from the general peritoneal cavity. On the removal of the gauze, which ought to be left in for at least five days, the local area has thus been transformed into what is virtually a superficial discharging wound. It is unnecessary to use a drainage-tube in combination with gauze if one has gently mopped out the offensive fluid. At the best the tube would drain for a few hours only, as the openings in it are soon closed by the omentum or by coils of intestine. The tube, also, is a source of danger from pressure necrosis, and may thus determine the occurrence of a fæcal fistula. Several cases of hæmorrhage from the external iliac artery from this cause have been reported.

If, however, the patient is so ill (for example, in a case of ruptured abscess) that great speed is necessary, and there is no time to mop out the pus, then one can insert a tube surrounded with gauze, the tube being withdrawn in twelve or twenty-four hours. The withdrawal of the tube by loosening the gauze allows of further drainage through the latter.

The only case that presents any real difficulty is the acute diffuse peritonitis in which the general peritoneal cavity contains offensive pus. It is impossible to drain the general peritoneal cavity effectively by mechanical means, and in these cases all that one can do is to employ local drainage, if that is called for by the local conditions, and enable the peritoneum to drain itself by the use of Fowler's position, supplemented by proctoclysis. Some advantage may be gained in these cases by leaving a tube in the pelvis (and this can easily be done in combination with the local gauze drain if that is employed), but at the best this drains for only a short period.

With the exception of the acute diffuse peritonitis, it is usually easy to decide at the time whether drainage is necessary, but in some cases it may be impossible to tell whether the bacteria or the cells are winning. The duration of the symptoms, the condition of the patient, may help one to form an opinion, but the method suggested by Wilkie, of Edinburgh, is the only reliable guide. In cases of acute diffuse peritonitis Wilkie examines the fluid during the operation. If the large mononuclear cells outnumber the polymorphonuclear cells, and are displaying their phagocytic activity in ingesting the latter, if the polymorphonuclear cells are not degenerated, and if the bacteria are largely intercellular, he concludes that the defensive forces have obtained the upper hand. This fluid is defensive, and ought to be left. If, on the other hand, there are few mononuclear cells, if there is little phagocytosis, if the polymorphonuclear cells are degenerated, and if there are a large number of extra-cellular bacteria, then he concludes that the bacteria are winning, and the fluid can rightly be treated as offensive and steps taken for its removal. Since reading Wilkie's paper I have employed his method in every case, and have found it a most useful guide to the character of the fluid and to the need for, or inadvisability of, drainage of the peritoneal cavity.

To those who advocate primary closure for all types of cases, and who point to the occurrence of a fæcal fistula or a ventral hernia as the disastrous result of drainage, one can truly answer that these complications occur not because, but in spite of, the employment of a gauze drain. These complications, also, are trivial when compared with the retro-peritoneal cellulitis, sub-diaphragmatic abscess, or even acute diffuse peritonitis, which occasionally do occur when cases— *e.g.*, localised abscesses—which demand local drainage are treated by primary closure.

These principles with regard to drainage have been followed in the treatment of the cases in this series. Several cases of Types I and II, in which local drainage was employed in 1911, would undoubtedly have been treated by primary closure had they occurred in 1912 or 1913. In 1911, also, I was more apt to use a drainage-tube in addition to a gauze drain, and I had not realised that the defensive pus was not only innocuous but beneficial, and that its removal was not only unnecessary but harmful.

Cases treated by primary closure.—In 27 cases of this series primary closure was employed. Sixteen of them were cases of Type I, in which there was pus inside the appendix, and in which the peritoneal conditions varied from a normal peritoneal cavity to a diffuse purulent peritonitis.

Ten were cases of Type II, in which the appendix was gangrenous, and in which the general peritoneal cavity contained serous, sero-purulent, or purulent fluid. The remaining case was one of Type VI, a case of acute free-spreading peritonitis of three days' duration with a large quantity of pus in the general peritoneal cavity. This patient was very ill with acute bronchitis, and I felt that his only chance was to close the abdomen in the hope that the peritoneum would be able to attend to its own drainage. The local conditions in this case did not call for any local drainage. This proved to be correct, and the fact that he had no open wound undoubtedly helped him to pull through the attack of acute double pneumonia which ensued.

Twenty-three of the 27 cases healed by first intention; in the others there was a bacillus coli infection of the sub-cutaneous tissues, which became evident at the end of about six days, and which delayed the healing of the wound.

The case already referred to under "mortality" who on his admission to hospital was in a moribund condition, and who died six hours after operation, is not included in these figures, although his wound was closed at the operation, as the closure was due not to his chances of recovery, but to the certainty of his almost immediate death.

Cases treated by drainage.—A. In 3 cases the wound was almost completely closed, *a drainage tube* being inserted for various reasons.

In 1 case (one of Type I) this was done because there was a large quantity of inodorous (and therefore not bacillus coli) pus in the general peritoneal cavity. The appendix, which was distended with pus, was covered with purulent exudation. The tube might have been dispensed with as little, if any, discharge came through it, and the wound healed by first intention. Had the pus been examined during the operation it would evidently have proved to be defensive in character.

In the second case (one of Type II) the drainage tube was also unnecessary; very little discharge came from it, but it led to infection of the wound which opened up on the sixth day, after which there was a copious purulent discharge.

In the third case (one of Type III) there was a very small abscess of five days' duration. This pus, although strictly speaking offensive, evidently contained few active bacteria, as there was little discharge through the tube, and the wound healed by first intention.

A local drain was advisable, but gauze would have been more suitable than a tube.

B. A gauze drain was used in 69 cases.

Type I.—Two cases of Type I were treated with a gauze drain, but if immediate examination of the peritoneal fluid had been made it would have been found to be defensive, and, as in neither case was local drainage called for, primary closure could safely have been employed. In the first there was free non-odorous pus which proved to be due to a staphylococcus; in the second the fluid, which was sero-purulent, was due to a pneumococcus.

In both there was very little discharge, either through the gauze drain or after its removal; and in both the wound, which had been almost completely stitched, healed without infection.

Type II.—Three cases of Type II were treated with gauze drainage. In the first the drain was used because the omentum was very œdematous, the pelvis was full of pus, and the patient was very ill (temperature 100° F., pulse 120); but immediate examination of the pelvic pus would have shown that drainage was unnecessary. There was little discharge, and the wound, which had almost completely closed, healed without infection.

In the second case the appendix, which was gangrenous, lay behind the terminal ileum, and during its removal the retro-peritoneal tissues were opened and infected with the contents of the appendix. Although the partially stitched wound healed without opening, the necessity for local drainage was shown by the copious purulent discharge which followed the removal of the gauze.

In the third case also the gauze drain proved to have been necessary. The wound was not closed because there was an area of local necrosis of the peritoneum on the right side of the pelvis some distance away from the gangrenous appendix, which was iliac in position. Although there was little discharge when the gauze drain was removed on the fifth day, a localised collection of pus formed at the brim of the pelvis which was evacuated on the eleventh day.

Thus, in 3 of these 5 cases of Types I and II in which a gauze drain was used, it might have been dispensed with if an immediate examination of the peritoneal fluid had been made.

Type VI.—In 16 cases of Type VI a gauze drain was employed chiefly for local drainage.

In 2 cases in 1911, and in 1 case in 1912 a tube was also used because of the very large amount of fluid present; it proved unnecessary in all 3, and would not have been used if immediate examination of the fluid had been made.

The remaining 48 cases which were drained with gauze were cases of *abscess,* either localised (26 cases), leaking (16 cases), or ruptured (6 cases), and I have absolutely no doubt that in all drainage was not only advisable but necessary.

In 10 of these cases, all in 1911, a tube was used in addition, usually because of the large amount of pus in the abscess, sometimes because the condition of the patient did not allow of time being taken to mop out the pus. In all the tube proved to be practically useless; and, as a fæcal fistula occurred in 2 of these cases, it was probably not only useless but harmful. The gauze drain in order to be efficacious must not be too tightly packed; it must be introduced right down to the seat of the local gangrene or necrosis, and it ought not to be removed before, at least, five days. If it is removed earlier the adhesions, which are shutting off the localised area from the peritoneal cavity, are disturbed, and a spreading peritonitis may be the result.

If the gauze is forcibly withdrawn too soon the clotted veins in its vicinity may be injured, and a septic clot, becoming loosened, may give rise to a sudden acute septicæmia or pyæmia. In 1 of my fatal cases in 1911 a fresh spreading peritonitis developed shortly after the gauze drain had been removed on the second day, and a large secondary abscess ultimately formed on the left side of the abdomen. I feel sure that the disastrous train of complications in this case which ultimately led to the patient's death arose directly from the too early removal of the gauze drain. In another fatal case, the patient's condition, which was satisfactory on the morning of the second day after operation, became rapidly much worse after the gauze drain had been removed on that day, and death took place two days later. In this case the early removal of the gauze did not give rise to a peritonitis, but to an acute septicæmia with petechial hæmorrhages on pleura and pericardium.

In one other case death took place with tragic suddenness within fourteen hours of the removal of the gauze, but in this case the gauze was not taken out until the fifth day, and the removal was accomplished so easily (with no disturbance of the local conditions) that it is hard to make its removal responsible. But at the same time the patient, whose pulse was 64, became ill a few hours after the removal, showing unmistakeable signs of acute toxæmia. The mesentery of the appendix was in a condition of septic thrombosis, and it would have been well to have left this gauze in even longer.

Leaving the gauze in for five days makes its removal easy (no anæsthetic is required except occasionally for children); it makes its removal safe (except perhaps in cases of septic thrombosis of the appendix mesentery in which it might with more safety be left longer); and it does away with the necessity of repacking. The wound is usually patent enough, after the removal of the gauze drain on the fifth day, to allow of free exit for the discharge. If there is any suggestion of it being dammed back one can easily introduce a *short* drainage tube for one or two days, but care should be taken that this does not protrude into the abdominal cavity.

Repacking of the wound was done in 9 cases, but besides being unnecessary, and unpleasant for the patient, this may be harmful by favouring the formation of a fæcal fistula (in 4 cases) or a ventral hernia (in 3 cases).

Partial stitching of the wound was done in 45 out of the 69 drained with gauze. In some the wound was almost completely stitched, the gauze drain being a very small one. Of these, 25 healed without the wound being infected—that is, more than 50 per cent. Thus, it is well worth while, in many cases, partially to close the wound, leaving of course sufficient exit for drainage, as besides shortening the convalescence, it lessens the chance of a ventral hernia.

Secondary stitching of the wound was done in 10 cases only, and in most of them only a few stitches were used to draw the edges together. In most of the cases it was found that the edges could be satisfactorily brought together by strips of adhesive plaster as soon as the discharge had ceased.

Post-operative treatment.—In many of the cases, especially in Types I, II, and III, very little post-operative treatment is necessary beyond the administration of small doses of a sedative during the first twenty-four or forty-eight hours to relieve pain.   On the other hand, the treatment of acute spreading peritonitis after operation is all important. Fowler's position ought to be employed in all cases in which there is a pelvic or a diffuse peritonitis.   In addition to this, vigorous effective proctoclysis ought to be instituted immediately after the operation, and, provided that sufficient saline is introduced into and absorbed by the bowel, I do not think that it matters much whether this is done by the continuous or the interrupted method.   If there is great collapse saline ought to be given subcutaneously or intravenously immediately after the operation.

For the relief of pain morphia (or omnopon) ought to be given in small frequently repeated doses.   If there is much post-operative distension physostigmine given in doses of gr. $\frac{1}{120}$ every six hours is usually very effective, and can be conveniently combined with gr. $\frac{1}{12}$ of morphia.   Turpentine or quinine enemata are sometimes helpful if flatus is not passed within twenty-four hours.

There is nothing to be said against, and a great deal in favour of, early purgation, and feeding should be commenced as soon as sickness has stopped.

Duration in bed.—The average duration in bed of my cases was 29 days.

Conclusions.—1. Every case of acute appendicitis ought to be operated on at once.

2. The operation ought to be of short duration—never more than quarter of an hour.

3. As little as possible should be done, and that little should be done very gently.

4. The gridiron incision is the best for almost all cases.

5. Local drainage ought to be employed when the local conditions demand it. The best drain is gauze, which should be left in for at least five days. The wound should not be repacked.

6. Partial closure of a drained wound is advisable.

7. Secondary stitching is usually unnecessary.

8. The peritoneal fluids are, broadly speaking, of two kinds—"offensive," which ought to be removed; "defensive," which ought to be left alone.

9. Drainage of the general peritoneal cavity, when required, is very ineffective by mechanical means; local drainage, with possibly a pelvic tube, must be supplemented by Fowler's position and proctoclysis.

Obituary.

RICHARD BURNS MACPHERSON, M.D.Glasg.,
Cambuslang.

WE regret to announce the death of Dr. R. B. Macpherson, which
occurred at his residence on 2nd June. Dr. Macpherson, who is
survived by a widow and a grown-up family, was born in Port-
Glasgow in 1852, and studied medicine in the University of
Glasgow, where he early made his mark, being the first Rainy
Bursar. He took the degree of M.B., C.M. with honours in
1876, when, as the most distinguished student of his year, he
carried off the Brunton Memorial Prize. After graduation he
served as resident physician in the Glasgow Royal Infirmary,
and afterwards as resident surgeon in the then recently
established Western Infirmary. From 1876 to 1877 he was
president of the Glasgow University Medico-Chirurgical Society,
and at the end of his term of duty in the Western Infirmary he
passed to active service, joining the surgical staff of the Turkish
army in the Russo-Turkish war of 1877-78. He served throughout the war, and at its close received the thanks of the Turkish
Government and the Imperial Order of the Medjidieh. His
experiences in the war are vividly recounted in *Under the Red
Crescent: or Ambulance Adventures in the Russo-Turkish War,*
a volume which he published after his return, when he settled
in practice in Cambuslang. He took the degree of M.D. in
1885, and in the course of his busy life he held many public
appointments. He was medical officer of health and parochial
medical officer for Cambuslang, and also certifying surgeon
under the Factories Act. Occupied as he was, he still found
time for literary pursuits, and was a well-known member of
the Scottish Society of Literature and Art. His interest in the
public affairs of Cambuslang was keen and constant, and he was
the first president of its Highland Society, which he did much
to found. His genial personality and his ready helpfulness
endeared him alike to his patients and to his professional
brethren, among whom his loss will be widely mourned.

JOHN GAREY, M.R.C.S.,
GOVANHILL.

WE regret to announce the death of Mr. John Garey, M.R.C.S., which took place on 19th June at a nursing home in Glasgow. Mr. Garey, who studied medicine at the Glasgow Royal Infirmary, took the degree of M.R.C.S. in 1880, and thereafter settled in Govanhill, where he conducted a large practice until the onset of his fatal illness. In addition to the attention which he devoted to his professional work, Mr. Garey was also keenly interested in public and political affairs. He took a prominent part in the annexation of Govanhill to the city in 1891, and was one of its first representatives upon the Town Council, of which he was a member for about fourteen years. He was an enthusiastic Radical, and acted as chairman at most of the Liberal meetings held in Govanhill. His death, which followed upon some months of failing health, was due to an internal malady, on account of which he had entered the nursing home for operation.

CURRENT TOPICS.

GLASGOW MEDICAL JOURNAL: NEW SERIES.—With the present number commences a new series of the *Glasgow Medical Journal,* in accordance with the announcement made in the previous issue. The alterations in the size of the page and in the general appearance of the *Journal* are so evident as to require little comment. It is believed that the increased size of the page and the wider spacing of the type will make the numbers easier to read, and that the paper which has been selected will reproduce. photographic and other illustrations more clearly than that which was formerly used. Subscribers will also notice another change to which attention may be directed, namely, that an Editorial Committee has been appointed to assist the Editors in the work of scrutinising the material sent for publication in the pages of the *Journal.* The names of the members of the Committee appear on the cover, and it will be seen that they have been chosen to represent the various special branches of medicine and surgery and the cognate sciences.

The history of the *Glasgow Medical Journal* is a long one, and at the beginning of a new series it may be of interest briefly to recall it. Dr. Wallace Anderson's paper on Dr. Andrew Buchanan, which appeared in the June number, was devoted to one of its earliest editors. The first series of the *Journal,* however, began in 1828, under the editorial auspices of William Mackenzie, who afterwards became Waltonian lecturer on diseases of the eye in Glasgow University, and who is still remembered as one among the most distinguished ophthalmologists. The series was issued in quarterly numbers, and five annual volumes were publised under a variety of publishers and editors, among the first of whom was Dr. Andrew Buchanan. A second series was begun in 1833, and like the first was published quarterly, but survived for only one year. A long hiatus followed, and it was not until the session of 1851-52 that a committee of the Medico-Chirurgical Society was appointed to take steps for the establishment of a periodical under the auspices of that body. At the close of the session of the Society in 1852 nothing had been decided, and it was left to private individuals (Drs. J. B. Cowan, George Buchanan, and Steven) to obtain a guarantee fund, and to secure an editor in the person of Dr. William Weir, to whom they were appointed assistant editors. The first number of the third series, which still maintained the quarterly form, was issued in 1853. The first year's working resulted in a considerable deficit, a change of publisher, and a grant_in-aid from the Medico-Chirurgical Society, after which publication was un-interrupted until the third series came to an end in January, 1866. During this period the editorship passed successively into the hands of Drs. George Buchanan and J. B. Cowan, Drs. Joseph Bell and William Leishman, and Dr. P. A. Simpson. It was under the editorship of Drs. Cowan and Buchanan that the names of the editors first appeared upon the cover, and this step was taken in response to an attack made by Dr. Lawrie, then Professor of Surgery in Glasgow University, upon an editorial on the monopoly of University teaching for graduation, which he denounced as "an anonymous article by two unfledged editors."

The fourth series, still under the editorship of Dr. Simpson, immediately followed the third, and inaugurated the issue of monthly numbers. After two years, however, the quarterly form was resumed in 1868, the change being the occasion for the beginning of the fifth series, which came to a close with the issue of our previous number. In 1878 the monthly form was once more adopted, and in 1879 the issue of two volumes a year began. Between 1869 and the present time there have been many editorial changes, and the *Journal* has been successively edited, separately or conjointly, by Drs. J. B. Russell, H. E. Clark, Joseph Coats, A. Napier, Lindsay Steven, John Carslaw, and T. K. Monro. In all, eighty-one volumes of the fifth series have been published, and, if we add to these the volumes of the previous series, the total number amounts to a hundred and two volumes, which have been issued in the course of sixty-seven years of publication.

It remains to add that the *Glasgow Medical Journal* was the first medical journal to be published outside of London.

APPOINTMENTS.—The following appointments have recently been made :—

W. Kirkpatrick Anderson, M.B., Ch.B. Glasg. (1902), to be Visiting Physician to the Eastern District Hospital, Glasgow.

L. C. Broughton-Head, M.B., Ch.B. Glasg. (1903), L.D.S. Eng., to be Dentist to the Royal Hospital for Sick Children, Glasgow.

John Brownlee, M.D. Glasg. (M.B., 1894), D.P.H., D.Sc., Physician-Superintendent of Ruchill Hospital, to be Medical Statistician under the Government Medical Research Committee.

F. J. Charteris, M.D. Glasg. (M.B., 1897), to be Visiting Physician to the Western District Hospital, Glasgow.

John Shaw Dunn, M.A., M.D.Glasg. (M.B., 1905), to be Director of the Clinical Laboratory in the Western Infirmary, and Lecturer on Clinical Pathology in the University of Glasgow.

C. H. Hall, M.D.Glasg. (M.B., 1890), to be Certifying Factory Surgeon for the Watford District, co. Hereford.

Thomas Kay, M.B., C.M.Glasg. (1893), F.R.F.P.S.G., to be Visiting Surgeon to the Glasgow Royal Infirmary.

George M'Intyre, M.B., C.M.Glasg. (1886), F.R.F.P.S.G., to be Physician for Diseases of the Skin, Glasgow Royal Infirmary.

Ivy M'Kenzie, M.B., Ch.B.Glasg. (1902), B.Sc., to be Lecturer in Mental Diseases in the Anderson College of Medicine, Glasgow.

Hugh Morton, M.D. Glasg. (M.B., 1907), to be Professor of Physiology in the Anderson College of Medicine, Glasgow.

R. M. Riggall, L.R.C.P. & S.E., L.R.F.P.S.Glasg. (1907), surgeon R.N., to be Assistant Medical Officer to the Queen Alexandra Sanatorium, Davos Platz, Switzerland.

J. Goodwin Tomkinson, M.D. Glasg. (M.B., 1901), to be Lecturer in Dermatology in the Anderson College of Medicine, Glasgow.

Archibald Young, M.B., C.M.Glasg. (1895), B.Sc., to be Visiting Surgeon to the Eastern and Western District Hospitals, Glasgow.

Army Medical Service: Surgeon-General William Babtie, V.C., C.B., C.M.G., M.B.Glasg., to be Honorary Surgeon to the King. Captain Reginald Storrs, L.R.C.P. & S.E., L.R.F.P.S.Glasg. (1898), to be Major.

THE LISTER WARD.—At a meeting of Glasgow University Court, held on 11th June, it was intimated by Sir David M'Vail, as one of the managers of the Royal Infirmary, that a request from the University Court had been considered on the previous day at a meeting of the Board of Managers. The Court, having learned that the Infirmary managers had decided to remove the Lister Ward, requested them to grant the University an opportunity of acquiring the materials of the Lister Ward and of the Lister operating theatre for the purpose of re-erecting them in the University grounds. After very full consideration, although some of the managers were loth to grant the request, the majority were of opinion that, in view of its situation, the ward would be detrimental to the new buildings in course of erection. They, therefore, decided to transfer the materials of the ward and theatre, which Sir David was sure would be a great asset to the University. Principal Sir Donald MacAlister intimated that the matter would come up at the next meeting of the Court.

GLASGOW UNIVERSITY CLUB, LONDON.—The half-yearly dinner of this club, held in the Trocadero Restaurant on 27th May, was notable for the occupancy of the chair by Emeritus Professor John Cleland, and for the large number of medical and other graduates of Glasgow University who assembled to do him honour. Among those present were Sir Henry Craik, M.P., Principal J. Yule Mackay, the Rev. Dr. John Smith, Govan; Sir W. B. Leishman, Mr. John R. Cleland, R.F.A.; Professor J. M. Thomson, Professor John Adams, Dr. Quintin Chalmers, Professor J. D. Cormack, the Rev. W. Parker Hanks, Professor G. B. Henderson, Mr. W. Craig Henderson, Mr. J. Keller, Dr. Norman M'Lehose, Sir John M'Call, Surgeon-General Sir Arthur Slogett, Professor W. R. Smith, Lieut.-Colonel Stonham, Lieut.-Colonel Legge, Inspector-General of the Australian Forces; Dr. Guthrie Rankin, Professor J. B. M'Ewen, Sir Thomas Oliver, Lieut.-Colonel Sir Newton Moore, Dr. Morris, Commonwealth Medical Officer in London; and Dr. Roxburgh and Dr. Alex. Macphail, hon. secretaries. Among the apologies for absence was one from Principal Sir Donald MacAlister.

Professor Cleland proposed " The University of Glasgow " in a speech in which he drew on personal reminiscences. He supposed that it was the *Alma Mater* of nearly every man in the room, and he would not be surprised if he were one of the very few of those present who were not thus connected with it. But he could say this, that he had spent a much longer time in the University than most of those present. He had performed the duties of Professor of Anatomy for thirty-two years, and he had been two years a demonstrator previous to that. His recollections, therefore, went back to a time long before their formation of the Glasgow University Club in London. Glasgow University had produced men of great mark—for example, Black the chemist, and Campbell the poet, and he was sorry that his active days in connection with it were past. His first connection with Glasgow was as demonstrator under Professor Allen Thomson, the father of a gentleman whom he saw present. A most genial man he was, and he did much for the study of anatomy. He raised its character to a height which it had never reached before. Besides that, he was the first man in this country to teach that very important part of his subject which went by the name of embryology. He was sorry to say that there were very few of the professors alive that were in Glasgow at the time he became a professor. There was only one who still remained in his chair, Professor Ferguson. He was glad, however, that some of the other professors with whom he had been associated in early years were still with them. As he looked round the room he would say "Long may the University of Glasgow flourish." His connection had been entirely with the medical school, and it had produced men who had distinguished themselves in a remarkable way, such as their friend, Professor Leishman. Professor Leishman had made himself famous in what were now known as "Leishman's bodies." The prosperity of the University in the past few years had been very rapid. The medical school in Glasgow might now set itself up as as good as any university in the kingdom.

At the close of the evening, Principal Yule Mackay, speaking as an old student and friend of Professor Cleland, proposed "The Chairman" in words expressing high appreciation of his personal and professional character. The toast, which was received with Highland honours, was drunk with great enthusiasm.

GENERAL MEDICAL COUNCIL.—A number of points of interest to the medical profession were dealt with by Principal Sir Donald MacAlister in his address as President of the General Medical Council in London on 25th May.

He mentioned that much attention was given by the Council at the end of last year to certain questions arising under the regulations for National Health Insurance. From time to time communications reached the Registrar vaguely alleging that medical men sometimes described as "panel" and sometimes as "non-panel" practitioners were disregarding the warning notices of the Council in respect of canvassing or advertising with the intent to attract patients or of issuing certificates of a misleading or inaccurate character. By direction of the Executive Committee the Registrar had made widely known that the Council took a grave view of such practices, and had intimated its purpose to inquire judicially into the conduct of any practitioner against whom a substantiated complaint of the kind might be brought. Certain complaints of this nature would, on the advice of the Penal Cases Committee, be submitted for judgment during the present session. But it was proper to say that a few general allegations had been sent to the office which were unsupported by tangible evidence, or were made by persons who declined to take the responsibility of formulating any specific complaint on which even a preliminary inquiry could be based.

The Midwives Act of 1902, under which certain duties were laid upon this Council, did not apply to Scotland. A Bill "to secure the better training of midwives in Scotland and to regulate their practice" had, on the initiative of Lord Balfour of Burleigh, passed the House of Lords, and now awaited consideration in the other House. Having in mind certain improvements on the English Act that had from time to time been desired by the Council, he ventured to suggest to Lord Balfour at an early stage that these might advantageously be introduced into the Scottish Bill, and he believed that nearly all of them had now been incorporated. The Lord President had sent to the Council a copy of the Bill as thus adjusted, with a request for their observations. The Executive Committee would, in due course, be ready to propose a convenient method of dealing with the subject.

The Pharmacopœia Committee and the editors had been busily occupied in forwarding the preparation of the text and appendices of the *British Pharmacopœia.* Before the end of the present session the committee would be able to lay on the table of the Council a copy of the revised proof, representing the completed work, which the committee hoped to have ready for issue during the summer.

MEMORIAL TO DR. COWAN, MAYBOLE.—A meeting of the committee having charge of the Dr. Maclure Cowan Memorial Fund was held on 1st June in Maybole. The hon. secretary and treasurer of the fund reported that the subscriptions received amounted to £573. Of this total Glasgow and Ayr subscribed £192, and the villages around Maybole about £140, while the Maybole district contributed about £240. The committee have resolved to purchase an annuity payable for 18 years on behoof of the widow and children, the annuity to cost £500. A monument is being erected at the grave of the late doctor in Maybole cemetery, and is to embrace a bronze medallion likeness of Dr. Cowan. No less than £190 of the total sum received has been subscribed by the medical profession.

THE EYESIGHT OF BRITISH SEAMEN.—The Board of Trade issued on 26th May a White Paper containing a report on the sight tests used in the mercantile marine and sea fishing service, covering the period from 1st April to 31st December, 1913. During that period the total number of candidates examined was 6,183, and of these 6,053 passed in form vision and 130 failed. There was a total of 5,799 candidates examined in the colour vision tests, of whom 283 failed at local examinations and 163 were referred for further examination. Of the candidates who failed 94 appealed for special examination, of whom 26 passed and 68 failed; while of the referred candidates 97 passed, 39 failed, and 36 had not been re-examined at the close of the period covered by the report. The total number of candidates who failed in colour vision between 1st April and 31st December was thus 287. The number of officers (including skippers and second hands of fishing vessels), already in possession of certificates, who on coming up for examination in the above period failed to pass the form vision test was 5,

1 holding a certificate as master, 1 as first mate, and 3 as second mate.

GLASGOW EAR, NOSE AND THROAT HOSPITAL.—The annual general meeting of patrons and subscribers to the Glasgow Ear, Nose and Throat Hospital was held in the institution at Elmbank Crescent on 10th June. Colonel Charles M. King presided. Dr. Thomas Barr, who submitted the medical report, said that 3,334 patients had been treated in the hospital, 1,830 males and 1,504 females, and, as each patient was seen on an average about four times, the attendances had been 14,258, or 48 daily. The figures showed an increase of 100 patients over the previous year.

The directors' report, which was read by Mr. Adam Sutherland, secretary, showed that the income was £1,220, 1s. 2d,. and the expenditure £1,033, 19s. 3d., leaving a balance of £186, 1s. 11d. The directors had received a sum of £100 from the residue of the estate of Mr. Jas. Clason Harvie; £100 from the estate of Mr. J. Carfrae Alston, a former director; and £200 from the estate of Mr. William Weir of Kildonan. In the matter of donations from patients and friends there was an increase of £96, 13s. 9d. as compared with the previous year, while many of the public works had responded to the appeal for a share of their charitable funds.

The chairman, in moving the adoption of the reports, said they all felt great pleasure at the steady advance the hospital was making in all its branches. They had always been lucky in finding money to keep them going, but they were becoming a little ambitious, and they might expend some in improving their premises.

Colonel Howie seconded, and the reports were approved.

Dr. Barlow, Dr. Fraser, Mr. D. C. Andrew, and Mr. Scott also took part in the proceedings. Mr. Wm. Cuthbert, of the Clyde Shipping Company, was appointed a director in room of Mr. Skinner.

DONATION FOR CANCER RESEARCH.—The treasurer of the Glasgow Royal Cancer Hospital (Mr. Thomson Brodie, C.A.) has received an anonymous donation of £1,000 towards the funds of the research department of that institution.

NEW CONVALESCENT HOME.—The Broomfield Convalescent Home, Shandon, which is intended for the treatment of recently confined women and their infants, was formally opened on 29th May. The home was founded and endowed by Mr. A. F. Yarrow, the well-known shipbuilder, who has presented it to his daughter-in-law, Mrs. Harold E. Yarrow. It occupies a picturesque site on the shores of the Gareloch, and the grounds surrounding it extend to about six acres. The home is under the care of Dr. Robert Jardine, with whom is associated Dr. Leonard Findlay, physician to the Royal Hospital for Sick Children, Glasgow. Dr. Arthur D. Downes, Helensburgh, is the visiting physician. Six mothers and infants are to be accommodated, and each mother, who will have a room to herself and child, will be entitled to remain for a fortnight. Preference will be given to patients from the Royal Maternity and Women's Hospital, Glasgow, and to the wives of the workmen of Messrs. Yarrow, but other deserving patients will also be received.

STATE INSURANCE: EXTRAVAGANT PRESCRIBING.—Dr. James R. Drever, Secretary of the Glasgow Medical and Panel Committees, has issued a circular directing the attention of medical practitioners to the serious position which has arisen in the local area in connection with the drug fund. The circular states that the committees view with alarm the increase in the average price per prescription, which in the present medical year has risen to 10·37d., as compared with an average of 9·1d. for last year, while at the same time there is a great increase in the number of prescriptions dispensed, and in the consequent charges upon the fund. The figures are not finally adjusted for the months of April and May, but the committees understand that the total charges are much in excess of the amount available for the period. The committees have no evidence that these increases are to be accounted for by any excessive sickness, nor have they evidence that there has been any increase in the efficiency of the service corresponding to the increase in cost. An investigation is proceeding into the incidence of prescriptions, as well as into the quantities and nature of the drugs, medicines, or appliances ordered, and the Panel Committee wishes to intimate clearly that it may be necessary to exercise the powers conferred on it by the medical benefit regulations of reporting to the Insurance Committee such cases as may appear to them to have been the cause of an excessive demand upon the drug fund. The committees are further of opinion that abuse of insurance funds in this direction may form a sufficient ground for recommending the removal of any practitioner concerned from the panel. The present condition of the drug fund is not only serious but alarming, and the committees earnestly ask that practitioners will exercise a wise discretion, consistently-with the interests of their patients, in so prescribing that economy may be effected.

SOCIETY OF MEDICAL OFFICERS OF HEALTH.—The annual provincial meeting of this Society was held this year in Glasgow on 30th May, under the presidency of Dr. A. K. Chalmers, and proved to be the best attended of all its provincial meetings. Surgeon-General Gorgas, Chief Medical Officer of the United States Army, and Principal Sanitary Commissioner on the Panama Canal, was elected an honorary fellow, and Drs. S. H. Dankes, Archibald Fairlie, O. M. Holden, Ada M'Laren, Elizabeth J. Moffett, and Olive Robertson were elected fellows of the Society. Professor Matthew Hay, of Aberdeen, delivered an address on "Public health research," in which he said that he noted with pleasure the Budget proposals to devote a considerable sum to the maintenance of laboratories in aid of medical diagnosis, and he presumed also in aid of the public health service. The question would be raised as to the manner in which the grant should be expended, and he was disposed to think that the work in contemplation should be mainly carried out in laboratories specially created, as in Glasgow, for the purpose. He also referred to the need for registration reform, and was inclined to favour putting registration under the control of the Local Government Boards. He would be glad to see the proposed statistical bureau of the Medical Research Committee helping to bring about uniformity of classification, and pressing for improved medical certificates.

The members of the Society were afterwards entertained to luncheon by the Corporation, under whose auspices they also took part in an excursion to Loch Lomond in the afternoon.

SECURITY OF TENURE FOR HEALTH OFFICERS:—Replying to a deputation from the British Medical Association and the Society of Medical Officers of Health at the House of Commons on 11th June, the Chancellor of the Exchequer said security of tenure to medical officers of health and sanitary inspectors must be an essential preliminary to any further legislation dealing with the housing question. Executive officers should be in a position where they could feel they could report without fear or favour upon actual conditions in their areas. Parliament could legislate, but the work must be done locally. When the Budget was being framed, and when it was a question of the distribution of grants, the Government felt there ought to be a specific grant for the payment of salaries of the officers concerned. That put them in a better position to demand better treatment from local authorities. It was very important that they should have a superannuation scheme, because it was the only way of getting rid of the hardship of men past their work. It also gave them a sense of security and independence so as to enable them to do their work. He invited members of both parties to support the measure which would deal with these problems.

THE HOUSING PROBLEM.—Under the auspices of the National Housing and Town Planning Council, a two-days' conference of representatives of Scottish local authorities was held in Glasgow on 26th and 27th May. The conference was called to consider "the practical administration of the Housing and Town Planning Act of 1909," and took place in the Trades Hall, the chairman on the first day being Mr. John Lindsay, Town Clerk of Glasgow, and on the second Sir Thomas Hunter, Town Clerk of Edinburgh. Mr. Lindsay on the first day reviewed the operation of the Act in respect of housing, and expressed the opinion that a drastic remedy for the existing state of affairs was called for which would either repose the power of closure and demolition of uninhabitable dwellings in the hands of the local authorities or give the right of appeal by the owner to the Local Government Board only. Sir George M'Crae, the Vice-President of the Scottish Local Government Board, emphasised the need of speeding up the housing machinery in order to participate in the increased grants that were coming to Scotland. The day's discussion had to do with the relative merits of tenements and cottages. The second day's conference was opened by a speech delivered by the Right Hon. T. M'Kinnon Wood, Secretary for Scotland, on the invitation of the chairman. Mr. M'Kinnon Wood said that the sympathy of the Government was with those engaged in the clearance of slums, in the proper provision of dwellings for the people, and in town planning, and that the Local Government Board for Scotland was heart and soul with them in these matters. They would find, when they came to consider the allocation of the money which came to Scotland under the new grants, that a very substantial sum—very, very largely in excess of anything formerly received—would be given for purposes of public health, and might be devoted by their town councils and county councils to the purpose of clearing away their slums and improving the health of the people. The day's discussion turned upon the question of development pending the completion of large schemes of town planning, rents for cottage houses, and subsidies for the poor, after which Mr. Bryce, of the Master of Works Department of Glasgow Corporation, explained the details of the Corporation Western District Scheme of 1913, which included a very wide avenue right out from Anniesland Cross in the direction of Bowling. At the close of the conference the Scottish National Committee of the National Housing and Town Planning Council was reappointed.

NOTIFICATION OF TUBERCULOSIS.—Regulations have been made by the Local Government Board, in terms of Section 78 of the Public Health (Scotland) Act, 1897, providing for the compulsory notification, as from 1st July, 1914, of cases of tuberculosis in Scotland. These regulations provide for the notification of all forms of tuberculosis, and supersede the previous regulations in regard to the notification of pulmonary tuberculosis. The local authority is required to send a copy of the regulations to each medical practitioner in their district. The local authority should also take steps to furnish medical practitioners, school medical officers, and medical officers of institutions situated in their district, in which persons suffering from tuberculosis are received for treatment, with a supply of forms set forth in the schedules. The regulations follow closely the form and requirements of the earlier Order. New requirements provide for the medical officers of institutions, in which persons suffering from tuberculosis are received for treatment, sending weekly admission and discharge lists to the medical officers of health of the districts from which the cases were admitted or to which they are going on discharge. Notification is to be made on the strength of evidence other than that derived solely from tuberculin tests. A fee of 2s. 6d. is payable to a medical practitioner in respect of each case occurring in his private practice, and 1s. if the case occurs in his practice as medical officer of any public body or institution. No fee, however, is payable to school medical officers. The Board repeat that it is unnecessary and undesirable that notification should involve publicity. The medical officer of health is required to keep a register of all cases of tuberculosis notified to him under the regulations. A school medical officer is required to notify all cases of tuberculosis occurring among children inspected by him. So far as the regulations touch upon the work of school medical officers, they have the concurrence of the Scotch Education Department.

LUNACY IN SCOTLAND: INCREASE OF PATIENTS AND COST.— The report of the Commissioners in Lunacy for Scotland for the year 1913 has been issued. As the Mental Deficiency and Lunacy (Scotland) Act is now in force, this is the last report which will be presented by the Board as Commissioners in Lunacy. It states that on 1st January of the present year, exclusive of insane persons maintained at home by their natural guardians, there were in Scotland 19,346 insane persons of whom the Commissioners had official cognisance, including the inmates of training schools for imbecile children and of the criminal lunatic department of Perth prison. Of these, 2,624 were maintained from private sources, 16,660 by parochial rates, and 62 at the expense of the State. As the total number at 1st January, 1913, was 19,188, an increase has taken place during the past year of 158.

In the past year decreases, amounting in all to 134, have occurred in 14 counties, or urban areas, while increases, amounting in all to 204, have taken place in 20 counties, or urban areas. Glasgow city and Govan districts, which showed an increase last year of 77, show a decrease this year of 19, while Lanark county shows an increase of 41, and Renfrew of 22. It should, however, be borne in mind that these increases are not necessarily due to a larger number of patients being sent to asylums. They may equally arise through accumulation, whenever a falling off occurs in the number discharged.

· ·The total number of patients admitted to establishments during 1913 was 3,682, which is 213 more than in the previous year, 121 more than in 1911, and 233 more than the average for the quinquenniad 1905-09. This is the highest number of patients admitted in a single year into establishments for the insane in Scotland.

·The Commissioners point out that the constant demand for additional accommodation for the insane, the large scale on which it has been found necessary in many cases to provide it, and the magnitude of the expenditure involved, have been the subject of much discussion. They have for long urged upon district lunacy boards that all asylum buildings should be of the utmost simplicity compatible with efficiency for their special purpose, and that no expenditure should be incurred on external ornament or in other similar directions which are contrary to a strict economy, and which in no way contribute to the amelioration of the condition of the insane.

In the year ending 15th May, 1913, for the maintenance of 19,139 pauper lunatics, who were under care for longer or shorter periods during the year, in asylums, lunatic wards of poorhouses, and private dwellings, and for other expenses connected with them, a total sum of £432,534 was paid by the parish councils, of which £346,422 was for maintenance in asylums (including institutions for imbecile children), £19,351 was for maintenance in lunatic wards of poorhouses, £54,492 was for maintenance in private dwellings, and £12,332 was for certification, transport, and other expenses. Of this expenditure, £23,378 was repaid by relatives and others, and £116,389 was contributed from the local taxation account. The net expenditure by parish councils on the maintenance of patients was thus £292,767, which is £3,871 more than the expenditure of last year.

THE WELLCOME HISTORICAL MEDICAL MUSEUM.—The historical medical museum, which was founded by Mr. Henry S. Wellcome in connection with the Seventeenth International Congress of Medicine, was reopened on 28th May as a permanent

institution in London. It is now known as the "Wellcome
Historical Medical Museum," and is open daily from 10 A.M. to
6 P.M., closing at 1 P.M. on Saturday; entrance 54A Wigmore
Street, Cavendish Square, London, W. Since closing last
October the collections in the museum have been considerably
augmented and entirely rearranged. Many objects of importance and interest have been added, which it is hoped will
increase the usefulness of the museum to those interested in
the history of medicine. Members of the medical and kindred
professions are admitted on presenting their visiting cards.
Tickets of admission may be obtained by others interested in
the history of medicine on application to the curator, accompanied by an introduction from a registered medical practitioner.
Ladies will be admitted *only* if accompanied by a qualified
medical man.

LITERARY INTELLIGENCE.—The fifth edition of Sir Patrick
Manson's *Tropical Diseases*, revised and enlarged, is announced
for early publication by Messrs. Cassell & Company.

Messrs. J. & A. Churchill have pleasure in announcing for
early publication the following new works and new editions:—
The Anatomy of the Human Skeleton, by J. E. S. Frazer, F.R.C.S.
Eng., Lecturer on Anatomy, St. Mary's Hospital Medical School.
With 219 illustrations, many in colour. As implied by its title,
this work is not a conventional account of the bony skeleton,
but aims at helping the student to master the connected parts
as they exist in the complete body. It is intended for use with
the skeleton and dissected parts, and the author has drawn a
large number of figures, many in colours, with the object of
enabling the student to follow the descriptions on the actual
specimens. *A Manual of Dental Anatomy, human and comparative*, by Charles S. Tomes, F.R.S., F.R.C.S. Seventh edition,
edited by H. W. Marett Tims, M.D., M.Ch.Edin., F.L.S., F.Z.S.;
and A. Hopewell-Smith, L.R.C.P., M.R.C.S., L.D.S.Eng. With
286 illustrations. The text has been completely revised and
many new illustrations have been added. *The Story of Plant
Life in the British Isles* (vol. ii), by A. R. Horwood, F.L.S.,
Member of the British Botanical, Ecological, Conchological
Societies, &c. With 71 illustrations from photographs and 7
diagrams.

REVIEWS.

Asthma and its Radical Treatment. By JAMES ADAM, M.A., M.D., F.R.F.P.S. London: Henry Kimpton; Glasgow: Alex. Stenhouse. 1913.

DR. ADAM is specially qualified to make a contribution to the elucidation of asthma. He is in the fortunate position of being able to view this disease, or symptom as probably he would prefer to term it, not only from the standpoint of the specialist in diseases of the respiratory tract, but also as one having a wide and accurate knowledge of general medicine.

Asthma according to the author is primarily a toxæmia which arises partly in the bowel and partly in the tissues, and is mainly due to an error in nitrogenous metabolism closely related to an excess of carbohydrates in the diet. The toxæmia tends to show itself first as catarrh, later as spasm in the respiratory tract.

In the elaboration of his thesis the author devotes chapters to the following aspects of the subject:—The acute attack, the chronic asthmatic, the periodicity of asthma, atypical asthma, asthmatic dyspnœa, the nose in relation to asthma, etiology, morbid anatomy, diagnosis, prognosis, and treatment.

The author considers that too much attention is paid to the most striking feature of asthma, the spasm, and too little to the predisposing and exciting conditions. He states that the nose is rarely normal, there being usually some obstruction, and he points out a connection which has not previously been referred to by writers, namely, that when asthmatic signs are limited largely to one lung there is greater obstruction in the ipsolateral nostril. The descriptions given by a number of our own patients would seem to confirm Dr. Adam's observation. By the way, we were not aware that "the importance of a nasal factor in asthma . . . was first recognised by Herck, of Freiburg, in 1844, and revived by Voltolini in 1872." We understood that Voltolini, in 1871, was the first to point out the association, and that *Hack,* of Freiburg, wrote a paper on allied matters in 1882.

The common notion that the asthmatic pulse is one of high tension is shown to be wrong; as a consequence, arterio-sclerosis is not a feature of the disease.

The skin affections associated with asthma are considered specially with the view of emphasising the toxæmic nature of the latter.

The week-end periodicity of asthma, especially in the working classes, is shówn to be related to increased feeding and diminished exercise on Saturday and Sunday.

The chapter on atypical asthma contains some valuable remarks on the recurrent bronchitis of children. "It results from the same evil—feeding, want of exercise, and defective metabolism as the typical asthma of adults. Yet how seldom are these poor little wretches treated on this rational basis! They are put to bed, coddled, steamed, poulticed, kept in pokey rooms, 'at an equable temperature,' fed on an atrocious dietary called 'milk foods' instead of 'slop poison,' that only makes them worse. What helps to blind us to this error is that in these cases the temperatnre is sometimes up, though in my experience this is the exception rather than the rule." Again, in regard to adults—"It is worth pointing out that in over-fed adults, especially in fat women, the wheezy bronchitis that is so common results from the dietary, want of exercise, and defective oxidation, and can be cured by attention to these points rather than by drugs. . . . The great point of interest both in adults and in children, is that first we have a catarrhal, then a spasmodic, process arising as the result of excessive carbohydrate intake and defective oxidation of food and tissue."

In the chapter on treatment careful instructions are given as to diet, the mode of cooking special dishes, exercise, drugs, &c. Nasal treatment is warmly advocated—"The nose and throat should be put in order." We think that the author might have indicated the class of case in which the asthma would almost certainly be benefited by nasal treatment, also that in which benefit would be doubtful; and he might have mentioned the possibility of seriously aggravating the disease by operative interference with the nose.

Dr. Adam has done good service in directing attention to the toxæmic conception of asthma. His book is a valuable and well written contribution to the subject, based on personal observation, and it contains many practical hints which cannot fail to be of value to those who have to deal with asthmatics.

The Principles and Practice of Medical Hydrology. By R. FORTESCUE FOX, M.D.Lond., F.R.Met.Soc.—London: University of London Press.

THIS is a clearly written and well printed book of 291 pages, with marginal headings which make reference easy.

Part I gives a very complete account of the physiological laws concerned with bathing with special reference to children.

Part II deals with the action of the various kinds of baths and of medicinal waters taken internally. The dangers attending the heroic reduction of temperature in fever by the use of too cold water are put very forcibly. It is only in robust subjects or when the pyrexial reaction is acute that Brand's point (65°F.) ought to be reached or exceeded.

Part III deals with medicinal springs and baths, and gives an account of those in Great Britain.

Part IV is for the medical practitioner the most important in the book, as it deals with the use of baths and waters in the various diseases likely to be benefited by their use.

A useful index of spas brings the volume to a close. This book will be found to give a satisfactory answer on any point concerned with practical hydrology, and will prove of service to all ranks of practising physicians.

Stammering and Cognate Defects of Speech. Two Vols. By C. S. BLUEMEL. New York: G. E. Stechert & Co. 1913.

THIS is an excellent book and might well be taken as a model upon which such works should be framed. From this statement it may be judged that the book is the antithesis of most works upon the same subject. It is a scientific monograph and not a catchpenny pamphlet. From the preface it may be gathered that the writer suffers under the condition which gives the name to the book.

The first volume deals with the physiology and psychology of stammering and, indeed, of normal speech as well. The reviewer has never found this difficult subject made so clear as in the present work. At the same time detail and accuracy are never sacrificed for the sake of obtaining that clearness of exposition which is so noteworthy a feature of the book. The writer's view in regard to causation is that the primary factor is auditory amnesia, while the secondary factors may be "fear, wavering of the will, multiple thought, distortion of imagery," &c.

The second volume deals with contemporaneous systems of treating stammering. In Chapter II (Vol. II) the relationship of respiration to stammering is discussed, and some caustic and fully justifiable hits are made at those who hold that the defect may always be cured by breathing exercises and attention to respiration.

In Chapter IV the influence of articulation upon stammering is considered, and the author indicates what is valuable in the various systems of treatment. His sense of humour is keen but kindly, and some of the remarks made in reference to various methods of treatment are worth remembering. At the same time he is always fair and gives each system credit for all in it that is really creditable.

Chapter VIII deals with "Stammering-schools" and speech-specialists. The extensive degree of fraud that attaches to many of these institutions and individuals is indicated. This is a most valuable chapter from the point of view of the stammerer, as it gives him ample warning of the many greedy and unscrupulous charlatans that are on the lookout for prey.

This is by far the best book on the subject with which the reviewer is acquainted. The style is delightfully clear, terse, and humorous. The writer holds out no panacea, but gives most judicious advice.

ABSTRACTS FROM CURRENT MEDICAL LITERATURE.

EDITED BY ROY F. YOUNG, M.B., B.C.

MEDICINE.

The Experimental Formation of Acute Gastric Ulcers. By T. R. Elliot (*Quarterly Journal of Medicine*, January, 1914).—Whilst experimenting with tetrahydro-β-naphthylamine on animals, the author noted that in guinea-pigs ulcers invariably occurred in the stomach. These developed with such certainty and rapidity that a series of observations was made on them alone, partly because the reaction illustrated well one of the modes in which acute gastric ulcer may be formed, and partly in the hope that chronic gastric ulcer might be formed and studied—a hope that was not fulfilled.

Sub-lethal doses of the drug were injected subcutaneously into the animals, and they were subsequently suddenly killed by decapitation so as to allow them to bleed freely and the vessels to be more or less emptied of blood. Within one to two hours after the injection ulceration was invariably visible in the walls of the stomach. This appeared as an irregular patch of hæmorrhage, with erosion on the surface. The lesions were confined almost entirely to the stomach. The epithelium surrounding the ulcerated area was degenerate. The cells stained badly, and were exfoliating. The appearance was that of necrosis and erosion spreading inwards from the epithelial surface. Within twenty-four hours the symptoms had abated, but on examination in all the cases deep ulcers with overhanging edges were found in the stomach ; the ulcers extended to the muscularis mucosæ. In three days healing had commenced if the ulcers remained aseptic. A thin layer of epithelium was seen to have spread over the ulcerated surface. This repair epithelium was probably derived from cells in the ulcerated surface which had escaped necrosis. In the septic cases the healing process occurred more slowly, and was complicated by inflammatory changes. In some of these septic cases the ulceration spread to the serous coat, but never resulted in actual perforation. By repeated injection of the drug the author failed to produce chronic ulcers. He thinks that the drug damages the gastric epithelium, and allows the gastric juice to digest it. He found that if the guinea-pigs were starved ulceration did not occur, while if the animals had been recently fed it invariably occurred. He considers that this was due to the absence of gastric juice in the starved animals.

The paper is illustrated with plates showing the morbid processes in the stomach.—G. B. FLEMING.

On Pneumo-pericardium. By Cowan, Harrington, and Riddell (*Quarterly Journal of Medicine*, January, 1914).—The authors report a case of pneumo-pericardium, a rare condition, there only being forty-three cases recorded in the literature. The case is of interest as it was somewhat atypical (the apex impulse and area of cardiac dulness did not disappear), and the diagnosis was only made on x-ray examination. The skiagrams are almost unique, as only one other case has been published with skiagrams, and in that case the pneumo-pericardium was produced artificially.

The patient, a boy of 8 years, was admitted to hospital with vague symptoms pointing to meningitis. Sixteen days after admission he developed symptoms of pneumonia. Skiagrams taken a month after admission showed the pericardial sac distended with gas, there being a clear area between the shadow of the heart and the pericardium, which appears as a dark stripe surrounding the left border of the heart. There is also a clear area between the lower border of the heart and the diaphragm. The apex of the left lung is seen to be affected, and there is an abnormal shadow immediately to the left of the heart. Fourteen days later skiagrams showed further distension of the pericardial sac with gas, but about three weeks later the distension had begun to diminish. At one time a tympanitic area was discovered surrounding the left border of cardiac dulness. Four months after admission the patient was dismissed from hospital well.

The authors think that there was a septicæmia which provoked a lesion in the mediastinal glands ; that this became disseminated first to the lungs and then to the pericardium, permitting the entrance of air from the lungs into the pericardium. They do not think that a gas producing organism was responsible for the condition, as there were no signs of pericardial friction, and the skiagrams exclude the presence of effusion. The literature is discussed, and the paper is illustrated with excellent skiagrams.—G. B. FLEMING.

SURGERY.

A New Method of After-Treatment of Prostatectomy. By J. W. Van Bisselick (*Zentr. f. Chirurgie*, 21st March, 1914).—This method of after-treatment of prostatectomy was introduced by Rotgans in order to shorten the period to be spent in bed by the patient. It depends on the continuous use of a catheter and the closing of the bladder except for a small opening through which a tampon is led. The prostate is removed in the usual way, and if hæmorrhage is severe the whole bladder is tamponed. The catheter which was used during the operation remains in the urethra. The bladder is partly closed in two layers, catgut being used for the inner and silk for the outer. A portion of the muscularis of the bladder wall is left open and a purse-string suture of catgut is applied round it, the ends of this being left long. The cavum Retzii is tamponed and the abdominal wall is closed except for an aperture through which the tampon and the catgut ends are brought. Generally this tampon is removed after twenty-four hours. The bladder is then washed out from above to remove blood-clot, and the catgut threads tied off after infolding the edges of the bladder wound. A tampon on the closed bladder wall secures drainage should the wound burst open. The bladder is washed out every two hours, and the catheter changed every day. After three or four days the catheter is left in only at night, while after seven or eight days its use is discontinued. The patient should then be able to urinate even at night. If there is infection of the bladder the tampon should remain for forty-eight hours. In case of very serious infection the operation is to be done in two stages.

Of nine patients treated this way, six were able to pass urine spontaneously, and could walk about the ward without leakage of urine. Of the remaining three, one had carcinoma of the prostate, and in the other two the catgut sutures, which were tied after forty-eight hours, gave way.—CHARLES BENNETT.

A New Method of Treatment of Chronic Gonorrhœa and Simple Urethritis with Lytinol.

By Edward Baumer (*Zeit. f. Urologie*, Bd. VIII, Heft I).—Non-gonorrhœal urethritis is a form of disease not nearly so rare as is commonly supposed, nor is its treatment so easy as might be thought from the term "simple" being often applied to it. The author separates simple urethritis into two groups—(1) those cases in which there has not previously been gonorrhœa, or where an early gonorrhœa has been completely cured. The usual history in this type is that about fourteen days after intercourse a greyish, ropy secretion appears at the orifice, and the subjective symptoms are those of a slight attack of gonorrhœa. The discharge will often be found to contain bacilli and cocci, among the latter being diplococci, in many respects resembling the gonococcus, but not with the characteristic concave contour ; (2) those cases in which gonorrhœa has been cured and all gonococci have disappeared, but a viscous greyish secretion remains. The author treats patients of these classes with lytinol, the discovery of Dr. Auerbach, of Russia. It is a preparation of iodine with the power of preventing and curing inflammatory hyperplastic processes in the mucosa and submucosa. He begins with 5 per cent lytinol and works gradually up to 10 per cent. Urethral injections are administered thrice daily. The treatment is completed by the use of a weak astringent injection, usually a preparation of zinc. The author recommends the remedy to urologists, gynæcologists, and rhino-laryngologists.—CHARLES BENNETT.

Direct Implantation of Nerve in Muscle.

By Professor Heineke (*Zentr. f. Chirurgie*, 14th March, 1914).—Attempts to restore the function of a paralysed muscle have up to the present always been in the direction of endeavouring to bring the motor nerve of the affected muscle into union with an adjacent healthy motor nerve. It occurred to the author that it might be possible to establish new functional union by directly implanting a healthy nerve into the muscle substance. Up till now he has tested the question only in an experimental fashion. The operations were carried out on the hind leg of a rabbit. In the thigh one or two cm. of the tibial were excised, thus throwing the musculature of the posterior part of the leg out of function. The peroneal was then followed downwards and cut through below the head of the fibula. Finally, with a blunt instrument a small tunnel was bored in the gastrocnemius, the end of the peroneal inserted into this and fixed by the overstitching of a small fold of muscle. The result was as imagined. After fourteen days galvanic and faradic excitation of the peroneal nerve produced slight twitchings in the gastrocnemius. In eight weeks the contractions of the muscle could not be distinguished from normal, not only in the gastrocnemius, but also in the other muscles of the flexor group. Experiments to determine whether the same results can be obtained when the muscle has been paralysed for a much longer time are not yet concluded, but progress so far has been encouraging. The author thinks that the method may, on occasion, be quite well applied to human beings.

—CHARLES BENNETT.

DISEASES OF CHILDREN.

Respiratory Infections in Infants' Wards. By Walter E. Chappell, M.D., and Alan Brown, M.D. (*Amer. Jour. of Child. Diseases*, May, 1914, p. 381).—These authors remark that while deaths from gastro-intestinal troubles have diminished much during the last decade, deaths from respiratory diseases, on the other hand, have greatly increased. Respiratory troubles are at present the great scourge of all infant hospitals and asylums, and a common cold in the head may rapidly travel all round a ward, and the subsequent broncho-pneumonia claim many victims. In hospitals it has been shown that the degree of susceptibility of a child to any infection bears a definite relationship to the length of residence in the institution; for this lowered vitality the term hospitalism has been introduced.

While it has been demonstrated that measles, scarlet fever, diphtheria, smallpox, and mumps are in reality contagious diseases, and that simply by placing the patients suffering from these different diseases in stalls cross infection is avoided, such prophylactic measures have little or no effect on the dissemination of coryza and bronchitis. It would thus seem that transmission of the pneumococcus and staphylococcus causing catarrhal conditions of the respiratory system is by the air. As it is a practical impossibility to eliminate completely this factor, these authors have practised post-nasal injections of boracic lotion or hydrogen peroxide, followed later by saline twice weekly, with very encouraging results. In one ward where this douching was practised there occurred during a period of six months 27 cases of infection, whereas in a control ward, where no such measures were undertaken, there occurred 57 cases of infection of the respiratory tract during the same period. Two cases of retropharyngeal abscess developed in the ward where the prophylactic measures were adopted, while not one was met with in the control ward. On the other hand, only 4 cases of otitis media developed in the ward where the post-nasal douching was practised, and 11 in the control ward.—LEONARD FINDLAY.

Congenital Malaria. By Murray H. Bass, M.D. (*Archiv. of Pediatrics*, April, 1914, p. 250).—The passage of the malarial parasite from mother to child *in utero* has always been looked upon as a possibility, but the majority of writers have been rather inclined to disregard it. In the present paper clinical histories of four cases from recent literature, along with one personally observed by the author, are recorded. In all the mother had suffered from malaria during pregnancy, and one of the children born prematurely during a paroxysm died within an hour; malarial parasites were found in fœtal blood. In two of the infants born apparently healthy, and developing fever at ten and seventeen days, examination of the blood revealed the parasite. In the author's case the child, healthy at birth, became fretful at three weeks with vomiting, undigested motions, and loss of weight; examination of the blood at seven and a half weeks revealed the presence of the tertian type of hæmamœba.—LEONARD FINDLAY.

Books, Pamphlets, &c., Received.

Appendicitis : Its History, Anatomy, Clinical Ætiology, Pathology, Symptomatology, Diagnosis, Prognosis, Treatment, Technic of Operation, Complications, and Sequels, by John S. Deaver, M.D., Sc.D., LL.D. Fourth edition, thoroughly revised, containing 14 illustrations. London: William Heinemann. (17s. 6d. net.)

The British Journal of Surgery. Volume I—July, 1913, to April, 1914, Numbers 1 to 4. Bristol : John Wright & Sons, Limited.

Preliminary Report on the Treatment of Pulmonary Tuberculosis with Tuberculin (King Edward VII Sanatorium, Midhurst), by Noel D. Bardswell, M.D. With a Prefatory Note by Professor Karl Pearson, F.R.S. London : H. K. Lewis.

The Medical Annual : A Year-Book of Treatment and Practitioners' Index, 1914. Thirty-second year. Bristol : John Wright & Sons, Limited.

X-Rays : An Introduction to the Study of Röntgen Rays, by G. W. C. Kaye, B.A., D.Sc. London : Longmans, Green & Co. 1914. (3s. net.)

Outlines of Zoology, by J. Arthur Thomson, M.A., LL.D. Sixth edition, revised, with 424 illustrations. London : Henry Frowde and Hodder & Stoughton. 1914. (12s. 6d. net.)

The Therapeutic Value of the Potato, by Heaton C. Howard, L.R.C.P.Lond., M.R.C.S.Eng. London : Baillière, Tindall & Cox. 1914. (1s. net.)

Riedel's Berichte und Mentor. 1914. London : The J. D. Riedel Co.

Pain : Its Origin, Conduction, Perception, and Diagnostic Significance, by Richard J. Behan, M.D.

The Prevention of Dental Caries and Oral Sepsis, by H. P. Pickerill, M.D., Ch.B., M.D.S.Birm., L.D.S.Eng. Second edition. London : Baillière, Tindall & Cox. 1914. (12s. 6d. net.)

Auricular Flutter, by William Thomas Ritchie, M.D., F.R.C.P.E., F.R.S.E. London : Longmans, Green & Co. 1914. (10s. 6d. net.)

Clinical Examination of the Blood and its Technique : A Manual for Students and Practitioners, by Professor A. Pappenheim, Berlin. Translated and adapted from the German by R. Donaldson, M.A., M.B., Ch.B., F.R.C.S.Ed., D.P.H. Bristol : John Wright & Sons, Limited. 1914. (3s. 6d. net.)

Spectrum Analysis Applied to Biology and Medicine, by the late C. A. Macmunn, M.A., M.D. With a Preface by F. W. Gamble. With illustrations. London : Longmans, Green & Co. 1914. (5s. net.)

A Manual of Surgical Anatomy, by Charles R. Whittaker, F.R.C.S.Ed., F.R.S.E. Second edition, revised and enlarged. Edinburgh : E. & S. Livingstone. 1914. (6s. net.)

Sclero-Corneal Trephining in the Operative Treatment of Glaucoma, by Robert Henry Elliott, M.D., B.S.Lond, Sc.D.Edin., F.R.C.S.Eng., &c., Lieut.-Colonel I.M.S. First edition, 1913 ; second edition, 1914. London : George Pulman & Sons, Limited.

Diseases of the Rectum and Anus : A Practical Handbook, by P. Lockhart-Mummery, F.R.C.S.Eng. London : Baillière, Tindall & Cox. 1914. (7s. 6d. net.)

Extraction of Teeth, by F. Coleman, L.R.C.P., M.R.C.S., L.D.S. Second edition. With 57 illustrations. London : H. K. Lewis. 1914. (3s. 6d. net.)

GLASGOW.—METEOROLOGICAL AND VITAL STATISTICS FOR THE FOUR WEEKS ENDED 13TH JUNE, 1914.

	WEEK ENDING			
	May 23.	May 30.	June 6.	June 13.
Mean temperature, . .	53·8°	50·5°	52·4°	56·5°
Mean range of temperature between highest and lowest,	13·2°	16·4°	18·9°	13·6°
Number of days on which rain fell, ...	4	3	1	3
Amount of rainfall, . ins.	0·40	0·21	0·02	0·12
Deaths (corrected), . .	358	311	354	300
Death-rates, ...	17·8	15·5	17·6	15·0
Zymotic death-rates, . .	1·5	1·5	1·2	1·1
Pulmonary death-rates, .	4·0	3·8	4·0	3·8
DEATHS— Under 1 year, . . .	77	52	76	58
60 years and upwards, .	79	86	93	71
DEATHS FROM— Small-pox, ...	...	...	...	...
Measles, ...	17	7	11	6
Scarlet fever, . . .	3	2	2	1
Diphtheria, . . .	1	2	...	2
Whooping-cough, . .	7	19	11	12
Enteric fever, . . .	1	...	1	1
Cerebro-spinal fever, . .	2	...	2	2
Diarrhœa (under 2 years of age),	10	4	8	3
Bronchitis, pneumonia, and pleurisy, . . .	59	50	61	52
CASES REPORTED— Small-pox, ...	...	....	...	...
Cerebro-spinal meningitis, .	1	1	3	3
Diphtheria and membranous croup, ...	19	20	25	21
Erysipelas, . . .	33	29	25	20
Scarlet fever, . . .	85	104	86	68
Typhus fever, . . .	...	...	...	...
Enteric fever, . . .	6	6	4	8
Phthisis, ...	51	46	51	36
Puerperal fever, . .	3	3	10	4
Measles,* . . .	214	185	134	124

* Measles not notifiable.

SANITARY CHAMBERS,
GLASGOW, 26th June, 1914.

CONTENTS.

Annual Subscription, 20s., payable to Dr. W. B. INGLIS POLLOCK, 21 Woodside Place, Glasgow.

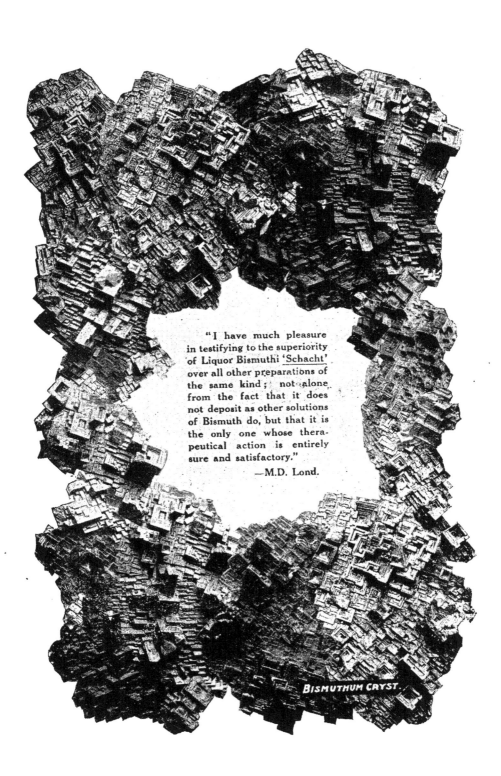

"I have much pleasure in testifying to the superiority of Liquor Bismuthi 'Schacht' over all other preparations of the same kind; not alone from the fact that it does not deposit as other solutions of Bismuth do, but that it is the only one whose therapeutical action is entirely sure and satisfactory."

—M.D. Lond.

BISMUTHUM CRYST.

THE

GLASGOW MEDICAL JOURNAL.

No. II. AUGUST, 1914.

ORIGINAL ARTICLES.

MALIGNANT GANGLIO–NEUROMA OF LEFT SUPRARENAL.*

BY T. K. MONRO, M.A., M.D.,

Regius Professor of Practice of Medicine in the University of Glasgow ;

AND

JOHN SHAW DUNN, M.A., M.D.,

Director of the Clinical Laboratory in the Western Infirmary ; Lecturer on
Clinical Pathology in the University of Glasgow.

Clinical report by Professor T. K. Monro.—James M'L.,
aged 3½ years, was seen with Dr. E. R. Weir on 17th
December, 1913.   His ill-health dated from July, when he
was noticed to be "hanging."   He improved for a time, and
then became worse.   He was first seen by Dr. Weir in connection with this illness about the second week of November.
At that time the skin was slightly yellow.   The temperature
was occasionally observed to exceed 100°, but it now varied
from about normal to 99°.

The boy's past health was good.   The parents and the two
other children of the family were all healthy.

* Read at a meeting of the Medico-Chirurgical Society of Glasgow
held on 1st May, 1914.

Condition on 17th December, 1913.—There is marked pallor of the face, and large veins are seen on the forehead. Nothing worthy of note is found in the skin. The limbs are emaciated, but the abdomen preserves its rotundity. There is no dyspnœa or œdema. There is no evidence of pain, and the patient permits free handling of the abdomen. The appetite is good. There has been no vomiting now for four weeks. The bowels are kept regular by medicine. The stools have the colour that might be expected from a milk diet. There has been no loss of blood.

A large mass is found in the situation which an enlarged spleen might occupy, but the anterior edge is thick and rounded, and the mass extends more transversely in proportion to its size than would be expected of an enlarged spleen. It is of firm consistence, and has a projection at the back. It is easily moved in an antero-posterior direction, and can also be moved horizontally. There is little, if any, enlargement of the liver. A systolic murmur is audible over the cardiac area generally.

It was considered that, on the whole, the relations of the tumour were probably with the kidney rather than with the spleen, and it was decided to examine the blood, and then, if necessary, have an exploratory operation performed.

The patient was accordingly admitted to the Western Infirmary on 18th December. It was then found that the hæmoglobin of the blood amounted to 48 per cent of the normal. The reds numbered 2,020,000, and the whites 4,000 per cm. The urine was normal. The boy was transferred to Mr. Edington's wards with a view to operation.

Note on operation by Mr. Edington.—On 24th December Mr. Edington attempted removal of the mass by laparotomy transversely in the left flank. The colon was found lying on the front of a large retroperitoneal swelling which occupied the renal fossa. At the lower end of the swelling was a reniform body, freely movable. The arrangement was that of a kidney pushed downwards by an enormously enlarged suprarenal body. Considerable glandular enlargements were present in the prevertebral and cæcal regions. The posterior parietal peritoneum was opened external to the colon, and the tumour had been partly separated from its bed when respiration ceased. Attempts to restore respiration were unavailing.

Pathological report by Dr. J. Shaw Dunn.—The *post-mortem* examination was carried out by Dr. John Anderson, and we are greatly indebted to him for the notes of the condition, and for permission to make use of the material.

A tumour the size of a large orange was found occupying the site of the left suprarenal body, and the remains of that organ were found stretched out over the upper pole of the tumour in such a fashion as to indicate that the tumour had developed inside the gland. The tumour was in part composed of firm pale tissue, and in part of soft hæmorrhagic tissue. Metastatic deposits were present in the retro-peritoneal, mesenteric, mediastinal, cervical, and inguinal glands. Tumours were present also in the ribs and in the bones of the skull. The liver and the spleen were free from invasion.

Histological examination showed that the firm, pale parts of the primary tumour in the left suprarenal were composed of nervous tissue. The cells present were mainly ganglionic nerve-cells, many of them being of typical structure, with conical protoplasmic processes running off from them to form nerve-fibres. Others were of more or less aberrant type, possessing several nuclei, or being of unusually large or small size. These cells were supported by fibrillar material, in which, by special staining, it was easy to demonstrate great numbers of naked axis-cylinders. No myelinated fibres were present. In addition to these fairly mature elements, there were present in some parts foci of smaller cells, which could be recognised as corresponding to the embryonic nerve-cells which form the sympathetic nervous system in normal development. These smaller cells were accompanied by knots of special nerve-fibrillæ, the so-called "rosettes" which represent embryonic nerve-fibres, and corresponding closely with similar structures which occur in the normally developing tissues. The soft hæmorrhagic areas of the primary tumour were composed almost entirely of the smaller type of cell, with comparatively scanty amounts of the embryonic nerve-fibrillæ. In these parts the type of growth was much more luxuriant than in the firmer parts first described, and was of obviously malignant character, and associated with much necrosis and hæmorrhage.

Examination of a large number of the secondary tumours showed that they were exclusively composed of the small-celled malignant tissue.

The main point of interest in this tumour lies in the fact that it is formed, in part, of mature nervous tissue, both cells and fibres, and consequently represents a tumour-growth of the highest type of cell in the body. Tumours of this description are of somewhat rare occurrence, and, although their existence has been recognised since 1880, up till the present only about thirty-six have been described. Of these the great majority have been associated with the sympathetic nervous system, chiefly with the main lateral chains, or with the suprarenal medulla, which is of sympathetic origin. Six have shown malignancy, but probably none so exquisitely as the present example.

The structure of the malignant parts of the present tumour is of great interest, as it closely resembles that of the "neuro-blastoma" of the sympathetic nervous system — a tumour composed only of the embryonic type of nerve-cell.

GANGRENOUS APPENDICITIS WITH COPROLITH, ABSCESS, SEPTIC PERITONITIS, INTESTINAL OB- STRUCTION, RUPTURE OF INTESTINE, AND FISTULA — COMPLETE RECOVERY — AND REMARKS ON VOLVULUS.

By SPENCER MORT, Ch.B., M.D.Glasg., F.R.C.S., F.R.S.Edin.,

Medical Superintendent, Edmonton Infirmary ; late_M'Cunn Research Scholar, and Assistant to Regius Professor of Surgery, University of Glasgow.

In a recent issue of the *Lancet* (9th August, 1913) appears a description of "A case of volvulus of the small intestine com- plicating general peritonitis—Recovery," by Dr. C. W. Cunnington. I have had experience of a case broadly similar in its pathological bearings, as a sequence of septic appendix mischief, with a few points of difference in effect. In this case volvulus was not present, but obstruction by inflammatory adhesions came on in the same fashion ; general peritonitis was marked ; and the fistula spontaneously closed without operation. A gangrenous destruction of the intestinal wall was responsible for the fistula, in contrast with that in the case described by Dr. Cunnington, in which the aperture was a necessary operative measure to relieve the intestinal stasis resulting from the volvulus. Two other cases are noted with obstruction from volvulus, probably consequent on old appendicitis with adhesions. The twist was in the pelvic colon.

William G. B., aged 15 years, was sent to me by Dr. W. E. Porter, of Wood Green, as a case of acute appendicitis, requiring operation. He arrived at 8 P.M. on 6th March, 1911, in a con- dition of serious illness, and the diagnosis was verified at once. Three days before he was suddenly seized with cramps in the abdomen, sickness, and vomiting. The succeeding day he went out to his work, hawking bundles of firewood from door to door ; later in the afternoon he was wheeled back on his barrow by his little sister, who had accompanied him on his rounds. He was then suffering from severe colic, with vomiting. Next day he remained at home ; the day of admission he was seen by

Dr. Porter, who immediately ordered his removal. His bowels moved the day before.

On admission he was found to be acutely ill, the condition being—flushed face, pinched toxæmic appearance (Hippocratic facies), abdominal pain, tenderness and swelling in right iliac fossa and rectus rigidity, tenderness at M'Burney's point on pressure on the *descending* colon, no generalised tenderness, retraction of the knees, characteristic pain running down the right thigh (referred from ilio-inguinal nerve); temperature, 101° F.; pulse, 110 and rapid; and white furred tongue.

On rectal examination there was pain on pressure upwards; no obstruction could be felt. The abdomen was prepared for operation, and a simple enema given, without result. Immediate operation was decided upon, as no abatement in symptoms had come on in the hour after admission.

Suspecting pus, the incision was made well towards the right side, and the œdematous muscles were separated, gridiron fashion. A gush of pus and brownish fæculent-smelling fluid, resulting from the action of the bacillus coli, followed opening of the peritoneum. After some search the appendix was located, and removed by sleeve amputation. The tip was black with gangrene, and greenish sloughs and fibrinous exudate covered it; its base was constricted; the whole organ was much swollen and injected, and the distal portion was distended by a coprolith the size of a small date seed. The stump was treated with pure phenol, and imbedded into the colon by a purse-string suture. Thereafter the colon was inspected and found to be studded with darkened patches which resembled commencing gangrenous perityphlitis. Leathery omental adhesions were tightly fixed round the septic area, and a fairly confident hope of recovery from death was therefore expressed, with a suspicion that a cæcal fistula might follow, requiring further operation. One portion of gangrenous omentum required to be removed; the wound was subsequently disinfected, packed, and drained, after partial closure with silk sutures (Fig. 1).

Ten minims of laudanum were given to ease pain and partially paralyse the gut, and the lad was put up in Fowler's position and treated with rectal salines. After a restless night pain appeared easier, and feeding by peptonised milk was started. Towards evening flatus was passed, he was still a little restless, and laudanum (15 minims) was given. The temperature and pulse are recorded.

The following records the nurse's summary :—

7th March (first day after admission).—Slept five hours ; bowels not opened : flatus passed per rectum six times, by mouth once ; 12 oz. of peptonised milk given ; 10 oz. of urine passed.

8th March.—Day report : Fairly comfortable day ; wound

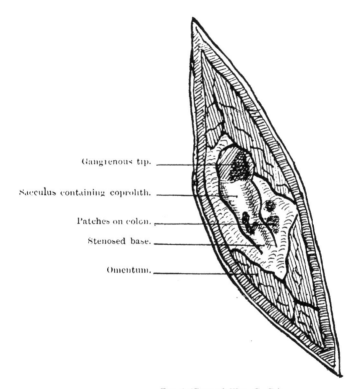

Gangrenous tip.

Sacculus containing coprolith.

Patches on colon.

Stenosed base.

Omentum.

FIG. 1 (Case of Wm. G B.).

Diagram of appendix *in situ* at first operation.

has been dressed ; slept four hours ; bowels not opened ; flatus per rectum twice ; 30 oz. of urine passed ; 12 oz. of peptonised milk given. Night report : Slept four hours ; bowels not opened ; flatus per rectum three times, vomited once ; 11 oz. of peptonised milk given, 2 oz. soda water ; 12 oz. of urine passed : and so on during the supposed convalescence.

On the third day ol. ricini was prescribed, 1 drachm every

two hours up to eight times if bowels had not moved, but being followed in fifteen minutes by a free motion it was discontinued. Pain was now absent, and the pulse and temperature had dropped. On the fourth day a troublesome cough had developed. On the fifth day Benger's food, Brand's essence, and bread and butter were given. On the tenth day (16th March) complications developed, and event followed event.

The temperature, which had been normal for a week, suddenly went up to 103° F., and the boy complained of pain over the wound, the pulse reaching 114. Next day there was a diminution in temperature and pulse (100° F. and 98 respectively), but there were remaining that pain, restlessness, and anxious look. Examination of the wound and the abdomen was negative. Troublesome diarrhœa with loose brown stools came on, accompanied by sickness, and vomiting of green fluid. The diet was again restricted, opium given, and whisky (2 drachms four-hourly) advised if necessary, aided by rectal enemata of a sedative nature. Enteric fever was discussed and dismissed from consideration.

On 18th March, twelve days after operation, disaster was imminent; absolute signs of peritonitis had developed, including abdominal distension, tympanites, rigidity and tenderness, sickness, and abdominal facies. The liver dulness was present. No flatus was passed per rectum, presumably on account of paralytic distension of the intestines. The temperature was 97° F., and the pulse about 140; in face of this another operation as a frail chance was performed at 6·30 P.M.

A focus of leakage was sought in the original lateral wound, but there the granulation barrier was sound and healthy. Consequently a large incision was made in the middle line between the umbilicus and the pubes. On cutting through the rectus fascia pockets of yellow pus were exposed; and on opening the peritoneum a small amount of ascitic fluid escaped.*

---

* In a moribund case of appendicitis and general peritonitis sent by Dr. Robert Gardner, Enfield, and operated on by me a few days before this, several pints of ascitic fluid gushed out. A *post-mortem* conducted later revealed an interesting condition; ascites due to portal obstruction from pylephlebitis and large sub-hepatic abscess, secondary to infective spread from a diseased appendix; no cirrhosis of liver. I have never noticed ascites

The intestines behind were in a condition of inflammation, matted up with new adhesions, and covered with green flakes of lymph. Between the coils were found sacculated collections of yellow pus. Hot saline lotion was poured into the abdomen, and the coils bathed thoroughly and separated, when a complication was discovered. Many coils of small intestine were much distended, but towards the right side there was collapsed and flaccid small intestine, one loop of which had fallen into the true pelvis. Thus, an obstruction was diagnosed in addition to peritonitis, and on following up the source, a band of omentum was found passing round and tightly gripping a loop of gut. At first I thought Nature had overstepped herself; that the cause of the boy's previous recovery—efficient consolidation and localisation by adhesions—had now sought to compass his death; but a little further examination vindicated Nature, for on removing the adhesion it was found to cover up and partially seal a rupture of two inches extent caused by gangrene of the wall of the intestine with sloughing; in doing so it sealed up also the natural lumen (Fig. 2, p. 90). There were thus three fatal conditions existing—diffuse septic peritonitis, acute intestinal obstruction, and rupture of the intestine. The band was ligatured and cut away, the rupture sutured by four layers of continuous Lembert silk stitches, a fenestrated loop of omentum of potential danger excised, and, after the usual cleansing, the peritoneal cavity was well packed with dry iodoform gauze, and two or three large loose silk sutures put in externally to prevent prolapse. Half a pint of saline lotion was purposely left in the abdomen to obviate shock, and as far as was possible the "quick in and quicker out" doctrine of Murphy was adopted. The boy was returned to his bed to be whipped up by stimulants as required, and dosed with morphia if necessary till the end would come. The nurses were instructed to cater to any of his desires, and supply him with whatever food he might wish for; strictness of dietary *régime* was to be abandoned, and the lad soothed in any way which would gratify him.

Restless, painful, and anxious hours followed. The pulse ran

remarked on as a complication of appendicitis. In another recent case the appendix, normally situated, was covered by a greatly enlarged liver, the dulness of which simulated a peritoneal abscess.

on in a flickering way. The bowels did not move, no flatus was passed, and it looked as if a mistake had been committed in suturing the rent gut, as I feared that other adhesions and obstructions might be present from a general matting up of the intestine. Preliminary shock was recovered from, the boy looked brighter and better, and the nurse was sanguine, only

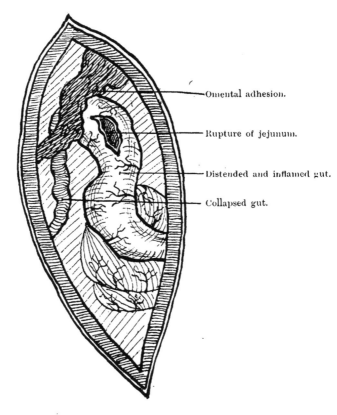

Omental adhesion.

Rupture of jejunum.

Distended and inflamed gut.

Collapsed gut.

FIG. 2 (Case of Wm. G. B.).

Diagram of condition at second operation. The ruptured portion was really partially covered by the omental band. The state of angry peritonitis is indicated.

dissuaded from hope on being assured that there could be no possible chance of recovery. Two days later the pulse reached 140, with a subnormal temperature of 97° F.; the boy was very ill. Three days after, the report read—"patient is slowly sinking." But still he lingered.

Next day the rotted portion of intestine ruptured again, and the intestinal contents poured abundantly from the upper part of the wound.

Five days, six days passed, and now *the boy was apparently recovering*, with yet a fistula in the small intestine. After this there was decidedly an added interest in the case.

That the fistula was high up, and probably in the jejunum, was presumed from the facts that milk or milky fluids exuded from the opening soon after each feed, the skin around rapidly became excoriated as if from pancreatic secretion, and bile was passed, while at the time of the operation, from the appearances noted, the affected part was presumably jejunum; also methylene blue introduced, *per rectum*, failed to appear through the fistula. As the boy had survived all the fatal conditions above noted, and seemed possessed of an extraordinary vitality, it was resolved to attempt to repair the fistula in order to prevent him from dying miserably by starvation—a bitter fate indeed—under the circumstances.

Before such operative procedure was adopted, the boy was obviously thriving, and the fistula lessening in size. All the wounds, including the fistula, closed spontaneously on 14th April, twenty-seven days after the last operation, and twenty-two days after the intestine burst.

Notes a month later read as follows:—" Getting obstreperous; up and fought a boy in the ward; a few days ago ran off with a nurse's bicycle and rode round the grounds!" On 13th May, 1911, he was discharged cured. The two abdominal scars had healed soundly, and there was no hernia.

Such a case presents a most interesting chain of complications worthy of recording. Each condition in itself might have proved fatal. The combination seems remarkable.

Remarks on volvulus.—With reference to occurrence of volvulus after peritoneal adhesions, I have recently operated on two such cases. One (25th July, 1913) was that of a man, John Wm. B., aged 39 years, who suffered from chronic constipation and intestinal toxæmia for years, with signs of old cured disease of the appendix seen in a matting of the structures in the right iliac fossa on operation. He had a previous history suggesting the " dyspepsia of appendicitis," and a volvulus of the pelvic colon was the cause of acute obstruction. This was untwisted, punctured to allow collapse, the puncture being buried in by stitches, and the distended colon was pleated and sutured down to prevent recurrence. Also there was an abundant velamentous peri-colitis resembling the veil of Jackson, with thicker fibrous strands in places. Recovery was straightforward. The other case was the unusual one of an old lady of 78 years (Harriett C.), who had had previous operations as follows :—

1. Abdominal section for obstruction (St. Barts. Hosp., 1897).
2. Another laparotomy (cause, date, and place unknown).
3. Relief of strangulated hernia, right side (Tott. Hosp., 1897).
4. Excision of left breast (Tott. Hosp., 1897).

She had the scars appropriate to the above history, and, in addition, an acute obstruction of an absolute nature of three days' duration, with fæcal vomiting, and pressed very much for operation. Laparotomy on 9th December, 1911, revealed a volvulus with many adhesions and excessive paralytic distension of the pelvic colon. In reducing the twist the intestine burst with a crack like a pop-gun and evacuated itself on the edges of the wound. Suture of the ruptured portion, followed by cleansing of the loop and the site of operation, with closure of the abdomen, was effectual in securing uninterrupted recovery, except for a suppurative parotitis developing three days after the operation. She walked home six weeks afterwards, to return on Christmas Eve, 1912, with a serious abdominal condition. There was obstruction with its usual signs, the skin of the abdomen was tightly stretched and glossy, but the recent scar was soundly healed and linear in form. There were thirteen cherry-red spots of telangiectatic appearance, such as are described in deep-seated visceral carcinoma, and in her dying state she asked again for operation which was not done.

A *post-mortem* examination was permitted and no tumour was found, the cause of death being extensive compression of the intestines from multiple peritoneal adhesions. The appendix had been removed. Surely it is extraordinary for a person to survive five major operations in succession in the seventh and eighth decades. She had a cheerful temperament, which undoubtedly helped her to a climax of "anoci-association" perfection.

Condensation-obstruction.—I believe adhesions to be very commonly associated with volvulus, as a preliminary in bringing two parts of a coil together and creating thus a pedicle for rotation, converting an undulating or sinuous loop of intestine into one with a sharp U-shaped curve which might readily twist, or into an Ω (omega) shaped loop; in each case there is a neck formed by a contracting adhesion. Volvulus occurs as a rule in patients who are approaching the age when sclerotic change and tissue fibrosis is in progress. Is it not possible, then, that adhesions may take part in this general tissue condensation process, and produce effects such as this, due to contraction of bands, which before have been less apparently noxious? I have suggested [1, 2] the name ", condensation-obstruction " as brief and descriptive.

These bands, be they developmental, embryonic, from " crystallisation of lines of stress," or inflammatory, would shrink, thicken, and harden with the age of onset of general arterio-sclerosis, and produce, in certain cases, gradual toxæmia and chronic obstruction from kinking as described by Lane, or, in other cases, sudden tragedy and disaster from an acute abdominal crisis with condensation-obstruction.

A definite hint for treatment is suggested in such cases. After reduction, with aspiration and evacuation if necessary, carefully investigate the condition of the *neck* of the loop, divide the bands, making them as short as possible by amputation of redundant tags, and cover over the raw stumps completely with a peritoneal fold fixed over as a plastic graft.

I must, finally, record grateful thanks to my assistants, Drs. C. K. Stevenson, A. W. Gregorson, O. B. Parry, and H. M. Rashbrooke, who were intimately associated with me in these cases, also to those of my nurses whose attentions were required and unstintingly given.

REFERENCES.

[1] Spencer Mort, "Intestinal kinks," *Lancet*, January, 1914.

[2] Spencer Mort, "Condensation-obstruction in relation to pericolitis and intestinal kinking," *British Medical Journal*, 1914.

ROUND-CELLED SARCOMA OF THE SCALP OF TWO WEEKS' DURATION, FOLLOWING AN INJURY.

By MILNE M'INTYRE, M.B.,

Dispensary Surgeon, Glasgow Royal Infirmary.

INJURIES are so frequent in the history of patients suffering from external malignant tumours that it is not surprising that trauma finds a prominent place among the suggested causes of

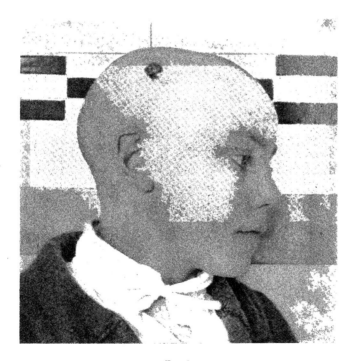

FIG. 1.
Sarcoma of scalp following an injury.

new growths. Sifted carefully there are few external malignant growths unassociated with a history of injury at sometime or other; but it has been reckoned (Thiem) that injury can only be considered a causal factor if the tumour develops at the very site of the injury, and when a continuous series of local phenomena intervenes between the injury and the appearance of the growth. The percentage of such has been reduced (Machol) to 2·06, the nature of the growth being more often sarcomatous than carcinomatous.

I venture, therefore, to think the following case of interest, since the growth appeared at the very site of an injury received two weeks previously.

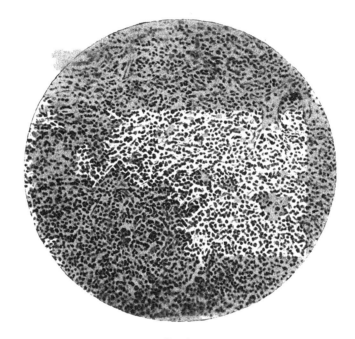

Fig. 2.

Sarcoma of scalp following an injury.

Summary.—*A wound of the skin, followed in two weeks by a round-celled sarcoma.*

The patient, a lad of 14 years of age, was admitted to the Glasgow Royal Infirmary, complaining of a small rapidly growing swelling on the scalp. Fours weeks previously he received a wound of the scalp from a small stone. The wound was stitched by his doctor, and thereafter healed, giving rise to no trouble for two weeks. A small swelling now appeared and was incised and dressed by his doctor; but two weeks later, the swelling increasing rapidly without any tendency to healing, he was sent to hospital.

In front of the right parietal eminence there was a small, red, soft tumour (Fig. 1, p. 94), the size of a chestnut, free from pain at all times, bleeding readily, and situated in the skin. The tumour was excised, and, on histological examination, proved to be a round-celled sarcoma. The structure is very cellular, the cells round and uniform in size, single in kind, and with many delicate thin-walled blood-vessels between them (Fig. 2, p. 95). Another feature in the section was the profuse proliferation of epidermal elements, apparently simple in nature.

The close association of the injury, and the development of the tumour, leaves no doubt as to the cause being primarily a wound of the tissues.

THE WESTERN MEDICAL SCHOOL, GLASGOW.

BY J. N. MORTON, M.A.,
Secretary to the School.

THE Western Medical School took its origin from a class in surgery, held by Dr. D. N. Knox in a hall over Mr. Stenhouse's bookseller's shop, in University Avenue, in the winter of 1878-79, and again in 1879-80. The students who attended in the first of these sessions were Messrs. Grier, Stanger, and Macvicar, and in the second Messrs. Guthrie Rankin, Anderson, and Macaulay. Dr. Knox's lectures were recognised by the Faculty of Physicians and Surgeons in January, 1879, as qualifying for their Licence, and by the University of Glasgow in May, 1879, as qualifying for degrees.

The University had removed from the eastern part of the city to the western in 1870; but Anderson's College, then the only extra-mural medical school, had not yet followed it, but was still housed in its old premises in George Street.

Before the winter session of 1880-81 began, Dr. Knox obtained as colleagues Dr. W. L. Reid to teach Midwifery and Diseases of Women, and Dr. (now Sir) David C. M'Vail to teach Practice of Medicine. Dr. M'Vail had been Professor of Physiology in Anderson's College, an appointment which he had resigned. An opening address, for this session, was given by Dr. Knox, with Dr. Scott Orr, the President of the Faculty of Physicians and Surgeons, in the chair. The number of students in attendance at the various classes was 16.

In the summer of 1881 a successful attempt was made to obtain efficient lecturers for the other branches of the curriculum. Mr. A. Ernest Maylard, M.B., B.S. Lond., formerly of Guy's Hospital, agreed to teach Anatomy; Dr. J. M. Milne, Chemistry; Dr. Neil Carmichael, Materia Medica; and Dr. Eben. Duncan, Medical Jurisprudence and Public Health. During the winter session 1881-82 lectures were delivered on chemistry, anatomy, surgery, practice of medicine, materia medica, and gynæcology; and during the summer session of 1882 on anatomy, operative surgery, midwifery, and medical jurisprudence. During this summer Dr. Duncan also delivered on Saturdays a course of lectures on public health, which was largely attended by both practitioners and students. In June, 1882, the staff was completed by the ¯election of Mr. William Limont, M.A., M.B., to the lectureship on Physiology.

Thus fairly launched, the Western Medical School pursued its way. The winter session 1882-83 was opened by an address from Dr. M'Vail on "Scottish Medical Teaching, Academic and Extra-Academic," Dr. J. B. Russell, Medical Officer of Health for Glasgow, being in the chair. The session proved on the whole a very encouraging one; but at the end of it the School sustained its first loss in the resignation of Mr. Maylard, who had been appointed assistant to Professor G. H. B. Macleod in the University. During the summer of 1883 the work of the anatomy rooms was superintended by Dr. Knox, who had the assistance, as demonstrator, of Mr. E. J. du Moulin, of the Edinburgh School.

Before the opening of the winter session 1883-84 a new occupant for the lectureship on anatomy was secured in the person of Mr. J. T. Carter, L.R.C.S.Edin., who was recommended by Mr. Symington, Lecturer on Anatomy, Minto House, Edinburgh. Dr. Carter came from New Brunswick to take up his appointment. In the summer of 1884, Dr. J. Walker Downie joined the staff to lecture on the Ear and Throat.

In this summer of 1884 the School sustained further losses in the resignations of Drs. Duncan, Carmichael, and Limont, and was faced with the prospect of Anderson's College coming west, to the neighbourhood of the University. As Anderson's College was appealing to the public for funds for its new building, the lecturers of the Western Medical School discussed the propriety of their making a similar appeal, but finally decided in the negative.

There is something of a hiatus in the records of the school for three years from 1884 to 1887, but when the curtain is again raised by the resumption of the minutes in November,

1887, it is found that Dr. Freeland Fergus is on the staff for the Eye, Dr. Hugh Murray for Skin Diseases, and Dr. T. Kennedy Dalziel for Anatomy. Drs. Reid, M'Vail, and Knox were still in their places. Dr. Carter, however, had died. He was a very successful teacher of anatomy.

At the end of the winter session 1887-88 Dr. Dalziel resigned his lectureship, having been only on the staff since the commencement of that session. In October, 1888, Dr. P. Caldwell Smith became Lecturer on Public Health. The winter session 1888-89 passed off successfully.

The autumn of 1889 saw the School nearly in the throes of dissolution. Indeed, it was stated in a London medical journal that the School had ceased to exist, but this was promptly denied. A crisis had arisen in this way. Dr. Reid had resigned his connection with the School on his appointment to the Chair of Midwifery in Anderson's College, which had migrated to Partick. Chiefly through the exertions of Dr. M'Vail, St. Mungo's College was founded in September, 1889, and to it Drs. M'Vail, Knox, and James K. Kelly (Dr. Reid's successor) transferred their services. In doing so they were no doubt influenced by the expectation that Anderson's College in its new situation would render any further successful career on the part of the Western Medical School impossible—an anticipation which has not been realised. Whatever their reasons, the arrangements which had been announced on the part of the Western Medical School for the winter of 1889-90 were abruptly cancelled.

Thus suddenly deprived of its principal teachers, the School would have closed its door but for the intervention of Dr. J. Stuart Nairne and Dr. R. Cowan Lees, whom the retiring lecturers obtained as successors. While these new men provided the "sinews of war" to keep the school going, it would be idle to pretend that they were fitted as teachers to make it a success. It was not till Mr. R. H. Parry joined the School in 1891 as Lecturer on Surgery that matters began to take a different turn. In 1890, however, Dr. John Edgar joined the staff as Lecturer on Operative Midwifery, and Mr. Robertson as Lecturer on Chemistry. Dr. Edgar only remained on the staff for one summer session, namely, that of 1890.

Dr. Walker Downie resigned his post in 1891. In the same year Dr. Harry St. Clair Gray joined the staff to lecture on midwifery, and Dr. A. Brown Kelly as successor to Dr. Downie; and Dr. P. Caldwell Smith resigned his post on his appointment to Anderson's College.

In 1892 Dr. A. R. Gunn joined the staff as Lecturer on Insanity and Diseases of Children—a somewhat odd combination of subjects. Early in 1893 Drs. Lees and Nairne retired from the School, and Dr. Freeland Fergus rejoined to lecture on the eye as before.

Dr. John Morton became Lecturer on Physiology in 1893, and was succeeded in that post by Dr. John Munro in 1894; in which year also Dr. G. Balfour Marshall, from Edinburgh, became Lecturer on Midwifery, and Dr. A. Brown Kelly resigned.

The records of the School again present somewhat of a hiatus from 1894 to 1897, but the School was all this time progressing towards a career of greater usefulness. A highly efficient staff of lecturers was being completed; Dr. G. H. Edington (Anatomy), Dr. Ernest Thomson (Physiology), and Mr. H. V. Craster (Chemistry) joining in 1896. Dr. R. M. Buchanan also joined the staff in this year as Lecturer on Pathology, remaining, however, only till 1897.

It may be noted here that following on his appointment in 1894, Dr. John Munro taught in the School other subjects besides physiology, conducting a plurality of classes on various parts of the curriculum. It is to be feared that overwork contributed to his death in 1896 at an early age.

The staff was augmented in 1897 by the joining of Dr. R. S. Thomson (Medicine), and Dr. James Rankine (Zoology). In the following year Dr. Frederick Dittmar became Lecturer on Physiology,* and Dr. John M. Cowan on Materia Medica; and in 1899 Mr. Hugh H. Browning, M.A., and Dr. Carstairs Douglas also became teachers, the former of physics, and the latter of Forensic Medicine and Public Health. Dr. Hugh M'Laren in the same year became Lecturer on Pathology.

It will thus be seen that at this period the staff had increased. Ten classes were taught in the winter session of

---

* In succession to Dr. Ernest Thomson, appointed to the Chair of Physiology in Anderson's College.

1899-1900, and nine in that of 1900-1901, and seven in the summer sessions of 1899, 1900, and 1901. The number of enrolments of students in winter and summer session combined was at this time between three and four hundred, Mr. Parry having especially large classes. This prosperity as regards numbers continued for several years further. Something in the shape of a constitution was given to the School by the adoption of a set of rules at a meeting on 2nd October, 1900.

It is not our purpose to pursue the roll of teachers further at present. Changes in the staff were tolerably rapid; those who became lecturers frequently doing so only as a stepping-stone to further advancement. In this way the School has supplied teachers to the University, to Anderson's College, and to St. Mungo's. Of the three gentlemen who may be looked upon as the pioneers or founders of the School, Dr. W. L. Reid, Dr. Knox, and Sir David C. M'Vail, two have filled the chair of President of the Faculty, and two became members of the General Medical Council—one attaining the double honour.

Without entering into invidious comparisons with more pretentious institutions, it may be said that the Western Medical School has, while undergoing occasional vicissitudes, had on the whole a successful and very useful career—a path in which it still continues. Such success as it achieves is simply due to providing the student with the teaching he requires from it. The teachers in their arrangements have never been hampered by the presence of laymen in their governing body, all affairs being managed by the teachers themselves, with the assistance of a lay secretary. The School is thus more on the lines of the Edinburgh School of Medicine than is either of the other Glasgow extra-mural schools.

In conclusion, it may be pointed out that the Western Medical School has never been indebted for any pecuniary help to the public, having been self-supporting from the beginning.

Obituary.

WILLIAM FORREST, M.B., C.M. Edin.,
POLLOKSHIELDS.

WE regret to announce the death of Dr. William Forrest, which took place at his residence in Pollokshields on 27th June. Dr. Forrest, who began the study of medicine in Glasgow during the last years of Lister's tenure of the Chair of Surgery in the University, followed the great surgeon to Edinburgh, where he completed his course, taking the degrees of M.B., C.M. in 1872. Settling in Glasgow after graduation, he rapidly built up, along with his elder brother, Dr. R. W. Forrest, who survives him, an extensive practice in the district of Crosshill. His interests were not confined to the practice of his profession. He was a man of much culture and wide reading, and he shared with his elder brother a bent to the practical applications of chemistry, which they turned to considerable profit by their discovery of a method of recovering gold from refractory ores. Dr. Forrest, who was unmarried, had retired from practice some years before his death.

CURRENT TOPICS.

APPOINTMENTS.—The following appointments have recently been made :—

John Macintyre, M.B., C.M. Glasg. (1882), to be Knight of Grace of the Order of the Hospital of St. John of Jerusalem in England.

D. J. Mackintosh, M.B., C.M. Glasg. (1884), M.V.O., to be Knight of Grace of the Order of the Hospital of St. John of Jerusalem in England.

W. B. Brownlie, M.B., Ch.B. Glasg. (1908), F.R.C.S.E., to be Assistant Ophthalmic Surgeon to the Blackburn and East Lancashire Royal Infirmary.

Randal Herley, L.R.C.P. & S.E., L.F.P.S. Glasg. (1903), to be Ophthalmic Surgeon to the Dewsbury and District Infirmary.

C. G. Mackay, M.B., Ch.B. Glasg. (1904), to be District Medical Officer to the Newport (Mon.) Union.

D. S. Richmond, M.B., Ch.B. Glasg. (1904), to be Medical Officer of Health to Cwmamman Urban District Council, and Medical Officer to the Post Office, Garnant and Glanamman.

Benjamin Hutchison, M.B., Ch.B. Glasg. (1908), to be Medical Officer for the Parish of Cambuslang.

J. P. Kinloch, M.D. Glasg. (M.B., 1909), D.P.H., to be Lecturer in Public Health in Aberbeen University.

J. Livingston Loudon, M.D. Glasg. (M.B., 1889), D.P.H., to be whole time Tuberculosis and Medical Officer for the Burgh of Hamilton.

Special Reserve of Officers, R.A.M.C.: Cadet Corporal Ian D. Suttie, M.B., C.M. Glasg. (1914), to be Lieutenant on probation.

Territorial Force, R.A.M.C.: Captain Samuel M. Sloan, M.B., C.M. Glasg. (1897), to be Major.

THE ROYAL VISIT.--The recent visit of their Majesties the King and Queen to Glasgow and its neighbourhood will long be remembered in the medical annals of the city. It was favoured with royal weather, it was accompanied by all the impressiveness of State ceremonial, and the programme of its first day included the opening of the reconstructed building of the Royal Infirmary, the opening of the new Royal Hospital for Sick Children, and a brief visit to the Western Infirmary, where a loyal address was presented by the managers. On the arrival of the royal train from Edinburgh the civic dignitaries were presented by the Secretary for Scotland, Mr. M'Kinnon Wood, and their Majesties, escorted by the Scots Greys, then drove in procession to the Royal Infirmary, where the King, then Prince of Wales, had in 1907 laid the memorial stone of the new buildings. Dr. J. D. Hedderwick, the chairman, was presented by the Lord Provost, and in turn presented the superintendent, Dr. J. Maxtone Thom; the architect, Mr. James Miller; the matron, Miss Melrose; and members of the board of management and medical staff. An address from the managers of the infirmary having been presented, the King handed his reply to Dr. Hedderwick. After prayer had been offered by the Very Rev. Dr. M'Adam Muir, His Majesty was presented with a gold key and formally opened the building, which the Royal Party entered, visiting some of the wards and special departments. In the course of their inspection Drs. John Henderson and Louise M'Ilroy, Professors Kennedy and Teacher, and Nurse Kate Bell were presented, and also a deputation from the Royal Faculty of Physicians and Surgeons of Glasgow, consisting of Dr. John Barlow, Dr. Ebenezer Duncan, Dr. W. G. Dun, and Mr. Walter Hurst, who presented an address from the Faculty, the King handing his reply to the president, Dr. Barlow. In the new King George V Electrical Institute Dr. John Macintyre was presented, and demonstrated the electro-cardiograph and other electrical apparatus. Their Majesties left the Infirmary after a visit of fifty minutes' duration.

The ceremony of laying the foundation stone of the extension of the City Chambers occupied the rest of the morning, and after receiving addresses from the Corporation, the Merchants' House, the Trades House, and the Chamber of Commerce, their Majesties lunched in the City Chambers, and then proceeded to the Royal Hospital for Sick Children. Here, in a pavilion erected before the main entrance, there were presented among others Mr. C. K. Aitken, chairman; Miss Simpson, matron; Sir J. J. Burnet, architect; Sir Hector C. Cameron, vice-president; and members of the board of management and medical staff. The Duke of Montrose, president of the institution, handed to the King an address from the managers thanking their Majesties for visiting and opening the new hospital, and the King, after handing his reply to the Duke, unlocked the door and declared the building open. In the course of the subsequent inspection Dr. George S. Middleton and Dr. T. K. Dalziel were presented, and the Queen unveiled the name-plate of the King George V and Queen Mary Ward.

Thereafter a brief visit was paid to the Western Infirmary, the royal carriage being drawn up in front of a stand occupied by the managers and medical staff, and facing the administrative block. Here were presented Sir Matthew Arthur, chairman; Mr. Arthur Hart, vice-chairman; Dr. D. J. Mackintosh, M.V.O., superintendent; Miss H. Gregory Smith, matron; and members of the board of management and medical staff. Sir Matthew Arthur, on behalf of the managers, presented an address to the King, who handed Sir Matthew his reply. On account of the limited time available, their Majesties did not alight from the carriage, and the day ended with a short visit to the University and the presentation of an address by Principal Sir Donald MacAlister.

THE HOSPITAL WORK OF GLASGOW.—*Apropos* of the recent visit of Their Majesties the King and Queen to Glasgow, the issue of *The Hospital* for 11th July devotes a leading article to the medical institutions which they opened or visited. The following extracts will be of interest to our readers:—

. "Tuesday last must have proved to their Majesties a day to remember, for they had the privilege of opening two splendid hospitals of the first importance to the city of Glasgow. . . . The King has by hard work and constant visitation acquired an exceptional knowledge of hospital construction and administration. We can well understand how gratified and surprised many of the Glasgow managers were at the proofs their Majesties gave during their visit to the two great hospitals referred to of their Majesties' appreciation and knowledge. . . .

"It is a remarkable fact that the managers of the Glasgow

Royal Infirmary should have boldly faced the rebuilding of the whole of this hospital, and so arranged matters that the work of the institution has been carried on with efficiency during the seven years it has taken to complete the work. Owing to the special care and business aptitude displayed by the managers, under the chairmanship of Mr. J. D. Hedderwick, LL.D., especial pains were taken to secure that not only the plans, but the whole of the internal arrangements should be entrusted to three experts, so that the new Royal Infirmary, opened on Tuesday last, has necessarily a peculiar interest for all hospital workers, architects, and hospital managers all the world over. We have no doubt that His Majesty King George was fully acquainted with these facts, and that this knowledge made the opening ceremony and inspection of the new hospital a source of real interest to him. This is a fine institution, and is one of the best and largest of the voluntary hospitals. Queen Mary, whose devotion to the interests of children has made her beloved by every mother throughout the British Empire, naturally took a supreme interest in the new Royal Hospital for Sick Children. We regret there was no time for their Majesties to inspect the Western Infirmary, but it was a signal mark of Royal favour that they should have found time to visit it on so busy a day. It is so extraordinary well managed as to make it just the sort of hospital King George would find pleasure in inspecting. . . .

"Glasgow has long aspired to be regarded as the second city in the United Kingdom, and the mere recital of the enormous sums spent upon the two hospitals which were opened by their Majesties on this day proves eloquently the deep hold the voluntary hospital system has upon Scotsmen as well as Englishmen. . . . It is indeed splendid evidence of a deep conviction that practically the whole of the money required to build and equip the Royal Infirmary and the Royal Hospital for Sick Children—approximately £700,000—had been provided prior to the date of the opening ceremony. Glasgow already has in the Western Infirmary a hospital of the first rank, full of up-to-date structural units, whose out-patient department has attracted visitors from all parts of the world. Dr. Mackintosh has proved himself to be a medical superintendent whose work constitutes a model of what a medical superintendent's should be. To Dr. Thom, the superintendent of the Glasgow Royal Infirmary, great credit is due for the fact that, during the nine years it has taken to rebuild this large hospital, containing 665 beds, the ordinary work of this great institution has been carried on with marked efficiency, without any complaint from the patients or their friends. The managers of the Royal Infirmary are entitled to feel proud that their long and arduous labours have culminated in the provision of so fine a hospital; and Mr. Hedderwick, their chairman, will, we hope, receive some adequate recognition of his public services, for he has been throughout the life and soul of one of the greatest hospital enterprises which have been undertaken and completed in recent years." . . .

In another part of the same issue there is an admirable photograph of Mr. Hedderwick, whose illness is referred to in sympathetic terms, and also a photograph of the "Florence Nightingale" window which he has presented to the Royal Infirmary Chapel.

Our contemporary returns to the subject in its leading article of 18th July, in which it regrets that their Majesties had not time to inspect some of the "administrative efficiencies" of the Western Infirmary, and suggests, in order that such efficiencies may not be missed by His Majesty, that he "should have on his staff a hospital equerry whose duty it would be to keep himself in touch with every matter of special interest which hospital progress may anywhere present."

"We have ventured to call attention to this suggestion of an extra equerry to the King," it continues, "because we greatly appreciate the genuine interest taken by His Majesty in our voluntary hospitals, and the surprising amount of information he has acquired about them and their management. King George is, in fact, a knowledgeable inspector of hospitals and kindred institutions. Indeed, effective changes have been introduced into the management of more than one institution as the direct outcome of the King's visits. . . . We feel, therefore, that King George might set an example for good to the whole of the governing authorities throughout the world should he ever see his way to appoint a knowledgeable hospital equerry. The King is the titular head of many things in this nation. Having identified himself closely with our voluntary hospital system, it would be but natural for His Majesty to desire to provide himself with first-hand knowledge of everything calculated to secure the interest and effectiveness of the voluntary hospitals."

THE LADY HOZIER CONVALESCENT HOME.—In commemoration of the visit of the King and Queen to Glasgow, Lord and Lady Newlands are giving £25,000 to complete the endowment of the Lady Hozier Convalescent Home at Lanark, an appanage of the Western Infirmary, Glasgow. This home, which was built and equipped in 1891 by the late Lord Newlands (then Sir William Hozier) in memory of his wife, was opened in 1892, and is said to have cost nearly £8,000. Three years later Sir William Hozier invested £10,000 in the names of trustees as an endowment fund towards the maintenance of the institution. His son, the present peer, has continued to take a deep interest in the welfare of the home, and last year made a donation of £516 to wipe out an adverse balance on the year's working. At present the endowment fund stands at £12,600; most of this is, of course, Sir William Hozier's original gift, and £2,000 more came from the estate of the late Mr. James Dick. The home accommodates 40 patients. Last year there were admitted 367 males and 213 females from the Western Infirmary, who resided on an average a fortnight each.

GLASGOW ROYAL INFIRMARY : RESIGNATION OF DR. HEDDER-WICK.—It is with much regret that we intimate that the condition of his health has compelled Dr. J. D. Hedderwick, LL.D., to resign the chairmanship of the Royal Infirmary board. Dr. Hedderwick, whose services to Glasgow and to the Royal Infirmary are known far beyond the bounds of Glasgow, took the chair in 1901 for the express purpose of carrying through the vast scheme of reconstruction which, under his guidance, has now been brought to so successful an issue. His labours being completed, it was his intention to retire at the end of this year, but he has found it necessary, in conformity with medical advice, to do so somewhat sooner. The sympathy of all those who are familiar with the arduous character of his undertaking and the triumphant success of his achievement will go with him in his retirement, and their good wishes for his speedy recovery will be no less earnest and cordial than their grateful thanks for his immense and disinterested labours.

DINNER TO DR. JOHN BROWNLEE.—A large company, mainly composed of Glasgow medical men, but representative also of the other learned professions in the city, met in the Grosvenor Restaurant, on 26th June, to do honour to Dr. John Brownlee, Physician-Superintendent of Ruchill Hospital, on the occasion of his appointment as Statistician to the Medical Research Committee under the Insurance Act Commissioners. Professor George A. Gibson presided, and the company included, besides the guest of the evening, Dr. Joshua Ferguson, Dr. T. K. Dalziel, Professor Stevenson, Mr. Barrett, Mr. A. Hood, Bailie Sloan, the Rev. William Brownlee, Dr. J. C. M'Vail, Dr. A. K. Chalmers, Dr. Hutchison, Bailie M'Connell, the Rev. Dr. John Smith, Sir David M'Vail, Dr. D. J. Mackintosh, Dr. Napier, Professor T. K. Monro, Mr. Paton, Professor Stockman, Dr. Neilson, Mr. Maylard, and Councillor Gemmell. Apologies for absence were received from the Lord Provost, Principal Sir Donald MacAlister, and others. The Lord Provost wrote stating that Dr. Brownlee's removal from Glasgow deprived the city of one of its most capable and distinguished public officials. He would be missed not only in the Health Department, but also in the various scientific institutes of the city.

The chairman, in proposing the toast of "Our Guest," sketched the elements in Dr. Brownlee's career which had led to his outstanding position as one of the recognised authorities in medical statistics. All through life he never was content with any text-book work or text-book solution—he always went to the root of things. Statistics had been the playthings of politicians as well as of doctors; it had almost seemed as if any theory in the universe could be equally well established out of the same set of statistics. Such a statement was, of course, a mere caricature of the actual position; but there was far too much reasonableness in the charge, and that was due entirely to the fact that not merely the ordinary statistician, but what might be called the expert statistician who took up the relation of statistics to special social problems, had never really faced the scientific study and correlation of these subjects. From the start they had had in Dr. Brownlee a man who had the equipment to tackle this problem successfully. Naturally he (the chairman) appreciated the value of mathematics, but he appreciated very much more a much rarer thing amongst statisticians, and that was a thorough knowledge of the data which medical studies were intended to unfold. He for one, with the knowledge he had of Dr. Brownlee's familiarity with statistical methods, from the knowledge he possessed of the medical facts upon which these statistics were based, would accept without question any statistical results that came forth from the office under Dr. Brownlee's signature. He was hopeful that a new era of statistical study was approaching. Dr. Brownlee's researches were original—he did not build on any man's foundation. It was exceedingly important, at the beginning of what he hoped was going to be a new career in medical statistics, that they had here a man who could look at the subject not merely as a mathematician, not merely as a statistician, but as the well-trained and ripe man of science looked at it. They had in Dr. Brownlee a man whose training, whose culture, whose general character fitted him admirably for the polished man of the world. Dr. Brownlee had an acquaintance with literary and historical facts that would do credit to many a professor of literature. They congratulated him upon the very responsible post to which he had been appointed, and they were certain that no better man could have been chosen for that post.

Dr. Brownlee said, in reply, that he had been very fortunate with regard to his home, his school, and his university. Glasgow High School had been a mágnificent training ground; and in the arts and medical faculties at Gilmorehill he had studied under men whose work and reputation had never been excelled. He felt a special pride that he, a Glasgow student purely, had obtained this appointment, open as it was to the whole country. In leaving the service of the Corporation after fourteen years spent between Belvidere and Ruchill Fever Hospitals, he felt he ought to say how fairly he had been treated. The next great step in medicine must come from the fever hospitals, and he trusted that they would waken up and realise their responsibility. In Ruchill Hospital he had a laboratory equipment such as not another in the country had, but unless the Corporation were willing to give men as well as laboratories, and thus develop the scientific side, this country was going to be left behind the other countries of Europe. There was no lack of men, and he would suggest that the Corporation should seek to attach to the fever hospitals for a much longer time the best of the medical men who passed through them. During the early years of their private practice many young doctors had sufficient time to continue their scientific study at the hospitals, and thus engage in work that would be of permanent value. It was of the utmost importance that the younger men should be associated with the fever hospitals for a few years, because the treatment of fevers was entering upon an entirely new epoch.

PRESENTATION TO DR. CASKIE.—At a meeting held in the Burgh Hall, Hillhead, on 29th June, Dr. A. T. Campbell presiding, Dr. W. A. Caskie was presented by the members of the Glasgow North-Western Division of the British Medical Association and by other members of the medical profession with an illuminated address and a cheque in recognition of the able manner in which he had discharged the duties of Secretary to the Division, and of his great labours in the interest of the profession during the past few years. Dr. John Lindsay spoke on behalf of the profession, and the presentation was made by the chairman, who referred in appropriate terms to Dr. Caskie's unwearying services.

JUSTICES OF THE PEACE FOR AYRSHIRE.—On the recommendation of the Earl of Eglinton and Winton, the following, amongst others, have been added to the Commission of the Peace for the county of Ayr:—Richard More, M.B., C.M.Glasg. (1882), Elistoun, West Kilbride; D. B. Campbell, M.B., C.M.Glasg. (1892), Saltcoats; Robert Allan, M.D. Glasg. (M.B., 1875), Ardrossan; G. D. M'Rae, M.D.Edin. (M.B., 1895), F.R.C.P.E., Ayr.

STATE INSURANCE IN GLASGOW.—The Insurance Committee for the burgh of Glasgow met on 8th July in the Burgh Court Hall, City Chambers, Mr. R. D. M'Ewan presiding.

The chairman, in the course of a review of the year's work, referred to the new medical benefit regulations, one important feature of which was the provision of a medical card to each insured person. Some 320,000 of these cards had been issued. During last year considerable interest was aroused in connection with proposals for the distribution of funds which, it was anticipated, would be left in the hands of the committee at the close of the medical year. On the basis of the provisional credit they had been able satisfactorily to settle with the medical practitioners in the area. Discussion had also arisen from time to time as to the maximum number of persons which should be permitted on any medical list, and the committee passed a resolution putting that at 2,000, while the local Medical Committee recommended 1,500. The committee had no powers summarily to limit the number upon a doctor's list, but the new medical benefit regulations made provision that, in the event of a practitioner being unable satisfactorily to treat the persons on his list, they might transfer from his list such number of persons as they might consider desirable in order to secure adequate treatment for the remainder. Out of 374 practitioners in the area, only 30 had lists exceeding the maximum number recommended by the committee, so that insured persons in Glasgow had a satisfactory freedom of choice. The attention of the sub-committee had also been directed to the increasing charges upon the drug fund. Not only had there been an increase in the number of prescriptions, but the price per prescription had also risen rapidly, particularly during the first quarter of the present medical year. An inquiry was at present proceeding into the incidence of the charges on the drug fund, with a view to ascertaining whether there had been any unnecessary extravagance, but it was hoped that with reasonable economy in the matter of prescribing it would not be necessary to resort to the drastic measure of discounting the chemists' accounts. On the whole, the medical benefit arrangements had proceeded most satisfactorily in the Glasgow area. The sub-committee on sanatorium benefit had dealt with about 1,700 applications, 1,300 being from males and about 400 from females. For various reasons—non-insurance, removal, &c.—some 400 had not been treated by the committee. Of the others, 1,237 had been recommended for institutional treatment,

28 for dispensary treatment, and 73 for domiciliary treatment. Of those recommended for institutional treatment, 1,135 had been admitted to various institutions, 552 being to institutions suitable for treatment of the "early" type of case, while the others had been treated for the most part in the hospitals of the Corporation, in institutions more suited to the advanced case. Out of the cases treated in institutions, 136 died there, while of those dismissed a number subsequently died.

STATE INSURANCE: PAYMENTS TO GLASGOW DOCTORS.—The minutes of the Insurance Committee for the burgh of Glasgow, submitted at the meeting held on 8th July, state that at a meeting of the sub-committee on 24th June the clerk submitted a statement showing the method of distribution of the total amount (£150,320) provisionally credited to the committee in respect of medical benefit for the year ended 11th January. It stated that £121,524, 5s. 9d. was paid to medical practitioners for medical attendance and treatment of insured persons on lists, including domiciliary treatment of tuberculosis; £1,272, 19s. 10d. paid in respect of insured persons permitted to make their own arrangements for receiving medical attendance and treatment otherwise than with doctors on the panel; and £27,522, 16s. 11d. paid to chemists, &c., for the supply of drugs, medicines, and appliances. The minutes also contain a statement showing, as at the close of the medical year, the distribution among the practitioners on the panel of the insured persons whose names appear on doctors' lists, and of the amounts paid in respect of the treatment of those persons. It is shown in the statement that one doctor for 4,468 persons on his list received £1,625, 8s. 1d.; one doctor, for 3,984 persons, £1,453, 8s. 8d.; four doctors, for an average of 3,275 persons, an average payment of £1,189, 8s. 1d.; seven doctors, for an average of 2,718 persons, an average of £986, 15s. 8d.; seventeen doctors, for an average of 2,223 persons, an average of £807, 17s. 9d.; forty-six doctors, for an average of 1,715 persons, an average of £618, 15s. 2d.; sixty-five doctors, for an average of 1,246 persons, an average of £447, 13s.; ninety-seven doctors, for an average of 725 persons, an average of £261, 2s. 8d.; and one hundred and thirty-six doctors, for an average of 191 persons, an average of £66, 12s. 4d. In addition, £1,097 was paid to nineteen practitioners whose names were withdrawn from the panel list during the year through resignation or death.

AYR SANATORIUM.—At a meeting of the Ayr Burgh Insurance Committee, held on 19th June, a minute of the Sanatorium Benefit Sub-Committee was submitted recommending that in view of the fact that the funds did not allow of further treatment the patients in sanatoria be brought home. A letter from the Commissioners, in reply to one sent by the Clerk, stated that the Commissioners would not be prepared to advance more than the proportion of funds applicable to each quarterly period, and suggested the expediency of exercising caution with regard to expenditure on sanatoria benefit. The Clerk stated that if they went on spending as they were doing at present his estimate would be exceeded by about £80 at the end of the quarter. Mr. Corrigan moved the approval of the Committee's recommendation. He knew that the proposal on the face of it looked revolutionary, yet they had no other alternative. He thought the local health authorities should now take up the cases. Mr. S. Hill, in seconding, said the committee were individually and collectively responsible for any deficiency they might cause. A counter-proposal that the matter be remitted back to the committee, with powers to continue the treatment of the more hopeful cases, and inform the Commissioners that the committee had been acting under a misapprehension, and that they were trying to bring their expenditure within the amount that would be available during the year, was defeated by 18 votes to 6, and the recommendation of the sub-committee was approved. The matter subsequently came under the notice of Ayr Town Council, who communicated with the Local Government Board, from whom the following statement was received:—(1) That where insurance committees, from want of funds or any other reason, discontinued the treatment of insured persons, it fell to the local authority to treat these cases if further treatment was necessary; and (2) that it rested with the local authority to determine the nature of the treatment, and in doing so they ought to be guided by the medical officer of health. In the view of the Board it was advisable that the patients should not be removed until it was determined what further treatment was to be given to them.

GLASGOW DENTAL HOSPITAL.— The twenty-ninth annual general meeting of the members and subscribers to the Incorporated Glasgow Dental Hospital was held on 30th June in the Merchants' House. There was a large and representative attendance, presided over by Deacon-Convener William Beattie. Mr. D. M. Alexander, secretary, submitted the annual report, which stated that during 1913 the number of patients treated in the hospital had reached a higher number than the record of any previous year. The total number of patients during 1912 was 13,443, while during 1913 there were 16,078. The total number of patients treated at the hospital since it was opened in May, 1885, had been 222,182. During the year 27 students joined the hospital for the full course of two years, and in addition 18 students for shorter periods, averaging three months each. The total number of students on the roll at 31st December, 1913, was 56, against 40 in the previous year. The Board acknowledged public annual subscriptions amounting to £136, 8s., and donations amounting to £218, 12s. 2d. This was the first year that the annual subscriptions had shown any marked increase, being an advance of £30 on the preceding year. The growing necessities, both of the hospital and school, had brought before the Board the need for increased accommodation. Their appeals for financial assistance had been generously responded to, and they were grateful to state that at the close of the year there was a balance in bank and on hand of £820, 12s. 7d.

PAISLEY: REPORT OF THE MEDICAL OFFICER OF HEALTH.— The annual report of the Medical Officer of Health for Paisley, Dr. G. Clark Trotter, issued on 19th June, refers to the number and causes of deaths in the burgh last year. The total number of deaths from all causes registered was 1,284, giving a death-rate of 15·0. After adjustment of the numbers, by interchange with other districts of deaths not in the usual place of residence, the corrected figures were 1,306—626 males and 680 females—giving a rate of 15·3 per 1,000 of the estimated population. In alluding to deaths which are uncertified, Dr. Trotter remarks that it is a most undesirable state of the law, especially where, as in towns, medical attendance is available, that registration of death is possible without a medical certificate. While doubtless death was nearly always due to natural causes, in these cases the cause assigned had not the same value as the opinion of a medical practitioner, and medical certification would remove any suspicion or doubt which might arise, as, for instance, in connection with the deaths of illegitimate children. In ·this connection Dr. Trotter quotes from the Registrar-General's last issued annual report, in which it was stated that in the larger burghs deaths uncertified as to cause were relatively most numerous in Paisley, the rate being 3·5 per cent.

"THE BRITISH PHARMACOPŒIA."—At a meeting held on 13th July the Executive Committee of the General Medical Council formally adopted as *The British Pharmacopœia, 1914*, the completed draft submitted by the Pharmacopœia Committee. It was resolved that copies, in advance of publication, should be made accessible to the public for inspection at the offices of the Council in London, Edinburgh, and Dublin, on Monday, 10th August, at 10 A.M., and thereafter from 10 A.M. to 4 P.M.

The official publication of the new *British Pharmacopœia* will be made by notice in the *Gazette* on Friday, 9th October, on which day, copies will be on sale by the publishers, Messrs. Constable and Co., Limited., 10 Orange Street, Leicester Square, London, W.C.

SOUTH AFRICAN INSTITUTE FOR MEDICAL RESEARCH.— Through the kindness of Dr. T. B. Gilchrist, of Johannesburg, an alumnus of Glasgow University who adds to his professional distinctions the merit of having been largely instrumental in founding the University of Glasgow Club of South Africa, we have received a copy of the first memoir issued by the South African Institute for Medical Research. It is devoted to an enquiry into the etiology, manifestations, and prevention of pneumonia amongst natives on the Rand recruited from tropical areas, and is from the pen of G. D. Maynard, F.R.C.S.E., statistician and clinician to the institute. Along with it there comes a copy of Sir Almroth Wright's report to the Witwatersrand Native Labour Association on prophylactic inoculation against pneumococcus infections, a report which is supplementary to the former memoir. Mr. Maynard's report, the result of a laborious statistical investigation, leads to the conclusions that the incidence of pneumonia is greatest immediately on the arrival of the natives on the Rand, that the length of the febrile period is somewhat less among natives than among Europeans, and that a termination by crisis is less common in the native, that pneumococcal meningitis is a commoner complication than in Europeans, that there is no evidence to show that pneumonia spreads from case to case, and that prophylactic inoculation reduces the incidence of pneumonia for a period of about four months, but has little influence on the case-mortality. The report of Sir Almroth Wright and his co-workers deals *in extenso* with the question of prophylactic inoculation, and claims a reduction in the death-rate of the inoculated varying from 31 per cent to 60 per cent upon an observation period of six months. They recommend the routine employment of prophylactic inoculation on recruitment of the native, the dose being 1,000 million cocci, and they consider that the dose should be repeated after a four months' interval. They consider that vaccine treatment in the form of small repeated doses is ineffectual, but they have had good results from a single large dose (250-1,000 millions) administered in the incubation period. They do not as yet advise the general use of therapeutic inoculation, but urge that further investigation should be given to the subject.

Both reports may be recommended as containing much of interest for readers in this country regarding the etiology and treatment of pneumonia.

MEDICINE AT THE PANAMA-PACIFIC EXHIBITION.—Recognising the large place which the modern achievements of medicine and sanitation have occupied in rendering possible the completion of the Panama Canal, the governing body of the Panama-Pacific International Exposition, which opens on 20th February, 1915, has attached much importance to a prominent representation of these two sciences, with the result that the medical visitor will find himself surrounded by material of engrossing interest. The Government of Cuba will show how the experience of the United States army in Cuba made possible the Panama Canal, and will exhibit model hospital wards as they are conducted in the tropics. Health exhibits will be shown from Argentina, Japan, France, Germany, the Philippines, and thirty other countries, and the British exhibits from Ghent will be shown in their entirety. Health and human welfare displays will be exhibited by the American Steel Corporation, the General Electric Company, the Rockefeller Foundation, the Russel Sage Foundation, Carnegie Institutions, and the Social Survey. Congresses will be held by many learned and scientific bodies, including the American Academy- of Medicine, the National Commission of Mental Hygiene, various societies for special diseases and for tuberculosis, and the Panama-Pacific Dental Congress. Nursing will be represented by many congresses and exhibits. A feature of the Exhibition will be the model emergency hospital, a working exhibit which is already open, and is in charge of Dr. R. M. Woodward of the United States Marine Hospital of San Francisco. Medical and surgical appliances, and anatomical, histological, and bacteriological instruments will be shown in the Palace of Liberal Arts.

TROPICAL DISEASES BUREAU.—We have received a copy of the Librarian's report on the library of the Tropical Diseases Bureau established in the Imperial Institute. The report, which was presented in April to the managing committee, shows that the library now contains 1,100 bound volumes, over 2,000 reprints, and 600 reports, departmental bulletins, and other unbound pamphlets. It possesses complete sets of forty-six of the more important tropical journals, and, in addition, many others of which the early volumes only have proved unprocurable, many important books of reference and standard works, and also a representative collection of recent books, which is constantly undergoing enlargement. It has also a large collection of reprints and of official medical and sanitary reports from India and the Colonies, and its usefulness is only limited by the fact that its advantages are not as yet widely known. It is evident that it must present valuable facilities to officers home on leave.

SCHOOL HYGIENE.—The Fifth International Congress on School Hygiene will be held in Brussels in 1915. The subjects for discussion will be grouped under the following heads:—The school building and its equipment; medical inspection in urban and rural schools; the prevention of contagious diseases in school; the teaching of hygiene to teachers, scholars, and parents; school hygiene in its relation to physical education; teaching methods, syllabusses, and school equipment in relation to hygiene; school hygiene in its relation to exceptional children; . school hygiene with regard to adolescents. The Congress will be under the patronage of His Majesty the King of the Belgians, and under the auspices of the Belgian National Institute of Pedology and of the Belgian Pedotechnical Society. The organising committee will be presided over by M. J. Corman, Director-General of Primary Studies in the Department of Science and Art, and by Dr. J. Demoor, Rector of the Free University of Brussels.

All communications and enquiries should be sent to Dr. H. Rulot, General Secretary, 66 Rue des Renticrs, Brussels.

NEW PREPARATIONS, &c.

From Messrs. The Bayer Company, Limited.

"Istin."—This is stated to be a synthetic product which is closely allied in chemical constitution to the active principles of the anthracene purgatives. It is supplied in 5-grain tablets, and the dose is said to be 1-1½ or 2 tablets before bedtime. It is claimed to be a mild but certain purgative that does not cause griping. The urine may be stained just as is the case when rhubarb is given.

The sample supplied was tried and found to act very efficiently in a case of simple constipation; no griping was experienced, and the urine showed a marked dark yellow discolouration for more than a day afterwards. The action was slow; the effects were not produced for about twenty hours.

There is one obvious advantage in the case of a synthetic drug of this kind—that it can be prepared always of exactly the same strength. In this way the uncertainty as to strength in the case of extracts of various samples of vegetable drugs is removed.

MEETINGS OF SOCIETIES.

MEDICO–CHIRURGICAL SOCIETY OF GLASGOW.

SESSION 1913-1914.
MEETING XI.—20TH MARCH, 1914.

The President, MR. A. ERNEST MAYLARD, *in the Chair.*

I.—THE RADICAL CURE OF HERNIA IN INFANTS.
BY DR. ALEX. MACLENNAN.

The treatment of hernia in infants is still a disputed matter. By the application of a truss or of a skein of wool, or by incessant reduction, a hernia may be made to disappear, but it is not cured. The sac of a hernia in an infant, though it becomes untenanted, nevertheless remains a sac, and the notice "To let" remains up. The presence of so many unoccupied sacs found in the cadaver and during operations goes far to prove the permanency of the sac, and, in view of the fact that the anatomy of hernia in infancy is identical with that of later life, it is clear that any form of treatment which does not obliterate the whole sac is useless. So many cases of hernia are met with in adults with a history of an infantile hernia said to have been cured, that it is very doubtful if such cases were cured, and it is practically certain that no one ever develops a hernia who has not had since infancy a sac ready formed.

The radical cure of hernia in the adult possesses a serious morbidity and some mortality, while the operation in infants possesses practically neither. In the majority of text-books, however, herniotomy in infants and young children is advised only in cases of irreducible or strangulated hernia, or in cases where truss treatment properly and continuously applied has failed to retain the hernia (*vide* Buford, Kirmisson, Willard, Kelly). Lange and Spitze, on the other hand, point out the disadvantages of truss treatment and the harmlessness of early operation, stating that "there is no single case known where an actual obliteration of the sac has followed the wearing of a truss, but there are many cases where, in spite of apparent cure, the hernia has reappeared later." With these views the writer is in complete accord.

That the early operation is absolutely safe has been proved by the wholesale radical treatment of hernias in infants attending the Royal Hospital for Sick Children (Out-patient Department). The credit for the initiative in operating on hernias in out-patients belongs to Dr. Jas. H. Nicoll; and the operation which the writer performs is so simple that the dangers associated with the radical operation have vanished.

The procedure adopted is as follows:—The cases selected are infants not over two years, in fair general health, with mothers of average intelligence, able and willing to give a little more attention than usual to the child. If phimosis is present the child is circumcised at least one month before the proposed radical operation, though in exceptional circumstances the circumcision and the radical cure may be done at the same sitting. Preparatory to operation, food is withheld for three hours, but the bowels are not interfered with. The neighbourhood of the groin is washed with soap and water while the anæsthetic (chloroform) is being administered. This is followed by a copious lavage with methylated spirit, and the area is then covered with sterile gauze. The hips of the child are well raised on a sand pillow. A "circumcision" towel (*i.e.*, a towel having in the centre a hole 2 inches in diameter, cut and hemmed) covers the child, and is placed over the gauze so that the hole exposes the operation area. When anæsthesia is complete the gauze is pulled through the hole, and the margins of the hole are clipped to the skin. The centre of the hole should be over the position of the internal ring. The incision is made over the internal ring, and should not exceed three-quarters of an inch. The skin

and subcutaneous fat having been divided, the deeper tissues
are raked apart by two blunt retractors. The sac and cord
being found are picked up with pressure forceps and drawn
out of the wound. The vas is identified by quickly tearing
through the various layers, and the sac is rapidly dissected
or wiped free by gauze from all attachments. To ensure the
necessary free separation of the neck of the sac and of the
parietal peritoneum in the immediate neighbourhood of the
ring, a pair of blunt-pointed scissors should be slipped along
the sac, and the attachments in the canal entirely separated
by gentle "digging." To facilitate the separation an assistant
should gently pull upon the cord while the operator pulls
upon the sac in the opposite direction. At the junction of
the sac with the peritoneum there is frequently a thickening
which shows as a white line or area: the sac should be freed
from all adhesions till this region is exposed. The sac is
treated as in Macewen's operation, care being taken to
make the last puncture through the neck of the sac
emptied of all contents. The sac, if long, should not be all
used, but only part of it. For the suture, No. 1 iodised
catgut (Salkinsohn process) is employed. The application of
a ligature to the neck of the sac high up, with removal of the
sac, is no doubt quicker and perhaps simpler than the
Macewen operation, but it is neither so safe nor so effective.
It involves risk of including in the ligature the bladder wall
or the ureter, whereas the sac when crumpled up at the
internal ring forms a scientific and efficient truss just where
the hernia originates. The suture used for puckering the
sac is used also for the closure of the deep wound, as in
infants there is no need of deep suturing, the structures
being in apposition once the sac has been removed. In older
children, however, with well distended canals and large
herniæ, adequate and careful suturing of the canal should be
carried out as in adults. The superficial wound is closed by
one or two silkworm-gut sutures, and dressed by a roll of
gauze made to cover little more than the wound, and retained
in position by a piece of adhesive rubber plaster, 3 inches by
2 inches in size. The skin is wiped with ether round the
wound, and the plaster heated to make it adhere instan-
taneously. Elaborate dressings are quite unnecessary and

only annoy the infant. After the lapse of a week the child is brought again to the dispensary to have the stitches removed, and a little powder sprinkled over the parts.

What happens in the interval between the operation and the removal of the dressing, as regards keeping the child from rising or twisting about or even crawling over the floor, is not enquired into and in any case does not signify. By far the greatest strain and risk to the success of the operation come from the sudden increase in intra-abdominal tension produced by the action of the diaphragm in coughing, vomiting, sneezing, and by resisting the mistaken kindness of restraint. The operation done rapidly through a small incision, with the minimum of manipulation, dissection, stitching, and without violence to the anatomy, entails little tax upon the vitality or amiability of the child, and indeed causes less distress than a simple circumcision.

In females the operation is even simpler than that described for males. In them the sac should always be opened, as otherwise the tube or ovary might be interfered with when the sac is puckered up. If this is to be done properly, it may be necessary in some cases to detach the broad ligament, at least in part of its extent, from the sac. Occasionally the ovary shows the presence of cystic changes, which require attention, or even call for oöphorectomy. The writer has twice found the uterus along with the tube and ovary of one side in the sac. In many cases the appendix is part of the contents of the hernia. In a large flaccid hernia in one infant the appendix was not only palpable, but visible, and was seen to share in the peristaltic action of the intestine. During the operation for hernia the appendix, besides presenting in the sac, has been adherent to it or otherwise abnormal, and in eight cases was removed. On two occasions the vas was accidentally severed, and repair was attempted by means of a strand of No. 0 catgut running along the lumen of the tube, and having its ends brought through the wall and knotted on the outside.

In estimating results it is proverbially difficult to trace hospital cases, but of those seen only one showed a recurrence. One or two of the infants showed some general disturbance from hæmorrhage distending the scrotum and spontaneously disappearing. One child died three weeks after operation, with symptoms of meningitis. None of the others were, so far as is known, at all upset by the procedure.

II.—ON MYELOID TUMOURS OF TENDON SHEATHS, WITH REPORT OF A CASE.

By Dr. Thos. P. Grant and Dr. Matthew J. Stewart.

Drs. Grant and Stewart's communication was published as an original article in our issue for May, 1914, p. 333.

III.—AN UNUSUAL CASE OF FRACTURE OF THE CARPAL SCAPHOID.

By Mr. Arch. Young.

Fracture of the carpal scaphoid is a type of injury which is now sufficiently well recognised, and its symptoms are known well enough to render it unnecessary to detail them here. As implied by the title, this case is brought forward in view of certain somewhat unusual features. These will be best understood if a brief account be given of the history of the case.

The patient is a lad, J. S., aged 21 years, an apprentice in a shipbuilding yard at Port-Glasgow. He consulted me, about three months ago, on account of pain in the left wrist, which had become so troublesome as to prevent him continuing at his work. The pain was felt chiefly when he attempted any movement involving pressure on the proximal part of the palm—especially on the thenar eminence—with the wrist extended. It became so troublesome that he could no longer exert the necessary pressure and grip in using his tools. There was no history at all of any recent injury, and the only clue one could get as to a possible cause was the story that, between two and three years before, when 'larking" with some friends, he fell rather heavily and hurt his left wrist and hand. In falling, the knuckles of the clenched hand forcibly struck the ground, and the wrist was then violently flexed. There ensued slight swelling of the affected wrist, which passed off altogether in a few days, and he had no great pain or discomfort at the time. So slight, indeed, did he at the time consider the injury that he was not off work at all, and he soon forgot all about it. About seven months ago, however, he began to have pain at his work when carrying out the movements already referred to. This gradually became worse, until it led, three months ago, to his having to stop work altogether.

When he consulted me I had difficulty in explaining the condition to myself. In the absence of any history of recent injury, the possibility of a fracture of the scaphoid did not at first suggest itself. On examination, however, I noted that there was definite tenderness and pressure pain over the scaphoid *en tabatière*, and in front; also, that forced extension of the wrist excited pain which limited the range of movement.

It was not, however, until an *x*-ray exposure was made that the true nature of the case became evident. The plate showed at once that the scaphoid was in at least two separate pieces—it will be noted later that there were in reality three fragments—and the diagnosis of fracture was made, in spite of the very unusual history of the original injury.

In view of the statement made by Dwight and others as to the not uncommon failure of union of the two portions of bone from which the scaphoid is formed, it naturally occurred to me that perhaps this might be a case not of fracture but of such failure of union. Dr. Wm. Rankin, who also saw the patient at this time, suggested that the other wrist should be radiographed; accordingly, an *x*-ray plate of the other wrist was obtained. It did not show any abnormality.

In view of the recognised fact that failure of union is a not infrequent sequel to such a fracture, the proximal fragment being intra-articular almost entirely, and thus apt to be cut off in great measure from efficient blood-supply, the failure of union in this case even after a lapse of over two years could be understood; but it was not altogether easy to explain the long absence of troublesome symptoms, unless on the assumption that the lad's work had been altered in the direction of increased or special strain at or about the time when symptoms first developed. Careful enquiry, however, failed to support such assumption.

I advised operative treatment; this was agreed to. Accordingly, on 12th February last, in the Broadstone Jubilee Hospital, Port-Glasgow, I exposed the dorsal aspect of the scaphoid through a short dorsal incision between the tendons of the long extensor of the thumb and the common extensor tendon of the fore-finger. These tendons were drawn aside, the posterior annular ligament was divided for a short distance, and two fragments were removed. My intention was, I confess, to remove the whole scaphoid, *i.e.*, both of the fragments into which I believed it had been broken; and I believed, on a perhaps somewhat superficial examination of the fragments after removal, that I had done so. An *x*-ray plate, however, taken about a fortnight after the operation, showed that a substantial part of the distal fragment remained in position. I can only suppose that, in addition to the usual cross break, the distal fragment must have been broken in a plane from side to side, *i.e.*, parallel with the dorsal surface of the wrist, and a further examination of the first plate seemed almost to bear this out.

After reunion of the divided annular ligament, and replacement of the tendons, the skin wound was accurately closed, and the hand and fore-arm were placed on a Carr's splint, with a rather narrower and lower cross piece than usual, and with fairly marked ulnar flexion of the wrist.

The after-course was uneventful. The splint was worn for two and a half weeks, massage, passive, and gentle voluntary movements being then instituted. At this date, just five weeks after operation, function is almost fully restored, and movements are practically free from pain or discomfort.

A further word is perhaps necessary regarding the operative treatment of such - cases. My intention was, as stated, to remove the whole bone. It should be admitted that this is not the generally accepted procedure. Most surgeons advise removal of the proximal fragment only. This fragment is undoubtedly the one which is most often displaced, and if displaced, removal, sooner or later, is likely to become necessary. The distal fragment is thought not to give substantial trouble and may safely be left.

One further point arises from consideration of this case. At the present time much is said and written about malingering, and about unjustifiable claims for compensation for accident. Here should surely have been an admirable opportunity for an unjust claim. A gross injury, such as this, producing a definite disability of a substantial kind, might easily have been claimed as due to a fictitious accident of recent date in the course of employment, and responsibility could with difficulty have been disputed by the employer. However, no such claim has been made. The lad quite honestly relates the condition to an old injury for which he alone is responsible.

Regarding the question of the occasional double condition of the scaphoid, the frequency of which is said by Professor T. Dwight to amount to 1 per cent of all cases, I can only say that except in fracture, caused by a definite injury, I have never seen the scaphoid in two parts. And, considering the frequency with which one now has occasion to examine x-ray pictures of the wrist region, it is difficult to believe that even a 1 per cent duplication could pass unnoticed.

[The patient was shown to the Society.]

IV.—LARGE SACRO-COCCYGEAL TERATOMA REMOVED FROM AN INFANT OF 11 MONTHS.

By Mr. Arch. Young.

The child, R. N., a female, aged 11 months, was admitted to the Broadstone Jubilee Hospital, Port-Glasgow, under my care on 23rd February, 1914. There was a large tumour springing from the right sacro-coccygeal and gluteal regions. The tumour had been present from birth, and the proportion of its bulk to the size of the child's body was the same then as it is now. Bulging out from the right gluteal and sacral region, it overhung the perineum and seemed to bulge into it, and it had similar relation to the upper part of the postero-external aspect of the thigh. At greatest width it measured 5 inches. The measurement from the sacral side of its base over the free extremity and back to the outer edge of the base was 12 inches. Over the greater part the skin was quite normal in appearance; over the lower part, however, it had a somewhat nævoid appearance, and in some places was thinned out and tightly stretched over fluid retained under some tension. There was no obvious increase in tension when the child cried.

The tumour was apparently free from the sacrum, though the lower end of this and the coccyx seemed projected abnormally backward, and there was a distinct suggestion that the latter was bifid in character. Bone-like material could be felt in the upper part of the tumour. This was verified by an *x*-ray plate.

The lower limbs could be moved freely, but the right was kept pretty constantly in a position of flexion at the hip, apparently by reason of the mechanical effect of the tumour mass. There was no obvious defect in bowel or bladder control.

The child seemed in every other respect well developed and quite healthy. The family history threw no light on the condition.

The question of operative removal of the tumour gave considerable thought, and operation was only resolved upon after full explanation had been given to the parents as to the grave risk involved in the removal of a mass with such important relations, and of such bulk from an infant of such tender age.

The parents, however, decided that operation should be carried out if feasible at all, and, accordingly, on 3rd March this was done. The child was anæsthetised by Dr. Alex. Butler, and, with less difficulty than I had anticipated, I succeeded in removing the main bulk of the tumour.

The removal was effected along with a fairly wide ellipse of overlying skin, by cutting freely between the tumour and the surrounding parts. The greater portion of the mass was cystic, and did not shell out easily, requiring to be cut away from its surroundings. At several points its wall was torn or cut, allowing of the escape of clear fluid, not unlike cerebro-spinal fluid in appearance. From one or two places the fluid contents which escaped had a different character, being rather of a pea-soup consistence and appearance, not unlike the contents of a dermoid.

The deeper part of the tumour passed underneath the projecting sacrum, and was attached to it by a narrow piece of bone or partly ossified cartilage, which had to be cut through

to permit of its detachment.   At the base of the tumour
there was some tissue which had a naked-eye resemblance
to nerve tissue, and on cutting into the tumour one mass of
this, in particular, was seen which had a strong superficial
resemblance to brain tissue.   There was found, however, no
obvious connection with the spinal canal, nor with any of the
larger nerve trunks of pelvis or hip.   When the tumour had
been completely removed, the posterior wall of the rectum
lay freely exposed.   There was moderate bleeding during the
operation.   This was controlled by pressure and ligation.
The wound edges were sutured completely, leaving a moderate
degree of redundancy of skin, which, it was hoped, would
soon subside.   No drainage was provided for.

The operation did not take a long time.   On account of
obvious shock to the child, it had to be considerably hurried.

The tumour, which was in great part cystic, but in part
solid, and which showed, here and there, small cysts containing buttery matter and hair, was sent to Dr. John Shaw
Dunn, who reported as follows:—

"The original size of the tumour has been much diminished
as a result of the escape of fluid from the interior, and now,
after fixation in 5 per cent formalin, it measures $4\frac{1}{2}$ inches in
length, $3\frac{1}{2}$ inches in width, and 3 inches in thickness.   A
longitudinal section through the mass shows that the lower
half is occupied by a large, irregularly shaped, cyst-like space.
The walls of this exhibit projecting ridges, and one fairly
large mass of tissue, of rounded shape, projects in from the
posterior wall.   The upper half is mostly solid, and appears
to be composed of white fibrous tissue, with a few small
cysts; some pieces of bone can also be distinguished here.

"*Microscopic examination.*—Sections from the upper part
of the tumour show an abundant stroma of ordinary fibrous
tissue, and closely mingled with this there are seen numerous
interlacing bands of nervous tissue, chiefly nerve-fibres and
neuroglia, with very few cells.   This nervous material is well
defined by the use of Van Gieson's stain, which colours it
brown; the presence of axis-cylinders is readily ascertained
by application of Levaditi's silver method, usually employed
for the demonstration of spirochætes in tissues; Weigert's
special glia stain is employed for the neuroglia.

" One of the small cysts in this part of the tumour is found to be lined by stratified squamous epithelium, and hair-follicles are present in its wall. In the neighbourhood of this cyst there occurs a large crypt, lined by columnar ciliated epithelium. A number of minute mucous glands are found surrounding this and evidently opening into it.

" The rounded mass of tissue, which has been mentioned as projecting into the large space, presents to the naked eye the appearance of brain-tissue of rather firm consistence. Sections of it confirm this impression, as it is found to be solid brain-like nervous tissue, containing only a few vessels and no supporting stroma. Numerous ganglionic nerve-cells, with large vesicular nuclei, and with long conical processes running out from them, are seen scattered about in a matrix of axis-cylinders and glia, similar to that described above.

" The tissues present in the tumour are all of quite mature type, and the individual elements correspond closely with those of normal tissues. Apart from ordinary fibrous tissue, the great bulk of the tumour is composed of nervous tissue of one kind or another. Other epiblastic elements are present in the form of squamous epithelium, resembling that of the skin, and hair-follicles. The crypt lined by columnar ciliated epithelium, and provided with mucous glands, closely resembles the mucous lining of the nose, or of a bronchus, and may fairly certainly be regarded as hypoblastic in origin. Mesoblastic tissues are represented by bone, cartilage, vessels, striped muscle fibres, &c.

" The tumour is made up of elements derived from all three germ-layers, and may be regarded as a teratoma, although it is one of comparatively simple constitution. The situation in which it occurred is one in which tumours of this class are not infrequently met with."

Following operation, the child was placed prone, and kept constantly so for several weeks, with the lower limbs separated widely. Shock was soon recovered from.

Two weeks after operation the wound was dressed for the first time, and the sutures were removed. The parts were already well consolidated, and the redundant appearance beginning to smooth off. A week later there was still further progress towards restoration of symmetry, and now (29 th

March) the result may be said to be in every respect satisfactory.

As regards the pathological position of this tumour there does not seem to be much difficulty. The whole appearance, the anatomical relations, and the histological components of the tumour seem to fully justify its being classed as a true teratoma. It is certainly not a simple dermoid. Neither its relations nor its histological characters are in keeping with a diagnosis of simple dermoid, either of the class of dermoids of the post-anal gut, or of the indefinite class of post-rectal dermoids, which are seldom of such a size and which are often overlooked in later life.

It would seem that this tumour almost certainly represents the result of an imperfect attempt at true posterior dichotomy, that it represents indeed a condition where the one fœtus (the parasite) "has been so suppressed as to form only a shapeless and ill-deformed lump" (Sutton).[1]

It is, in fact, an example of true "filial teratoma," which may be defined as "derived from groups of cells capable of developing into a fresh individual, either cut off from the parent by dichotomy" [as in this case]—as, *e.g.*, "sacral teratoma—or derived from the aberrant growth of the germinal cells—so-called ovarian dermoids, or mixed tumours of the testis" (Russell Howard).[2]

Photographs, an *x*-ray picture of the tumour and lower end of the trunk prior to operation, and the tumour itself laid open, were exhibited to the Society; also (by Dr. Dunn) microscopic preparations of the tumour.

REFERENCES.

[1] Bland-Sutton, *Tumours, Innocent and Malignant*, p. 448.
[2] Russell Howard, *Practice of Surgery*, p. 245.

MEETING XII.—3RD APRIL, 1914.

The President, MR. A. ERNEST MAYLARD, *in the Chair.*

I.—DR. JOHN BROWNLEE read a short paper on "The Cardiac Complications of Diphtheria."

II.—RADIUM IN THE TREATMENT OF MALIGNANT DISEASE.
BY DR. J. R. RIDDELL.

Dr. Riddell's communication has appeared in the *British Medical Journal.*

III.—LANTERN DEMONSTRATION OF PHOTOGRAPHS IN COLOURS OF CASES OF SURGICAL INTEREST.
BY DR. A. G. FAULDS.

Dr. Faulds showed cases of rodent ulcer, epitheliomas of the nose, of the lower jaw, and of the neck, in their natural tints, and quite easily diagnosed; these cases having been treated by him by radium. He also showed a carcinoma of the jaw in a woman under radium treatment at present in the Royal Infirmary. Another case was one of malignant pustule of a woman's neck, and several cases of lupus in the face, showing the remarkable results attained by radiopathy. He also showed the photograph of a lad with a fractured skull, displaying the sub-conjunctival hæmorrhage and petechial hæmorrhage in his shoulder in their natural tints. He showed the coloured photograph of amputation of the penis for malignant disease, and a case of cancrum oris in a woman's face.

Dr. Faulds made several remarks on the process of taking these coloured photographs, and emphasised the fact that they were very valuable for - teaching purposes. After commenting on the cost of these productions, he said that the preservation of the spoiled photographs and the re-using of the plates by re-coating them with a sensitive film greatly reduced the expenditure of beginners.

He has promised to give another exhibition next year.

SCOTTISH OTOLOGICAL AND LARYNGOLOGICAL SOCIETY.

THE Society met in the Western Infirmary, Glasgow, on Saturday, 6th June, Dr. Walker Downie, President, in the chair.

The PRESIDENT showed a patient, a girl, with lupus of the soft palate, fauces, pharynx, and larynx. Considerable improvement had followed the use of chromic acid locally and syrup of the iodide of iron internally. Dr. Logan Turner suggested the treatment of such cases by nascent iodine with electrolysis, a method of treatment which can be easily carried out with the aid of suspension laryngoscopy.

The President also showed a man, aged 57 years, who has had leucoplakia of the tongue and buccal mucous membrane for over sixteen years. No malignant change has taken place. Dr. Kerr Love, however, referred to a case in which he had watched leucoplakia of the tongue for a longer period, and in this patient malignant disease had occurred within the past year necessitating removal of the tongue.

Dr. Walker Downie also showed a man whom he exhibited a year ago with carcinoma of the ethmoid. The disease has very slowly progressed, though the patient himself has kept in very fair health.

DR. THOMAS BARR showed a patient, a young man in whom, as the result of an accident, the auricle was almost completely torn off. As a result it became permanently displaced forwards, and the meatus became entirely occluded. Two years later a thin fœtid fluid began to escape from a minute opening behind the auricle. After five years, during which time he had had attacks of pain, vertigo, and vomiting, he came under Dr. Barr's care. After milder measures had failed to effect a cessation of the discharge the radical mastoid operation was performed seven months ago. The result of this was satisfactory, a dry cavity resulting. There exists, however, a tendency to epithelial disquamation which necessitates occasional syringing. Various remedies for this were suggested, but probably the condition will, of itself, disappear in time.

DR. J. GALBRAITH CONNAL showed (1) a case in which acute middle-ear suppuration had been followed by a Bezold's mast-oiditis, from which a pure culture of streptococcus was obtained. (2) A patient, a coal miner, whose tympanic membranes were of a dark blue colour. No doubt the colour is due to coal dust in the tympanic cavity. The interest of the case lies, as Dr. Kerr Love remarked, in the point that as coal dust gets into the tympanic cavities, so may other dust, and it is an interesting speculation how far dust may be a direct factor in the causation of adhesive processes in the middle ear. (3) A man, who, when boxing, received a blow on the larynx causing swelling of the inside of the larynx on the left side. The cord was more or less fixed, and there was marked hoarseness. The condition is gradually passing off. The thyroid cartilage was not fractured. In this connection Dr. Walker Downie referred to four cases of fracture of the larynx from various causes, direct and indirect, which had come under his observation. (4) A man on whom he had operated for chronic middle-ear suppuration with labyrinthine and meningeal symptoms. On admission the caloric tests showed that the function of the left (the diseased ear) was destroyed. The radical mastoid operation was performed. The footplate of the stapes was absent. The labyrinth operation was, however, not carried out. Three days after operation meningeal symptoms showed themselves; lumbar puncture gave exit to turbid fluid under considerable pressure. The fluid contained abundant polymorphonuclear leucocytes but no organisms. An injection into his spinal canal of his own blood serum collected from blood withdrawn from a vein in the arm was made, on the suggestion of Dr. Shaw Dunn. Lumbar puncture was performed on several occasions and the patient ultimately recovered. An interesting discussion took place as to the indications for opening the labyrinth in aural suppuration.

DRS. HENRY WHITEHOUSE and J. GALBRAITH CONNAL showed a patient operated on for cerebellar abscess, the result of chronic middle-ear suppuration. Dr. Whitehouse also showed a patient, a woman of 30, with epithelioma of the hypopharynx.

DR. MACKENZIE BOOTH submitted a short report on the treatment of certain forms of deafness by Maurice's kinesiphone, and described the results in three cases in which it had been used. He was inclined to think this method had some value in the treatment of certain intractable aural conditions, though it remained to be seen whether the improvement, which certainly did occur in some cases, continued. Dr. Porter supported Dr. Mackenzie Booth in his attitude, and referred to a case in which marked improvement had followed this method of treatment. On the other hand, several members condemned the treatment as useless, and savouring of charlatanism. It is hoped that at a future meeting members will bring forward records of cases in which treatment by one or other of the forms of apparatus for auditory re-education has been used.

DR. LINDSAY HOWIE showed a man with a thyreoglossal cyst. The cyst was about the size of a pigeon's egg, and had been present since childhood.

DR. BROWN KELLY showed (1) a man with endothelioma of the maxillary antrum, and (2) a man suffering from tuberculosis of the nasal mucous membrane, chiefly in the region of the posterior part of the septum and of the middle meatus.

DRS. BROWN KELLY and J. F. SMITH showed some cases of ozœna treated by vaccine of Perez' bacillus. Though relapses had occurred, the vaccine seemed to have a specific action, and to be of more value than any of the multitudinous methods which have been used in the treatment of this affection.

DRS. BROWN KELLY and WM. WHITELAW showed a patient with chronic recurring aphthæ of the mouth, and recommended the use of arsenical compounds in this condition.

DR. JAMES ADAM showed a patient in whom a cholesteatoma had practically performed the radical mastoid operation, and Dr. Neil Maclay showed a very large cholesteatoma removed from a patient by operation.

Dr. Adam also showed (1) a boy under orthodontic treatment to improve the width of the palate and of the nasal fossæ.

Instead of the split plate actuated by a screw, the pressure is continuous by means of a spring of annealed gold wire tied to the teeth. (2) Two cases of Plaut-Vincent infection of the external and middle ear.

Dr. Adam also showed a case of malignant disease of the hypopharynx and ostium of the gullet in which apparent cure had taken place under radium. Dr. Logan Turner, who also saw the patient before the radium treatment was commenced, was inclined to doubt the diagnosis. One well-known pathologist described it as definitely malignant, whereas another declared that he could not so describe the portion submitted to him. There is now no trace of growth to be seen.

DR. KERR LOVE reported two cases of sudden non-syphilitic deafness in young children, and took the opportunity of impressing upon the members the extreme importance of immediately beginning the teaching of lip-reading to these children while they still have some speech.

Dr. Love showed three interesting cases of recovery after operation for intracranial complications of middle-ear suppuration—one of sinus thrombosis and two of temporo-sphenoidal abscess. In one of the latter the abscess opened spontaneously some days after the performance of the radical mastoid operation.

DR. W. S. SYME showed a patient in whom no recurrence has taken place after an operation nine months ago for primary malignant disease (endothelioma) of the mastoid. Pain was the chief symptom; there was no aural discharge.

Dr. Syme also showed a patient whose maxillary antral cavities were found, on operation, to be filled with a very thick viscid material which the pathologist described as probably pure myxoma, but which may have been (as Dr. Brown Kelly suggested) unusually thick mucin.

Dr. Syme also showed a patient on whom Killian's frontal sinus operation had been carried out. At the operation a very large and diseased fronto-ethmoidal cell was found, extending much further outwards than the floor of the sinus, a condition which, as Dr. Logan Turner remarked, made it impossible that intranasal treatment could have been successful. A fortnight after operation tenderness, with some œdema, showed itself over the left side of the forehead well beyond the limit of the sinus, and the temperature rose to 102·8° with oscillations, and the patient complained of shivering. It was feared that osteomyelitis of the frontal bone was developing. In two days, however, the condition subsided, and the patient made an uninterrupted recovery.

Dr. Syme also reported a case operated on for malignant disease of the ethmoid and antrum, with no recurrence after five years; and he also demonstrated by means of suspension laryngoscopy a case of dislocation of the arytenoid, probably congenital.

Mr. T. K. Dalziel showed a patient on whom he had operated for tubercular glands in the anterior mediastinum causing severe pressure on the trachea and bronchi. The sternum was removed, a small portion of the upper part only being left to maintain the shoulder girdle. The base of the heart and the large vessels were exposed and a large tuberculous abscess found beneath the arch of the aorta. Tuberculous material to the amount of about half a pint was removed, to the great relief of the patient, who appeared before to be in *extremis*. Mr. Dalziel referred to two other similar cases on whom he had operated with satisfactory results.

Pathological specimens, &c., were shown by Drs. Walker Downie, Connal, and Syme.

F. V. Adams and G. B. Eadie, both of Glasgow, were admitted members of the Society.

REVIEWS.

The Early Diagnosis of Tubercle. By CLIVE RIVIEKE, M.D.,
F.R.C.P.   Oxford   Medical   Publications.   London: Henry
Frowde and Hodder & Stoughton.   1914.

AT a time when so much stress is laid upon the necessity for
the early treatment of phthisis pulmonalis if the best results are
to be obtained, a book such as Dr. Riviere's appears very
opportunely.   Its contents are not quite co-extensive with its
title, for it discusses only the pulmonary form of tuberculosis,
as it appears in adults and in children; but it is after all in
phthisis pulmonalis that the greatest difficulties in diagnosis
arise, and that the importance of early diagnosis is most obvious.
Other forms of the disease, for the most part, affect at worst the
sufferer alone; the pulmonary form is chiefly responsible for
the dissemination of tuberculosis.

Dr. Riviere takes a very complete survey of his subject, and
neglects no means of diagnosis which may act even as an adju-
vant in the attainment of certainty.   Yet it is the chief of the
many services which his book performs that it insists so
emphatically upon the value of skilful physical examination.
To that all other diagnostic methods are subservient, and those
who wait for the detection of tubercle bacilli in the sputum
before they venture to pronounce must often miss the moment
for successful intervention.   The modern methods of physical
diagnosis are the old methods, but they have acquired an extension of their delicacy through recent elaboration and refinement;
and the author is to be thanked for calling attention to the
value of Krönig's method of percussing the supraclavicular and
supraspinous fossæ, and to the paramount importance of a light
percussion stroke.   He speaks, however, as if light percussion
had been introduced by Moritz and Röhl in 1907, and had
subsequently been popularised by Goldscheider.   It is perhaps
the thickness of our hyperborean mists that conceals our doings

from the eyes of the dwellers in the more favoured south; but that such a statement can seriously be made betrays a complete ignorance of the work of Gairdner. That great teacher insisted upon light percussion during the thirty-eight years of his professorship in Glasgow, which came to an end in 1900, and so impressed its value upon his disciples that both during his life and after his death the method has been the continuous tradition of the Glasgow school. Nor was his teaching oral only; the principles of light percussion are expounded at some length in an article he published in the *Medical Times and Gazette* of 19th December, 1885, an article which he quotes in his last paper, contributed to the *Edinburgh Medical Journal* in 1904, where it appears on pp. 408-413. It is to be hoped that in the subsequent editions which may confidently be looked for Dr. Riviere will correct what is no doubt an involuntary misstatement.

The care which the author devotes to his exposition of the physical signs both of apical phthisis and of hilus tuberculosis, a condition common in children and too apt to be overlooked, is equally conspicuous in his analytical discussion of the value of the various accessory methods of diagnosis. The interpretation of skiagrams, the significance to be attached to the results of tuberculin tests, the bacteriological and cytological examination of the sputum, all receive from him judicial handling, while the labour of reading is lightened by his possession of an easy and attractive style. His book is heartily to be commended as a very real aid to the early diagnosis of tubercle.

Diseases of Children. By JOHN M'CAW, M.D., R.U.I., L.R.C.P., &c. London: Baillière, Tindall and Cox. 1914.

As the author remarks in his preface "it cannot be said that there is a scarcity" of books on this subject, but he believes that there is room for a book of moderate dimensions specially designed for the needs of the medical student and busy medical practitioner, and for such a purpose he has written this textbook. The author has completely fulfilled his task, and has supplied us with a book of some 500 pages covering the whole

field of pædiatrics. Within these pages the reader will find
mentioned, if not discussed in great detail, all the points of
interest to the student of diseases of children. In fact, if we
have any fault to find with the work, it is that of being too
comprehensive, and we would have been better pleased, and at
the same time would perhaps have gained more real instruction,
if the volume had been more a personal production drawn from
the author's own ripe experience. In a work entirely devoted
to pædiatrics, and which the writer is attempting to make as
concise as possible, we are inclined to think that some valuable
space might have been saved by leaving out of consideration
the specific fevers. In most text-books on general medicine the
student will find them discussed in sufficient detail for his
purpose, and the space could have been used here for the discussion of some more specialised questions.

Anatomy, Descriptive and Applied. By HENRY GRAY,
F.R.S. Eighteenth Edition. Edited by ROBERT HOWDEN,
M.A., D.Sc., M.B., C.M. Notes on Applied Anatomy revised
by A. J. JEX-BLAKE, M.B., and W. FEDDE FEDDEN, M.S.
With 1,120 Illustrations, of which 431 are Coloured.
London: Longmans, Green & Co. 1913.

IT says not a little for the intrinsic value of any work,
medical or otherwise, that it has lived to an eighteenth edition.
The fact is one which would at once arrest our attention,
even if we were not already aware of the popularity of the
work with many successive generations of students.

If we ask ourselves the reason of such popularity, the
answer is that the author tried, and successfully, to simplify
both in the text and by the aid of illustrations a subject
which, view it how we will, is found difficult by the large
majority of students. In the course of time successive
editors took up the task of issuing fresh editions, and that
they have succeeded in carrying on the policy of the author
is abundantly evident from the popularity which the work
continues to enjoy. And be it noted that in simplifying
the subject of anatomy neither the author nor editors have

produced a "cram-book." Its 1,200 and odd pages are sufficient refutation of such a suggestion.

The work is already so well known that it is unnecessary for us at the present day to draw attention to its peculiar features. There are certain points, however, in the new edition which call for mention. First of all we note the use of English translations of the Latin terms of the Basle nomenclature. Where this nomenclature differs materially from the older terminology the latter has been added in brackets, and to minimise inconvenience a glossary has been provided; this the reader will find of great-service.

Another new feature in the present edition is the bringing together into a special chapter of the paragraphs on surface anatomy, which formerly were scattered throughout the text.

Some of the older figures have been replaced by new drawings. Many additional drawings, the majority of them from original preparations, have, however, been added.

This edition maintains the high standard of the work, and we venture to prophesy for it the wide circulation which it merits.

A Companion to Manuals of Practical Anatomy. By E. B. JAMIESON, M.D. London: Henry Frowde and Hodder & Stoughton. 1913.

THIS book has been written to provide an account of naked-eye anatomy, expressed in terms of the Basle nomenclature. Its small size necessitates the use of condensed language and contractions—*e.g.*, lig. for ligament, inf. for inferior—but this is an advantage, as the book is intended for use in the dissecting-room.

It is written for use as a companion to a manual of practical anatomy, especially for revision during dissection of a "part." The various structures have been described under their systems, but a detailed account of the relations in the more important regions has been included. At the end a very brief *résumé* of the embryology, according to prevailing ideas, of most of the organs has been inserted.

The Basle nomenclature, or an equivalent English translation, has, with a few exceptions, been used throughout,
but the old terminology has been inserted in brackets. The
fact that the author has had considerable experience as a
lecturer and demonstrator of anatomy ought alone to ensure
the book's usefulness to the student of practical anatomy.

———

Contributions to Clinical Medicine.   By Sir JAMES SAWYER,
    M.D., F.R.C.P.   Fifth   Edition.   Birmingham : Cornish
    Bros. 1912.

BUT few words are necessary to recommend Sir James
Sawyer's well-known *Contributions to Clinical Medicine*
to the notice of the profession. That a book has reached its
fifth edition is a better testimonial to its popularity and
usefulness than many commendatory expressions, and it will
suffice to say of the present issue that those who are already
familiar with the volume in its earlier shape will find in it
all those qualities which first attracted their favourable
attention, and that the added material, which includes, among
other essays, the substance of Sir James Sawyer's Lumleian
lectures on diseases of the heart, will make it amply worth
their perusal in its newer form ; while to those unacquainted
with the author's writings it will commend itself as containing,
in many departments of medicine, valuable observations
derived from the wide practical experience of a thoughtful
physician.

———

The Essentials of Chemical Physiology.   By W. D. HALLI-
    BURTON, M.D., LL.D., F.R.S.   Eighth   Edition.   London :
    Longmans, Green & Co. 1914.

THIS is the eighth edition of a very excellent practical book.
The matter has been thoroughly brought up to date, a good
selection, on the whole, being made of the most modern .
analytical methods. The present writer whole-heartedly
endorses Professor Halliburton's dictum that "it is far better

that a student should know thoroughly one method for estimating sugar than have an imperfect smattering of several." It is a pity, however, that in the description of methods, although van Slyke's method for the estimation of amino-nitrogen is given in detail, the admirable micromethods of Folin are not dealt with—methods which can readily be adapted for clinical use, as they permit of the examination of the urine for total nitrogen and urea being done without a fume chamber. The section devoted to respiration and blood gases gives a most clear and succinct account of the most recent findings.

The book is well suited for the use of both the junior and the advanced student.

———

The Biology of Tumours: The Bradshaw Lecture, 1912. By C. MANSELL MOULLIN, M.D., F.R.C.S. London: H. K. Lewis. 1913.

MR. MANSELL MOULLIN'S Bradshaw lecture, which has been published by request of the Council of the Royal College of Surgeons, deals with the interesting subject of the biology of tumours.

At the outset the lecturer expresses the opinion that there is no hard and fast line between innocent and malignant tumours. Metastasis, a prominent characteristic of so-called "malignant" tumours, is merely an accident of growth. In benign tumours the cells have reached a more advanced stage of organisation, and can no longer exercise their primitive power of detachment and autotransplantation. From a general consideration of tumours he looks upon them as leading a parasitic existence, but not as being caused by parasites. In considering the question of their biology it is necessary first of all to try and form a clear idea of the nature and origin of the laws controlling the growth and development of the body, these being the laws that are set aside by tumour tissues.

The force regulating and controlling the development of the organism is the mutual influence of germ cells and somatic cells upon each other and upon their fellows.

Tumours do not obey the laws framed by this force; they spring from, and live on, the parent body. And as the parent body consists of both germ cells and somatic cells, so tumours may arise from either of these groups. Germ-cell tumours are comparatively rare, the vast majority of tumours arising from the somatic cells, or from structures developed from them. Such tumours usually arise long after the early stages of life, and they become more and more common as age advances. The great power of multiplying possessed by tumour cells may be due to the force which, properly, should raise the differentiation of the cells being now available for growth.

How is it that the tumour cells are able to assert themselves and shake off allegiance to the other tissues? The force controlling development ceases to act, while growth continues unimpaired, and the result is a tumour. "Evolution stops when the power of hereditary transmission fails; but so also does involution." In this way fragments of organs which should disappear persist, and by growth become the nucleus of tumours. Further, just as the transmission of some special feature may be seen in a family, so in a family the controlling force may fail, and in several members of the same family for generation after generation we may find tumours growing.

Why does controlling power fail? From mere exhaustion, or from excessive action, as when enormous production of young cells occurs with great rapidity in response to some persistent chronic irritation.

Such are the views which Mr. Moullin elaborates in his *brochure*, and those who are interested in the subject will find in its pages much matter for thought.

The Administrative Control of Small-pox. By W. M'C. WANKLYN, B.A., M.R.C.S. London: Longmans, Green & Co. 1913.

ESSENTIALLY this book should be read in conjunction with the author's previous volume on "How to diagnose small-pox," but even by itself there is much interesting material on the question of how best to prevent or stop an outbreak of this disease. From long immunity from serious outbreaks we are perhaps inclined to think too little about this disease, but with the increasing percentage of the unvaccinated population of these islands the danger of an epidemic of considerable extent and virulence is becoming more and more apparent. Certainly the policy of "locking the stable door after the steed is stolen," at any time futile, is even more disastrous when we are dealing with a disease which, should it again become epidemic, may have a heavy mortality list appended. The 83 pages comprising this volume contain all the essentials for meeting any threatened outbreak of the disease, and therefore the book should be in the hands of all who are dealing with the public health in any of its many branches.

The book is commendably free from statistics or tables, and is eminently readable and informative on just those points which are essential.

———

St. Thomas's Hospital Reports. New Series. Edited by Dr. J. J. Perkins and Mr. C. A. Ballance. Vol. XL. London: J. & A. Churchill. 1913.

THE fortieth volume of the *St. Thomas's Hospital Reports* contains—besides the statistics and abbreviated case summaries from the medical, surgical, and gynæcological departments, and from the various special services of the hospital—a series of reports on subjects of surgical interest, such as recurrent hernia, the after-results of gastro-jejunostomy, cases of imperforate anus, and the results of laminectomy for special caries with paraplegia, which are of considerable statistical value. It also includes the Salter Research Report for 1911, by Dr. W. W. C. Topley, who has investigated "the action of certain drugs, toxic bodies, toxins, and micro-organisms on the fragility of the red blood corpuscles of man and animals." The effects of arsenic, mercury, and the Roentgen rays were studied with uniformly negative results; bile salts altered the fragility only in doses so large as to cause almost immediate death; injections of various pyogenic organisms increased it to a moderate extent; but the increase was much most notable in connection with injections of specific hæmolytic sera.

The hospital statistician will find much to interest him in the analysis of the wealth of clinical material afforded by St. Thomas's Hospital.

———

Protein and Nutrition: An Investigation. By Dr. M. HINDHEDE. London: Ewart, Seymour & Co., Limited.

THIS book is one of very considerable interest both to the scientific and lay reader, but it falls between the stools of popularity and science. Dr. Hindhede, as the result of his own personal experience in Denmark, very early came to the conclusion that the existing system of dieting, with its high protein content, was faulty, and, owing to some success with experiments on the feeding of the milch cows of the West Jutland farmers, he was eventually put in charge of a special Government laboratory for research in nutrition.

The book is devoted to the praise of the nutritive value of the homely potato. Dr. Hindhede makes it the staple article of diet in his own home; he does not exclude meat entirely, but uses it very sparingly. He preaches the doctrine, initiated by Chittenden, of the low protein intake, although not to the extent advocated by the American worker—a perfectly sound position to take up in the light of modern research.

Unfortunately the book suffers, from the scientific point of view, from three marked defects—(1) it is written in rather a popular style, and large parts are devoted to quite unnecessary discussions which have no direct bearing on the question under review; (2) it gives no full data of his· experiments, from which alone the true scientific value of his work can be deduced; and (3) it is marred by a bitter attack on other workers in the field of metabolism. His attack on the work of Voit is particularly to be· regretted. Dr. Hindhede seems to forget that it was due to the genius of Voit that the problem of protein metabolism assumed so early a definite form, that it was due to Voit's efforts in attacking this problem in so dogged and sincere a fashion that further research, including that of the writer of the book under review, was possible. Although it is true that some of Voit's dogmatic statements have had to be discarded, this does not suffice to render his memory open to the vicious onslaught of such a worker as Dr. Hindhede.

The translation has been, on the whole, efficiently done.

A Manual of Practical Chemistry. By A. W. STEWART, D.Sc. London : John Bale, Sons & Danielsson, Limited. 1913.

THIS little book has been compiled for students of public health, and is arranged especially for those studying for the D.P.H.

Essentially the book consists of short descriptions of the chemical processes, a knowledge of which is required by students in practical public health laboratory work, and it may be found useful where such work is undertaken without proper instruction and supervision. On the other hand, the descriptions as a rule are too condensed for the student to follow without supplementary instruction, and the *raison d'être* of the book is thus largely neutralised.

The student is recommended (page 3) to use a tared watch-glass with the balance when weighing substances, but in all probability the author really means that *two* watch-glasses of exactly equal weight should be employed ; this is certainly the routine in most laboratories. On page 6 the test for acetic acid is not well described, and there are other and better tests. On page 13, in the estimation of oxygen in the atmosphere, the student is told to "place the two tubes under the same pressure " ; how this is done is not stated.

On page 73 appears "Part VI—Microscopical work." It is not clear why microscopical work should appear at all in a book ostensibly on practical chemistry.

The interleaving for additional notes will be found quite essential. There is no index.

ABSTRACTS FROM CURRENT MEDICAL LITERATURE.

EDITED BY ROY F. YOUNG, M.B., B.C.

MEDICINE.

The Mechanism of Recovery in Pneumonia. By Ludvig Hektoen, M.D. (*The Journal of the American Medical Association*, 24th January, 1914).—Hektoen discusses this question with special reference to the crisis. The early explanations, he says, are connected with the doctrine of critical days, a pet dogma of the Galenic system, and appear to us as fanciful and of only historical interest. After the discovery of the pneumococcus, the Klemperers explained the crisis as the result of a rapid detoxication, due to the antidotal action of substances similar to diphtheria antitoxin; but this idea that the cure of pneumonia is the effect of a direct antitoxic action remains without experimental support. The hypothesis was abandoned, and eventually the attention of investigators became focussed on reactions which are antimicrobic rather than antitoxic. In some diseases destruction of the invading microbes is accomplished principally by direct solution or lysis, while in others, notably the streptococcal and pneumococcal infections, the phagocytic reaction appears to predominate. The author examines the evidence which has accumulated in the last ten years, and concludes that crisis does not mark a point at which the invading pneumococci suddenly become avirulent, but rather the point at which a more or less complete and rapid destruction of the organisms is accomplished. It coincides with the height of a wave-like increase of anti-pneumococcal substances in the blood. In rapidly fatal cases the defensive reactions are inadequate to destroy the pneumococci which persist and multiply in the lungs and blood, and free antibodies have not been demonstrated in the blood. In favourable cases, on the other hand, the pneumococci are destroyed more or less rapidly when the anti-pneumococcal reactions reach a certain height, and here the blood contains an excess of free antibodies.—ADAM PATRICK.

Erosion of Tissues by Aneurysms. By Allen J. Smith, M.D. (*New York Medical Journal*, 7th March, 1914).—No fixed tissue of the body, the author says, can permanently resist the eroding influence of an aneurysmal sac. He thinks that erosion is partly due to pressure atrophy, but that the dominant factor in its causation is the accompanying inflammation in and about the wall of the aneurysm. He explains the inflammation as a reaction due to the presence of particles of dead tissue which have necrosed in the process of degeneration. The writer believes that whatever atrophy is actually attributable to the pressure is secondary to the tissue changes induced by the inflammation, and that without such coincident inflammation true erosion is impossible. In each case the attachment of the aneurysmal sac to the surrounding tissue precedes the process of erosion. Syphilitic endarteritis, often with the formation of minute gummata, is most frequently the basis for the production of aneurysm, and possibly the extension of the inflammation from the wall of the sac to the adjacent tissue may be due to migration of spirochætes.—ADAM PATRICK.

Shock. By Eugene Boise, M.D. (*New York Medical Journal*, 16th May, 1914).—Boise summarises the principal views which have been held as to the nature of shock, and gives his own opinion on the matter. In 1869 Erichsen wrote of it as a "derangement of the harmony of action of all the great organs of the body." Gay (1888) said that "experimental physiology has demonstrated that in shock there is a reflex paralysis of the heart and abdominal vessels, through the medium of the vasomotor system," and that there is "a reflex inhibition, probably in the majority of cases general, affecting all the functions of the nervous system, and not limited to the heart and vessels only." Fisher (1890) thought that "traumatic shock is virtually a vasomotor paralysis, especially of the splanchnic vessels, the vascular disturbance is the primary and chief factor, and the other symptoms are caused by the resultant anæmia." Crile (1899) agreed with Groeningen that "the apparent vasomotor paralysis is in reality exhaustion from over-stimulation by traumatic impulses," but stated further that "failure of blood-pressure is the primary and principal (if not the sole) cause of all the symptoms of shock." Howell (1903) advanced the theory that there are two forms of shock—a cardiac and a vascular—neither due to an exhaustion of the medullary centre, but that there is an inhibition of the tone of the vagus and of the vasomotor centre. Porter and also Malcolm were certain that the vasomotor cells are, in shock, neither depressed, exhausted, nor inhibited, and Seelig and Lyon (1910) proved experimentally that the peripheral vessels are contracted, a condition incompatible with vasomotor paralysis. They showed also that the vasomotor centre is not only not exhausted, but is on the contrary more active than normal to stimulation. Henderson advanced the theory that shock is due to a diminution of the amount of carbonic acid in the blood. Gray and Parsons (1912) concluded from experiment that exaggerated or violent impulses cause exaggerated responses. The stimulation of the vasomotor centre results in efferent stimuli to the entire sympathetic system resulting in rise of blood-pressure from general vaso-constriction, acceleration of the pulse rate, and diminution in the size of the pulse because of contraction of the arteries. They attribute the fall of pressure in shock to fatigue of pressor fibres, the pressor fibres becoming exhausted earlier than the depressor. Boise has maintained for twenty years that the pathological condition in shock is a hyper-irritation of the whole sympathetic system. He believes that the one and only cause of the low blood-pressure is strong stimulation of the augmentor nerves of the heart, by reason of which there ensues a condition of cardiac hypertonus, the heart contracting strongly in systole and relaxing very imperfectly in diastole. The heart and arteries are imperfectly filled because the heart cannot relax sufficiently to receive blood from the engorged veins.—ADAM PATRICK.

SURGERY.

The Mathematical Calculation of Prognosis in Fractures at the Ankle and Wrist. By E. H. Skinner (*Surgery, Gynecology, and Obstetrics*, February, 1914).—The object of this paper is to show that, though anatomical reduction of fracture with displacement is advisable, the functional result depends on the correct relation of the joint surfaces and on the lines of the weight-bearing forces. The author relies on two axioms in fractures of the ankle and wrist.

"The functional result of an ankle fracture depends upon the proper reduction of the astragalus so that the line of weight-bearing force which passes through the centre of the tibia also passes through the astragalus at its centre."

"The entire styloid process of the lower end of the radius is constantly distal to a line which touches the tip of the ulnar styloid, which line is at a right angle to the longitudinal axis of the radius. The functional result of fractures at the lower end of the radius depends upon the reduction of the radial styloid to this position."

The prognosis as to the functional result is made from x-ray photographs, a number of which illustrate the paper.—Roy F. Young.

Evil Results of Colles' and Pott's Fractures, and how to avoid them. By R. Hertzberg (*American Journal of Surgery*, May, 1914).— The author explains the mechanical processes producing these fractures in some detail, and then proceeds to describe the methods of treatment from which he has obtained the best results.

The principles applied to Colles' are (1) to continue the extension of the wrist which resulted in fracture, thereby freeing the fragments; (2) to flex the wrist, and, by fixing in this position, to maintain the fragments as nearly as possible in normal line.

For Pott's fracture he adopts the usual methods of inversion, dorsi-flexion, and pulling forward of the foot. For fixation the box method with sheet and lateral splints is used. Inversion is kept up by strips of adhesive plaster fastened near the outer edge of the dorsum, passing under the sole and continued up the leg in spiral fashion.

He advocates the use of general anæsthesia for examination and reduction of these fractures.—Charles Bennett.

Subacromial Bursitis. By L. W. Littig (*The Journal of the Amer. Med. Assoc.*, 21st March, 1914).—Littig agrees with Codman, who first drew attention to this affection, that inflammation of the subacromial bursa causes more shoulder-joint disability than all other shoulder disorders combined. Trauma and sepsis are most frequently the cause of this bursitis.

Three stages are recognised—the first, in which abduction and rotation are limited by muscular spasm, and in which there is marked tenderness external to the acromion when the arm is lying by the side; the second, in which abduction and rotation are limited by adhesions; and the third stage, when adhesions have been sufficiently stretched or absorbed so that movement may be relatively or completely unimpeded, unless the bursa be distended with fluid and so limit abduction by being caught between the tuberosity of the humerus and the acromion.

Treatment, in the first stage, is rest ; in the second stage, persistent but mild stretching of adhesions ; in the third stage, continuation of movement, with possible excision of the bursa, though many surgeons do not advise this owing to its widespread attachment.—ROY F. YOUNG.

Some Uses of Fat in Surgery. By J. F. Binnie (*Surgery, Gynecology, and Obstetrics*, March, 1914).—In spite of the reputation which fat has acquired as a tissue of poor resisting power it is well suited for transplantation. Binnie enumerates a number of conditions in which fatty transplants are of service—

I. As a tamponade to produce hæmostasis in wounds-of-the liver and similar parenchymatous and vascular organs. In such cases free omental grafts are used, and it is found that the omental plug becomes adherent to the raw surface of the liver wound, and ultimately becomes converted into fibrous tissue. It does not become adherent to the intact peritoneum.

2. In cases of traumatic epilepsy with adhesions between the meninges and the skull Rehn found that, forty-five days after a cranial defect had been filled with fat, a clear and distinct basal connective-tissue sheet spanning the dural defect had developed in the transplant. This sheet was elastic enough to permit of expansion. Binnie also suggests the use of a plug of fat as a suitable tampon in cases in which a cavity is left in the brain after removal of a tumour or evacuation of a cyst.

3. In depressed scars of the face if, through a suitable incision, the adhesions are thoroughly divided, and a suitable mass of fat (autoplastic) is gently insinuated through the cut to fill up the depressed area, an ideal result may be obtained.

4. Some surgeons after excising the breast for non-malignant disease have planted a fatty graft (lipoma, omentum, fat from thigh) in the bed left by the mammectomy with good æsthetic result.

5. Krabbel, from a study of ten cases, has come to the following conclusions:— (*a*) In chronic osteomyelitis without sinus implantation of fat has succeeded. If sinuses are present implantation is contra-indicated. (*b*) Sharply delimited, easily accessible, tuberculous foci are suitable for fat implantation, even when they are situated near the articular ends of the bone. Diffuse tuberculous lesions of bone and widespread diseases of the soft parts may only be plugged with fat after the most careful removal of all the disease. If healing per primam does not ensue, or if a sinus forms, the implanted fat must be removed.

6. In arthroplasty, in order to prevent adhesions reforming.

7. After tenorrhaphy or neurorrhaphy, to prevent the line of union becoming adherent to neighbouring structures.

8. Tuffier has successfully grafted voluminous masses of fat between the mobilised parietal pleura and the ribs in bronchiectasis.—ROY F. YOUNG.

OBSTETRICS AND GYNÆCOLOGY.

Nine Observations on Ovarian Autografts in Women.

De Rouville, Montpellier (*Arch. Mens. d'Obst. et de Gynécol.*, February, 1914), records his experience in nine women in whom he implanted grafts of ovarian tissue removed from their own bodies by operation. He is somewhat optimistic, though he confesses frankly that only one woman, from the clinical standpoint, received any benefit; other operators have done better than himself.

In all the cases the portion of ovary was embedded under the skin of the abdominal wound, as this permits of easy access for observation or for removal should this be found necessary. The results of the grafting can be controlled in three different ways—by direct examination of the ovary *in situ ;* by observing the re-establishment of its functions ; and by microscopical examination of the graft. To carry out the direct examination satisfactorily the graft must be under the abdominal skin, when its changes of volume—gradual or periodic—are visible and palpable ; but it must be noted that an ovary which has apparently retained its normal size may be completely atrophic and consist of only fibrous tissue. The observation of function is of great interest ; when not atrophied the ovary swells usually from five to twelve days before the onset of the period, and is painful and tender ; it is possible to doubt that the grafted ovary, after a bilateral oöphorectomy, really keeps up menstruation, for we know that pregnancy has followed such an operation even when grafting was not performed ; but even if menstrual functions are maintained, they may be so in an irregular and troublesome fashion, with menorrhagia, dysmenorrhœa, and so on. Such hæmorrhages are comparable with those set up by uterine fibroids, and cease when the ovary has been removed. The microscopic examination of the ovary was made only once, and the ovary, though still living and maintaining menstruation, was obviously in process of degeneration.

The woman No. 1 received no benefit, but was not inconvenienced ; No. 2 received no benefit and was inconvenienced by the painful periodic swellings ; No. 3 was decidedly benefited ; No. 4 would have been better without grafting ; No. 5 suffered from perverted internal secretion (due to degeneration of the corpus luteum), causing hæmorrhages which ceased on removal of the ovary ; No. 6 received no benefit ; No. 7 progressed just as if no graft had been made ; No. 8 received a very temporary benefit, and the rapid atrophy of the ovary makes it doubtful if any benefit really accrued from the presence of the ovary ; No. 9 showed only negative evidence, but the ovary was infected and should not have been grafted.

Rouville concludes that more observations are required to enable indications to be laid down as to cases and conditions favourable to the performance of this operation successfully.

The article is illustrated with two micro-photographs.—E. H. L. OLIPHANT.

Tubal Pregnancy Associated with Atypical Evolution of the Corpus Luteum.

—Schil, working with Professor Bar in the clinique Tarnier (*Arch. Mens. d'Obst. et de Gynécol*, February, 1914), was examining a series of ovaries, and was struck by the observation that the abnormal corpora lutea came from women who had suffered from tubal pregnancy. Conversely, of six tubal pregnancies, four showed cystic degeneration of the corpus luteum, and the remaining two showed sclerosed ovaries (the operations were unilateral), with no trace of corpus luteum. Ten years ago Fraenkel had already suggested a causal connection between the two conditions and had been supported by others.

Schil concludes from his observations that the causation of the tubal pregnancy is the absence of peristalsis in the tube during the passage of the ovum. The determining factor accordingly is the same as that which causes the cessation of the peristalsis, but as this peristalsis is normally maintained by the corpus luteum, cessation of peristalsis is due to one of two conditions, either some affection, such as cyst formation, which modifies the physiological activity of the corpus luteum, or extra-ovarian factors which are capable of inhibiting the action of the internal secretion of the corpus luteum.

In the first two ovaries examined the corpus luteum was found to contain no blood-clot, but a fibrinous fluid distending it in a cyst-like manner and causing atrophy of the peripheral tissues. The third case showed a layer of connective tissue lining the interior of the cyst inside the line of the lutein cells. The fourth case was a more completely formed cyst, lined apparently by endothelial cells. Schil discusses the normal and the atypical evolution of the corpus luteum, and also the modifications of the tubal epithelium under the influence of the corpus luteum of pregnancy. In particular he draws attention to the observation of Moreaux that the absence of ciliated epithelium at the time of the dehiscence of the ovary and at the beginning of pregnancy prevents one attributing the passage of the ovum to the action of cilia. Three micro-photographs are given.—E. H. L. O.

Prolapse of the Umbilical Cord (*Arch. Mens. d'Obst. et de Gynecol.*, December, 1913).—In the wards of the clinique at Lund, under Essen-Möller from 1900 to 1912, there were 35 cases of prolapse in 7,518 deliveries—that is, 1 in 215. These cases are related briefly as well as one from Professor Essen-Moller's private practice.

As regards etiology, it is noted that at least 20 per cent of the cases occurred in flat contracted pelves, but as internal pelvimetry was not systematically carried out the figures cannot be taken absolutely. The relative frequency in multiparæ is double that in primiparæ. The fœtuses were mostly very large or very small. Prolapse occurred more frequently in abnormal presentations and where limbs prolapsed in front of the head. Twin births seem also a predisposing cause. Liquor amnii is reported as abundant in about 18 per cent of the cases, and in some of the cases observed the prolapse occurred at the time of rupture (artificial or natural) of the membranes. In general the cord was longer than the average. Placenta prævia with version and marginal attachment of the cord are noted once each. In four cases the cord was looped round the child.

Two of the patients were admitted with dead children. The rest of the cases are tabulated according to results of treatment along with those of other reporters. Essen-Möller's own cases were as follows:—

	Living Children.	Dead Children.	Mortality.
Version,	7	1	14·3
Retropulsion,	...	...	...
Forceps,	7	2	28·6
Version in shoulder presentations,	3	2	66·6
Footling deliveries,	11	3	27·2

The prognosis is naturally worse where the prolapse occurs early in labour, and where from any cause rapid delivery is impossible. Expectant treatment is bad, and Dr. Johanson recommends in head presentations with undilated os the incision of the cervix and delivery by forceps where this can be done without risk to the mother.—E. H. L. O.

The Effects of X-Rays on the Ovaries (*Arch. Mens. d'Obst. et de Gynécol.*, December, 1913).—This work is from the thesis of Lacassagne, of Lyons, 1912-1913. The observations were made on rabbits with single doses of hard filtered x-rays up to tint iv of Bordier's radiochromometre. Sometimes the radiation was unilateral, so as to use the sound ovary as a check. Examinations at various dates showed that degeneration begins a few hours after irradiation and is completed in about fifteen days, with disappearance of the follicles. In spite of this, sterilisation is rarely complete, for follicles in their primary stage remain. During a second stage, from the second to the third month, the interstitial gland regresses, and the epithelium becomes cubical, then flattened, resembling an epithelium.

After the fifth month there is some amount of recovery ; a new interstitial gland arises ; the follicles begin to grow from the sixth month, with the epithelium becoming cylindrical. This does not always occur, and there is no reserve of follicles, so the animal's sexual life is shortened, and some animals are permanently sterilised ; but to ensure sterilisation the dose of irradiation must be so large as to risk the life of the animal. Photographs are given of the various stages in the interstitial gland and follicles.

It is concluded that it is impossible to sterilise a woman by x-rays ; the effects on fibroids are due to the destruction of the corpora lutea and to direct action on the fibroid.—E. H. L. O.

DISEASES OF THE SKIN.

Malignant Pemphigus Cured by a Single Intravenous Injection of Blood. By G. Praetorius (*Münch. Med. Woch.*, 22nd April, 1913, No. 16, p. 867).—This was a case of severe pemphigus of eight months' duration, cured by a single intravenous injection of 20 c. cm. of non-defibrinated fresh normal human serum. Salvarsan injection and all other means had failed. The patient refused to go into hospital, and as it was found impracticable to carry out the original method of Linser with 'defibrinated blood, Praetorius injected 20 c. cm. of untreated blood, which was withdrawn immediately before, from the veins of the patient's husband. The eruption was rapidly disappearing on the third day, and within a week it had entirely disappeared. After eight months' duration there had been no return, and the patient had gained 18 lb. in weight. The author hopes for further proof from other sources.—WM. BARBOUR.

On the Therapeutic Employment of the Patient's own Serum. By B. Spiethoff (*Münch. Med. Woch.*, 11th March, 1913, No. 10, p. 521).—The author relates some successful results from injections of the patient's own serum.

Blood was taken from a vein, centrifugalised, and the serum again introduced by injection. Two to three times weekly, 10 to 25 c. cm. were injected. From two to six injections were given.

The reactions were similar to those observed with "human serum." The best results followed when there was a general and a local reaction, and if there were no reaction with "native serum," the author found that it might be brought about by foreign serum or by mixed native and foreign serum. Dermatitis herpetiformis, the prurigo of Hebra, chronic urticaria, pruritus, psoriasis, eczema, chronic and acute, were treated with good results. As it might be thought that the withdrawal of blood could account for the results, a number of control cases showed that although some improvement often took place from a small bleeding it was not comparable with the excellent results of serum injection, and even Bruch's method of repeated bleedings and subsequent saline injections did not give such good results.—WM. BARBOUR.

Researches on the Vaccine-Therapy of Wright. By R. Sabouraud and H. Noiré (*Ann. de Derm. et de Syph.*, 1913, No. 54, p. 257).— This paper gives the results of the authors' experiences with vaccines prepared from the pyogenic staphylococci, the coccus cutis communis, and the acne bacillus. The staphylococcus vaccines are prepared from cultures from cold abscess, carbuncle, folliculitis, and sycosis, grown on peptone agar, to which is added 0·5 per cent urea. Subcultures grown for forty-eight hours at 38° C. are used. At intervals of eight days injections are given of 500, 1,000, 1,500, up to 2,000 millions, which dose is never exceeded.

The first dose gives a definite though variable local reaction, and subsequent injections much less so. Very favourable results have been obtained in cases of furunculosis, not a resistent case has been seen, and cases treated over a year ago have remained cured. In folliculitis of the sycosis type the results are not so good ; improvement occurs up to a point, but a few isolated pustules are prone to persist.

Cultures of the coccus communis are obtained from the scales of pityriasis capitis et steatoides. The authors find that vaccines made from the coccus communis never give a local reaction, and that they have no action in folliculitis and furunculosis. They state that it is too early to say whether the vaccine has any action in conditions thought to be due to this organism. They think that it may be necessary to combine it with the vaccine of another organism.

The acne bacillus is obtained by embedding comedones in Sabouraud's glycerin-acid-agar medium. Subcultures are then made on a new medium, the basis of which is whey, to which acetic acid, peptone, and saccharose are added, and an aerobic growth is obtained which can be used after about ten days.

The following results were obtained :—(1) In some cases marked improvement was noticed in four to five weeks after progressive injections of the same doses as with staphylococci ; (2) some cases, especially of acne furunculosis and acne necrotica, which show no improvement with progressive doses of acne bacillus vaccine in four or five weeks, improve rapidly if progressive doses of staphylococci are then given; (3) with simultaneous injections of the acne bacillus vaccine and the coccus communis vaccine no definite results were obtained, as might have been expected in cases of seborrhoeic pityriasis ; (4) no definite results were obtained in the case of simple seborrhoea of the face and scalp.

—WM. BARBOUR.

DISEASES OF THE EYE.

"The Relation of Ophthalmology to General Medicine"

is the title of a paper by Dr. C. O. Hawthorne printed in the *Ophthalmoscope*, September, 1913, and the substance of a paper read before the Oxford Ophthalmological Congress in July, 1913.

Dr. Hawthorne considers that there are some grounds for complaint regarding the relative usefulness of the ocular signs and symptoms associated with some systemic diseases to, first, the general practitioner, and, second, the ophthalmic surgeon.

In the first place, the writer considers that the general practitioner does not make full use of the ocular symptoms as aids to diagnosis. This may be the result of imperfect teaching or of lack of confidence on the practitioner's part, and it is, indeed, a very difficult matter to have students so well instructed in eye disease that they can recognise the import of some comparatively slight alteration in the fundus or in the subtleties of corneal and iritic lesions.

The poor student has so much to cram into his head in five years that he has but little time to devote to study those small variations which offtimes require much consideration on the part of a man who has spent years in close contact with them.

On the other hand, it is complained of the ophthalmic surgeon that he has under his care cases which are really general disease, with an eye symptom prominently in the foreground. Such, mayhap, is diplopia or optic nerve atrophy in a case of spinal disease, or some change in the fundus oculi which denotes systemic disease, such as Bright's disease or arterio-sclerosis.

It is the duty of the ophthalmic surgeon to transfer such cases to the physician or the surgeon as the case may be, and one would say that the ophthalmic surgeon is usually only too anxious to do so at once.

Dr. Hawthorne's paper is a plea for the routine examination of the fundus oculi and external parts of the eye in all cases, and also for the transference of all cases of general or visceral disease from the ophthalmic surgeon to the care of one who can and will devote more skill and time to it than he can.

In regard to the first proposition, it is a little hard on the physician to expect him to give all the time and care which are requisite to obtain a satisfactory knowledge of all the eye conditions which may or should influence his diagnosis. It is only possible, in many cases at all events, to learn to say when it is advisable to have the eye condition looked into thoroughly, and we presume that this is all the author desires.

With regard to the second proposition, it is, we would imagine, the rule for ophthalmic surgeons who see at the clinic cases of systemic disease to refer such cases to the care or guidance of a physician or surgeon as desirable.

—LESLIE BUCHANAN.

A **Case of Ocular Torticollis** is recorded by Dr. M. C. Pierola, of Lima, and, as the condition is not very frequently seen, a short description of it may be given here.

The patient was a lad of 17 years when first seen in Lagrange's clinique,

Bordeaux. It had been noted shortly after birth that the left eye deviated upwards from the level of the right, and a year or so later it was noticed that the head was habitually inclined to the right. There was evidently some faulty development of the left inferior rectus muscle from or even before birth. There was little probability of birth injury, as the birth was quite easy and rapid, and no instruments were used.

There was no diplopia so long as the head was inclined to the right, but whenever the head was held vertical the diplopia began to be evident. The movements of the eye up, down, in, out, &c., were normal. The inclined position of the head was evidently the result of experience acquired early in life, which showed that if diplopia was to be avoided some artifice must be resorted to, and the amount of the inclination of the head was proportioned to the faulty muscular development of the eye.

In order to correct the upward tendency of the left eye, the surgeon (Lagrange), operated upon the inferior rectus of the left eye by advancement, thereby procuring an excellent result. The eyes were now on a level, and only if the head was inclined was diplopia developed, so the patient speedily learned to keep his head erect, with the result that he could be dismissed cured in three months.

It is to be noted that the condition here described is a comparatively common accompaniment of the squint which follows errors of focus of the eye (concomitant squint), but is not common in paralytic strabismus.

In a case lately under care of the abstractor, an elderly man had a slight degree of torticollis, due to slight concomitant strabismus, and had been provided with suitable glasses many years ago. Recently the patient developed a strabismus due to a paralysis of the left superior oblique, and it was very interesting to see that the torticollis very notably increased in amount when the diplopia was at its worst, and gradually diminished as the muscle recovered its power. It happened, in this case, that the inclination required to correct the faulty position of the images due to the squint was one of exaggeration, but it might have been the opposite.

The rapid recovery of the erect position of the head in Pierola's case after the operation is rather interesting considering the duration of the distortion.

—LESLIE BUCHANAN.

"Specimens of Experimental Glasses Prepared by Sir William Crookes, O.M., P.R.S."—This is the title of a communication to the Royal Society of Medicine, Section of Ophthalmology, on 3rd December, 1913, by Mr. J. Herbert Parsons, which led to some very interesting remarks from members present.

The experimental glasses were prepared by Sir William Crookes, with the co-operation of Mr. Parsons, with the object of finding which combination of metallic salts with glasses cut off most heat rays and most ultra-violet rays. The research was undertaken, as Mr. Parsons says, "for the Glassworkers' Cataract Committee of the Royal Society, and the results were communicated to a recent meeting of that Society."

Special care was taken to measure accurately the transmission of heat, luminous and ultra-violet rays, a special radiation balance being invented to allow of accurate estimation of the heat transmitted, whilst the ultra-violet rays were estimated by photography, using a quartz spectrograph.

A great variety of the rarer metals were used in the experiments, and over three hundred varieties of glass were prepared. Cerium salts assisted in the cutting off of the ultra-violet rays and also heat rays. Chromium salts prevent the passage of ultra-violet rays principally, whilst iron especially and, to a less extent, copper and lead salts prevent the passage of heat rays.

No glass could be prepared which cut off all heat and ultra-violet rays completely without diminishing the transmissibility of luminous rays.

The best result for heat rays was a cutting off of 96 per cent, which is surely extremely good.

In the discussion which followed, Dr. T. M. Legge, H.M. Inspector of Factories, made a useful and interesting statement. He had special facilities, of course, for examining men engaged in glass work and kindred occupations, and had studied the subject as a member of the Departmental Committee which sat to enquire into compensation for industrial diseases under the Compensation Act of 1906. He had been specially struck by the number of men who, possibly unknown to themselves, suffered from the typical glass-workers' form of cataract, and stated that it did not appear to matter much at what branch of the trade they were working so long as they had to face the white light and heat of the furnace through the "glory-hole."

The president asked Dr. Legge if he had seen cases in which the cornea was affected as well as the lens, since he understood that Italian glass-workers, as at Venice, who were very close to the heat and glare, were subject to this form of change, but Dr. Legge had no specific information to give upon the subject.

It is an extremely interesting and important fact that this condition, glass-worker's cataract, has been recognised for over a century now (Wenzel, in 1806, mentioned it specially), and yet no satisfactory preventive has been brought to light, or at least nothing in the way of a serious effort to prevent the occurrence has been undertaken.

Robinson, writing in the *British Medical Journal* in December, 1903, stated that azure blue glass, used as goggles, would prevent it, but seemingly very little has been done further. We may hope that now, when the matter has been taken up by the Royal Society, a determined effort will be made to compel masters and men alike to provide and use the best means procurable in order to prevent the occurrence of this slow but sure loss of sight amongst a class of worthy industrial workers.—LESLIE BUCHANAN.

Books, Pamphlets, &c., Received.

Tropical Diseases : A Manual of the Diseases of Warm Climates, by Sir Patrick Manson, G.C.M.G, M.D., LL.D Aberd. With 12 colour and 4 black and white plates, and 239 figures in the text. Fifth edition, revised throughout and enlarged. London : Cassell & Co. 1914. (12s. 6d. net.)

Why Early Death ? By M. C. Sykes, M.D., D.P.H.Lond., F.C.S. London : The St. Catherine Press. (6d.)

Dietetics, or Food in Health and Disease, by William Tibbles, LL.D., M.D. (*Hon. Causâ*), Chicago. London : Baillière, Tindall & Cox. 1914. (12s. 6d. net.)

The Pocket Formulary for the Treatment of Disease in Children, by Ludwig Freyberger, J.P., M.D.Vienna. Fourth revised and enlarged edition. Adapted to the *British Pharmacopœia*. With an Appendix on Poisons : Their Symptoms and Treatment. London : William Heinemann. 1914. (7s. 6d. net.)

Physiologie Normale et Pathologique des Reins, par L. Ambard. Paris : F. Gittler. 1914.

Manuel de Cystoscopie, par E. Papin. Preface par M. le Professeur F. Leguen. Paris : F. Gittler. 1914.

Notions Pratiques D'Electrothérapie Appliquée a L'Urologie, par Le Docteur Denis Courtade. Paris : F. Gittler. 1914.

St. Thomas's Hospital Reports. New series. Vol. XLI. Edited by Dr. J. J. Perkins and Mr. C. A. Ballance. London : J. & A. Churchill. 1914.

A Practical Handbook of the Tropical Diseases of Asia and Africa, by H. C. Lambart, M.A., M.D. With 6 coloured plates and 82 other illustrations. London : Charles Griffin & Co., Limited. 1914. (8s. 6d. net.)

The Ileo-Cæcal Valve, by A. H. Rutherfurd, M.D.Edin. London : H. K. Lewis. 1914. (6s. net.)

Aids to Forensic Medicine and Toxicology, by William Murrell, M.D., F.R.C.P. revised by W. G. Aitchison Robertson, M.D., D.Sc. Eighth edition. London : Baillière, Tindall & Cox. 1914. (2s. 6d. net.)

Salvarsan Treatment of Syphilis in Private Practice, with some account of the Modern Methods of Diagnosis, by George Stopford-Taylor, M.D., M.R.C.S., and Robert William Mackenna, M.A., M.D., B.Ch. London : William Heinemann. 1914. (5s. net.)

Insanity in Every-day Practice, by E. G. Younger, M.D.Brux., M.R.C.P.Lond., P.P.H., &c. Third edition. London : Baillière, Tindall & Cox. 1914. (3s. 6d. net.)

Gas Poisoning in Mining and other Industries, by John Glaister, M.D.Glasg., D.P.H.Camb., F.R.S.E., and David Dale Logan, M.D.Glasg., D.P.H. With plans, coloured plates, and 36 other illustrations. Edinburgh : E. & S. Livingstone. 1914. (10s. 6d. net.)

GLASGOW.—METEOROLOGICAL AND VITAL STATISTICS FOR THE FOUR WEEKS ENDED 11TH JULY, 1914.

	WEEK ENDING			
	June 20.	June 27.	July 4.	July 11.
Mean temperature, . .	62·0°	56·7°	54·5°	59·0°
Mean range of temperature between highest and lowest,	20·1°	12·7°	16·8°	13·8°
Number of days on which rain fell, ...	1	2	6	0
Amount of rainfall, . ins.	0·04	0·07	1·28	0·00
Deaths (corrected), . .	306	265	305	283
Death-rates, ...	15·2	13·2	15·2	14·1
Zymotic death-rates, . .	1·4	1·3	1·0	1·1
Pulmonary death-rates, .	3·4	2·3	2·8	2·5
DEATHS—				
Under 1 year, . . .	65	57	50	52
60 years and upwards, .	81	53	72	62
DEATHS FROM—				
Small-pox, ...	...	...	...	...
Measles, ...	8	5	4	6
Scarlet fever, . . .	3	3	...	2
Diphtheria, . . .	1	3	3	2
Whooping-cough, . .	16	15	10	9
Enteric fever, . . .	...	2	1	2
Cerebro-spinal fever, . .	...	...	...	1
Diarrhœa (under 2 years of age),	9	2	4	6
Bronchitis, pneumonia, and pleurisy, . . .	42	29	34	27
CASES REPORTED—				
Small-pox, ...	...	...	...	...
Cerebro-spinal meningitis, .	2	3	1	1
Diphtheria and membranous croup, ...	23	23	32	27
Erysipelas, . . .	31	29	31	17
Scarlet fever, . . .	60	78	74	80
Typhus fever, . . .	...	...	...	1
Enteric fever, . . .	8	5	6	6
Phthisis, ...	53	56	31	49
Puerperal fever, . .	4	4	3	1
Measles,* . . .	106	78	84	35

* Measles not notifiable.

SANITARY CHAMBERS,
GLASGOW, 3rd August, 1914.

THE

GLASGOW MEDICAL JOURNAL.

No. III. SEPTEMBER, 1914.

ORIGINAL ARTICLES.

PRACTICAL POINTS IN ABDOMINAL SURGERY, BEING
THE "JAMES WATSON LECTURES" DELIVERED BEFORE
THE ROYAL FACULTY OF PHYSICIANS AND SURGEONS,
11TH AND 14TH MARCH, 1913.

BY T. KENNEDY DALZIEL, M.B., F.R.F.P.S.,
Surgeon to the Western Infirmary, Glasgow.

GENTLEMEN,—I must first thank the trustees of the James
Watson Prize Fund and the Fellows of the Faculty for the
honour they have done me in asking me to deliver these lectures,
and the trustees in particular for having suggested the subject.

One does not require to dwell on the continual advance which
is being made in surgery generally and in abdominal surgery
in particular. The changes are almost daily, so that statistics
for one year are not applicable to the next. So much is this
the case that I feel it is futile to discuss statistics as indicating
the dangers in any particular operation. There are few
surgeons who, knowing their patient, appreciating the principles
which underlie all surgical technique, and availing themselves
of the special knowledge of the physician, can not form a fairly
accurate opinion as to the probable issue in any particular case.
The result in any operation varies within a considerable range

in the hands of different surgeons.   Quite recently a surgeon of great fame, worthy of every honour, told me he did not consider gastro-enterostomy a justifiable operation.   And so we find the widest diversity of opinion amongst skilled surgeons as to the technique to be followed in given cases.   As there are many roads which lead to Rome, and some that don't, so there may be numerous ways of attaining a satisfactory issue, or otherwise, in a particular surgical problem.

I do not, then, propose to advance my own or any other person's statistics in the brief *résumé* of the following practical points in abdominal surgery, and I wish as far as possible to avoid alluding to the details of surgical technique.

As it is not possible to overtake even in a brief *résumé* the wide field of abdominal surgery, I shall merely endeavour to bring before you some points which, during the last quarter of a century, have struck me as important, many of them perhaps not fully appreciated, and some which I believe to be new.

Neuralgias simulating visceral lesions.—In regard to the retaining wall of the abdomen, I would venture to draw attention to neuralgias simulating visceral lesions.   Of these the most important, and, I fear, little recognised, is that of the twelfth dorsal nerve (occasionally the ilio-hypogastric), on which I have operated more than thirty times.   These cases were for the most part sent to my clinic either on account of the obscurity of the symptoms or with a diagnosis of some internal complaint—*e.g.*, on the right side, affections of ovary, appendix, ureter, and kidney; on the left, those of the kidney, ureter, sigmoid and ovary.   Indeed, quite recently I saw a lady whose ovary and appendix had been removed and her kidney excised, but whose only complaint evidently was neuralgia of the right twelfth dorsal nerve.   One is familiar with intercostal neuralgia, but the clinical significance of that of the twelfth (or ilio-hypogastric) nerve does not seem to me to have been sufficiently appreciated.   Why the twelfth nerve should be specially affected is probably owing to its liability to injury—leaving the spine and pursuing its course in the flexible flank where the rib may impinge on the crest of the ilium.   It is certainly liable to muscular pressure, and the branch which passes over the crest of the ilium to direct pressure.   The main trunk pursues its course to the abdominal wall in front of and above the pubes. In several of my cases direct pressure on the dorsal branch from carrying burdens resting on the haunch bone seemed the determining cause. We have in this way conditions which closely enough resemble those found in the sciatic nerve, and the resulting neuralgia may be as serious as in the latter case, in so far as incapacity to work or enjoy life is concerned.

The first case I saw was sent me twelve years ago by Dr. Stewart, then of Maryhill. The patient, a man of 40 years, had for fifteen years spent the greater part of his time as an invalid. He was a working man who, in his occupation, had frequently pressure on his left haunch. The pain at times was excruciating, with intervals of comparative comfort, but never such as to allow him to get into the full swing of work. He was on his way to the Poorhouse when sent to me for an opinion. There being no other apparent reason for his suffering apart from a neuralgia, I for the first time exposed and destroyed the twelfth dorsal nerve, with relief so immediate and complete that within six weeks he was once more at work, and has continued well.

Quite recently I had in my wards a case with a history of one year's pain, so severe as to render life almost a burden. This pain extended from the floating rib to above the pubes, with a well-marked area of tenderness on the dorsum ilii. He was sent in as a case of appendicitis, and, truly, he had pain sufficiently near M'Burney's point to arouse suspicion; but on palpating the course of the twelfth nerve it was found to be extremely tender, while nothing suggesting appendix mischief could be discovered. The twelfth nerve being mostly a sensory one, there need, happily, be no hesitation in dividing it, and though the patient complained subsequently of a feeling of numbness in the region supplied by the nerve, this soon passed off.

The following cases merely illustrate the condition :—

Joseph C., stoker, admitted 13th May, 1907, complaining of pain in left side along lower ribs. Eighteen years ago he was struck on the side by a case, and since then has had neuralgic pains along the side and down the crest of the ilium.

The twelfth dorsal nerve was exposed and 3 inches excised. Dismissed on 24th May, 1907, well.

James S., aged 28 years, admitted on 20th November, 1912, complaining of pain in the right side of one year's duration. Pain comes on at any time, and is not worse during or after micturition, but at some times is worse than at others. It comes round crest of ilium towards pubes and back of hip, following course of twelfth dorsal nerve. The course of nerve is tender to palpation.

The nerve was exposed and divided. Dismissed on 13th January, 1913; no pain.

Eliza L., aged 15 years, admitted on 5th January, 1911, complaining of pain in right side of five years' duration.

History.—Five years ago she was kicked in the right groin; sickness and vomiting occurred, and she was confined to bed for a fortnight. There was pain on micturition during the act, but no story of hæmaturia. At times she has noticed a swelling in the right iliac region. Menstruation began at 12 years; at each period pain increases in severity, so much so that she has to stay in bed a day or so.

Examination.— Abdomen normal except over M'Burney's point, which is tender on pressure.

28th January, 1911.—Pain now confined to right lumbar region and right buttock. No pain in right iliac region.

7th February.—Resection of twelfth dorsal nerve.

22nd February.—Dismissed well.

In regard to the areas of pain in such cases, generally they will be found in three points: a strip of pain from outside M'Burney's point above the brim of the pelvis, a tender spot near the root of the twelfth rib, and frequently a tender area, or, at least, an area complained of, corresponding to the dorsal branch of the twelfth after it passes over the crest of the ilium. As in sciatica, one finds complete freedom from pain for a time, or it may be recovery under dietetic and medicinal treatment. This affection of the twelfth nerve and sciatica are, as far as I can see, highly comparable, and we are compelled to have recourse to surgical interference in cases resisting other treatment.

The operation for the division of the nerve is a comparatively simple one. An incision by the outer border of the erector spinæ muscle below the twelfth rib will expose the nerve with its accompanying blood-vessel; it has been my practice to stretch the nerve until it gives way; a few minutes suffice for the operation, and the wound may be expected to heal in a week. The results have been extremely satisfactory. In only one case have we failed to obtain a complete recovery, and that in a case where the kidney had been explored, rendering the search for the nerve a difficult task.

I am aware that much scepticism has prevailed in regard to this condition and the necessity for operation; but those practitioners who have had their cases operated upon have no doubt whatever of its value.

Another condition which may give rise to difficulty in diagnosis in abdominal conditions is the occurrence of abdominal pain and rigidity of the muscles due to pleurisy affecting the lower zone of the chest, and no doubt due to the involvement of the intercostal nerves directly or reflexly. Such cases when first seen may present all the appearances of the "acute abdomen," a term much in vogue in some parts of the world; but which, while it may serve a purpose, does not suggest either accuracy of diagnosis or precision in treatment. In such cases we have not only rigid muscles, but frequently tenderness on pressure, and a temperature and pulse which may readily lead one to look upon the case as abdominal in origin. Some years ago I was led to explore the abdomen in such a case, and since then a number of cases have come within my knowledge. The point which most strikingly impresses one is the absence of the abdominal facies, a very important point which every surgeon will fully appreciate, as seen in cases where peritonitis exists, and the presence of which is the usual indication for treatment in the acute abdomen. In such cases it may not be easy to hold one's hand. Such reflex influences through the lower intercostal nerves are to be remembered, and may be recognised by careful examination of the chest.

Ventral hernia of extra-peritoneal fat.—These herniæ are found about 2½ inches above the umbilicus, generally in the middle line. They may be multiple, as in the case of a colleague from the Western Isles from whom I removed three, one in the middle line and one on each side about an inch from the centre. The first case of this kind coming under my observation occurred many years ago in the practice of Dr. Snodgrass, with whom I saw a patient suffering from profound gastric disturbance; the history being that he had attacks of vomiting without apparent cause, the vomiting being urgent and the disordered peristalsis leading to regurgitation of bile, which lasted for some days. At no time was pain complained of. In the interval the patient was well, had a fairly good digestion, and was unable to account in any way for the sudden onset of this abnormal gastric peristalsis. On careful palpation a small diffuse swelling could be detected in the region indicated. There was no history of this becoming larger, suggesting strangulation prior to his attacks, nor was the patient aware of its presence. On operating we found the swelling to consist of a mass of fat, simulating a lipoma, but evidently extruded through a small aperture like the lumen of a quill through the aponeurosis. The pedicle being ligatured and the piece of fat removed, the aperture was closed by a silkworm stitch; marked relief from the symptoms followed.

In such cases the clinical features are the occurrence of vomiting, usually becoming bilious. There is no dilatation of the stomach, probably no error in dietary, and no other condition accounting for the upset. The symptoms suggest a neurosis, and from the result of the removal of such hernia it seems probable that the neurosis originates in traction on the peritoneum reflexly acting on the stomach.

It is a condition well worth looking for in cases where we suspect gastric symptoms are due to some peripheral origin.

The origin of these herniæ is rather obscure. Similar protrusions are met with in the neighbourhood of the inguinal canal, not only descending the canal and apparently determining the visceral hernia by dragging a pouch of peritoneum with them, but also penetrating the tendon of the external oblique. One can only suppose that the fat finds a slight gap in the aponeurosis through which it grows. They are generally found by the lower margin of the fold of Douglas. The condition is not a common one, but as I see several cases each year, and have been able to give great relief by operation, it is one well worthy of attention. While not found in every text-book it has been described by other workers.

William K., admitted 25th February, 1908, for some months complaining of weight about epigastrium when at work. Five weeks ago he noticed swelling in epigastrium which was painful on pressure. No other symptoms. When he turns on his side and strains a small lump protrudes between recti, midway between sternum and umbilicus.

19th March, 1908.—Small extra-peritoneal lipoma removed.

10th April.—Dismissed.

John W., aged 61 years, admitted 10th January, 1912, complaining of pain in epigastrium of four weeks' duration. While at work in garden four weeks previously he was seized with sudden acute pain. Pain decreased and he worked on for four days, but had to give up then and send for his doctor, who discovered swelling in epigastrium. Never had pain previously though he has had flatulence and pyrosis occasionally.

Examination.—No pain. Abdomen flat and flaccid. Midway between xiphoid and umbilicus there is a small tumour, measuring 2 inches by 1 inch, soft and evidently fatty in nature. No impulse on coughing. During past fortnight tumour has increased in size.

16th January, 1912.—Excised tumour found to be composed of two lipomata. Wound closed by mattress sutures and wire filigree.

26th January.—Evidence of thrombosis of saphena vein.

24th February.—Dismissed. To wear elastic bandage from foot to thigh.

Donald M'C., aged 29 years, admitted 10th October, 1912, complaining of bilious vomiting off and on of two years' duration. Headache has been troublesome. No loss of appetite and always ready for his food. At times he felt "full" after eating.

Examination. There is a small protrusion of extra peritoneal fat midway between xiphoid and umbilicus. Stomach slightly enlarged.

18th October, 1912.—Opening closed.

1st November.—Dismissed well.

Other hernias.—Regarding other hernias through the abdominal wall it is unnecessary to speak, since they have for the last century been constantly under consideration. I would only venture to state that in hernia in infants it is probably unnecessary to pay so much attention to the stitching of the ring as has been customary. Within the last two years in the Children's Hospital well nigh one hundred cases have been operated on, the sac alone being dealt with. In only one case, where the ring was exceptionally large, was a retaining stitch necessary, and so far as I know there has been no recurrence.

If stitches are to be used it seems better to use silk or silk-worm-gut rather than catgut, which softens much earlier than seems generally to be supposed, and loses its retaining power. The period at which catgut is absorbed is no indication of the time for which it may be trusted to hold parts together. This applies not only to hernias, but also to the closing of laparotomy wounds in large ventral hernias, especially in fat people. Much benefit may be obtained by the use of the silver filigree inserted between the peritoneum and the muscular wall, which in all cases ought to be closed by overlapping.

In femoral hernia I have been quite satisfied with the use of the metallic staple as recommended by Roux, and in few cases has there been recurrence of the hernia or trouble from the staple.

An interesting hernia is that through the diaphragm, of which only two cases have come under my observation, but one of which is so interesting that it is well worthy of being put on record.

The case was that of Mr. B., who was stabbed from the back through the lung and diaphragm by a native of Portuguese East Africa. He sustained other injuries, but after a fortnight in hospital was able to travel. He ultimately returned to this country, and two years after the assault presented all the symptoms of intestinal obstruction in the neighbourhood of the splenic flexure. He complained of much pain on breathing, and his abdomen was much distended, particularly the transverse colon. In the absence of any history pointing to the origin, because the true course of the knife was not then known, I determined to remove the obstruction by operation, when it was found that a portion of the stomach and the splenic flexure of the colon had passed through an aperture readily admitting four fingers, the colon being adherent to the lung. The margin of the ring was incised sufficiently to draw the lung into view, and the colon liberated; there was naturally considerable oozing from the lung surface.

The aperture in the diaphragm was closed with numerous silk stitches, one of the most difficult tasks conceivable owing to the extremely powerful muscularity of the diaphragm; one had to wait one's chance, and during a brief spell of relaxation quickly tighten suture after suture.

The patient subsequently had a hæmopneumothorax and suffered for a week the worst agony I have ever seen, and I had to aspirate the chest several times; but he subsequently made a good recovery, and is to-day in the best of health.

Gall-bladder.—The surgery of the gall-bladder resolves itself, for the most part, into that of the removal of gall-stones and their complications. While typical cases of gall-stone disease may be readily recognised by the character of the pain and the evidence of obstruction of the ducts, there is a large class where the symptoms are so atypical as to render the diagnosis a matter of some difficulty. The most frequent difficulty in diagnosis is with affections of the pylorus and duodenum; affections of the head of the pancreas and the pancreatic duct; malignant disease in the vicinity, with affections of the right kidney; and, lastly, with colic of the gall-bladder from kinking by adhesions along the hepatic mesentery.

Undoubtedly gall-stones may exist without symptoms, and apparently without doing harm. Only when they endeavour to leave the gall-bladder or when catarrh sets in do they give rise to symptoms. But it is undoubted that a person with gall-stones may have pain and reflex disturbance without reference directly to the gall-bladder region. We now know so well the gall-stone dyspepsia, where two or three hours after food the patient complains of flatulence, discomfort, and a sense of fulness, occasionally passing on to actual gastric spasm. On the other hand, the symptoms may be much more vague, as in a patient in the Western Infirmary recently under my care, sent by Dr. M'Kenzie, of Larbert, who had pain in her appendix region, but in addition aching pain from the level of her fourth rib to her thigh. This pain, being more or less constant, was especially bad at night, but generally worst a few hours after food. Her suffering was so considerable that she pleaded to have something done, and as the presence of a gall-stone was suspected, an incision was made through the right rectus muscle and three large gall-stones removed from a gall-bladder remarkably normal in appearance, with complete relief from all symptoms.

Similarly, one may have merely pain in the right shoulder. In many persons with such vague symptoms local tenderness may be induced by causing the patient to stoop forward and relax the abdominal muscle, when the hand may be introduced under the liver and the stones pressed upon.

Serious disease of the gall-bladder may be present with very obscure symptoms.

Quite recently a patient was brought to me complaining of loss of flesh, with increasing weakness, and the presence of a tumour in his right hypochondrium. This tumour, occupying the region of the gall-bladder, was slightly sensitive to pressure, and very clearly represented a dilated gall-bladder. He could not recollect any pain, although his wife subsequently informed us he had had an attack of pain sixteen years before; his pulse and temperature were normal.

The diagnosis was probably malignant disease, originating in the gall-bladder, and determined by the presence of a stone. Operation revealed a gall-stone about the size of a hazel nut embedded in the cystic duct, and surrounded with cancer, while the gall-bladder was distended with foul pus, and the surrounding parts adhering owing to long-standing pericystitis.

Even in the gall-ducts stones may exist, and grow to a remarkable size, with a singular absence of urgent symptoms, especially when the duct becomes dilated, as in the case of a patient (Miss T.) whom I saw with Dr. Alexander. She had been confined more or less to bed for years with symptoms of dyspepsia, and only occasionally a very mild suggestion of jaundice. She had, however, become so emaciated that one was able to palpate the stone, as may be understood since it was found to measure, after removal, $1\frac{1}{4}$ inches in length and 3 inches in circumference. In this case the gall-duct was dilated somewhat like the small intestine, and one had no difficulty in removing the stone by a longitudinal incision. So free were the walls of the duct that suture was a matter of ease; no drain was inserted, and the patient got married within a year.

A striking feature in most cases of obscure gall-stone symptoms in differentiating them from gastric conditions is the fact that, while food in a general way determines symptoms, patients are often surprised that they can eat heartily at times without discomfort. Also, they have a somewhat characteristic complexion, perhaps understood by the term "a bilious complexion." Often, however, the diagnosis must be arrived at by a process of exclusion.

When inflammation of the gall-bladder and ducts sets in a new train of symptoms arises, not only of local evidences, such as the enlargement of the liver and tenderness, but also constitutional disturbance due to septic intoxication, in some cases of a profound character.

Where the septic catarrh is of the gall-bladder and bile-ducts, or extends to the pancreatic duct, there can be no doubt whatever that drainage of the gall-bladder is the correct line of treatment; but it is particularly important to make sure that any stones resting in the ducts, whether gall-ducts or pancreatic ducts, should be removed. Some years ago my practice was to remove the stones from the ducts either by incision or by dilating the cystic duct; but now for some years I have without hesitation incised the duodenum, dilated the ampulla, and so made sure of the complete evacuation of the ducts; in any case establishing an orifice sufficiently large to enable any fragments which may have been left to escape.

In two cases where pancreatitis was present it was found necessary to incise the pancreatic duct through an opening in the posterior wall of the duodenum, the opening in the duct being stitched to the margin of this intestinal wound. The fear that possibly such a wound might permit sepsis to persist in the pancreatic duct was not realised, both patients making excellent recoveries, and remaining well to this day.

Where the gall-bladder is grossly diseased with thickened wall and contracted lumen, I believe it to be good practice to excise it; and after many years experience I have concluded this proceeding to be, on the whole, more satisfactory, and not less safe than mere drainage. In no case have I ever inserted a drain into the cystic duct, and in no case have we had trouble from leakage of bile or peritonitis. In this respect I am aware that my opinion is at variance with that of many distinguished surgeons; but one can only speak, as I do now, from one's own findings, and I have no hesitation in removing the gall-bladder if the pathological condition seems to demand it. The suggestion made some years ago that such an operation deprived one of the possibility of draining the gall-bladder should pancreatitis or cholangitis demand it, does not seem to me to have much weight, since one must look on the gall-bladder as the source and origin of most, if not all, such conditions.   .

In addition to these few remarks on gall-bladder and gall-stone disease, in which I have by no means attempted to overtake a tenth part of the whole subject, but merely to suggest some points of importance in practice, I would like to draw attention to a condition of the gall-bladder itself, which gives rise to symptoms analogous to gall-stone colic, namely, a pendulous and elongated gall-bladder associated with congenital adhesion to the duodenum. The clinical features are merely those of a mild degree of gall-stone colic, without jaundice and with slight or no local tenderness. The secondary symptoms, in the way of sickness and disordered intestinal peristalsis, are just those met with in gall-stone colic; and, as in such, vary according to the temperament of the individual.

Perhaps the most striking case of this kind was one I saw with Dr. James Carslaw some years ago. The condition only being recognised when the abdomen was opened, was remedied by stitching the fundus of the gall-bladder to the parietal peritoneum, and dividing the congenital adhesion which was found extending from the gall-bladder to the duodenum.

Surgery of the kidneys, ureter, and bladder: incision in acute inflammation of the kidney, and in suppression of urine.—While the surgeon has brought under his notice certain well-defined affections which are only amenable to operative interference, it seems to me possible that advantage might be obtained by the physician by incision of the organ in cases of acute inflammation. Though in recent years somewhat fallen into disrepute, it seems probable that venesection was of great value in acute Bright's disease, as it undoubtedly is in sthenic pneumonia. It seems probable that greater good may be obtained in the case of the kidney by direct depletion.

I have only had an opportunity of doing this in two cases. When we consider that the operation is by no means one of severity and does not materially injure the organ, it seems worthy of further trial, as is being done in other parts of the world.

Acute inflammation of the kidney is interesting from another surgical point of view, namely, that it may give rise to all the symptoms of an acute abdomen, as happened in a case which came under my observation some years ago in Belvidere Hospital. The patient, suffering from enteric fever, developed acute abdominal pain and a degree of muscular rigidity, giving rise to the suspicion of perforation of an enteric ulcer. From the absence of tenderness I was inclined to doubt the diagnosis, but consented to perform an exploratory operation, when it was easily determined that no peritoneal mischief existed. The kidneys were found to be enlarged, and a catheter was passed, when a small quantity of urine was obtained, which contained some blood and excessive albumen, clearly pointing to acute nephritis being the cause of the condition. In supression of urine, also, it seems probable that the vasomotor derangement can be materially modified by incision of the organ.

Hæmaturia.—Apart from calculus, ulceration, malignant or tubercular lesions, and papilloma, we have more obscure lesions causing hæmorrhage.

First, Mr. A., a patient of Dr. Young, of Slamannan, was brought to me suffering from hæmaturia so continued as to cause profound anæmia. The hæmaturia had continued for six weeks, with all the characteristics of a renal hæmorrhage. He complained of pain over his left kidney, but neither organ was tender on palpation. He had at no time pain suggesting calculus. Examination of the ureteral effluent by cystoscope proved that the blood was escaping from the right kidney, the blood being in such amount as to form a splendid demonstration of the rhythmical ejaculatory action of the ureter.

I formed the opinion that there was probably a small hypernephroma in the right kidney and advised operation, which was performed by the anterior route. This method seems to me much preferable to the lumbar incision, as it affords an opportunity of more thorough diagnosis and of examining the other kidney at least by palpation, and of carrying out a more detailed and complete surgical technique.

On exposing the kidney in this case I was rather shocked to find not a single evidence of abnormality. In size and in consistence it was apparently normal, as was also the ureter. I was thus faced with the removal of an organ apparently normal, or the continuation of a hæmorrhage which was clearly killing the patient. Supported by an accurate observation through the cystoscope, I had no hesitation in excising the kidney. Anxious to discover at once the source of the hæmorrhage I laid it open, and, after considerable difficulty, found a small portion on the apex of one of the pyramids differing somewhat in consistence and colour from the normal. This portion was kindly examined for me by Dr. Shaw Dunn, whose description of the specimen is as follows:—

"*Specimen from kidney.*—The portion of tissue sent for examination consists of a medullary pyramid, with adjacent areas of cortical tissue. Towards the apex of the pyramid there are seen in sections a number of thin-walled vascular spaces filled with blood. They are of considerable size, and are scattered somewhat irregularly through the tissue of the pyramid, some being near the pelvic surface. The condition is such as would be likely to give rise to copious hæmorrhage at some time or other, although an actual point of rupture is not detected."

The condition is a rare one. It may be that a number of these cases are due to this condition, which has not been frequently described, and classified as "essential hæmaturia."

Varicose veins.—Sarah G., 32 years, transferred from Ward II on 20th March, 1912, complaining of intermittent hæmaturia and increasing anæmia of nine years' duration. During last nine years, at varying intervals, there has been hæmaturia, the attack lasting for a month, while for three or four months urine appears normal. No history of renal colic, no pain during micturition, and no frequency. On admission patient pale; dicrotic and rapid pulse; abdomen is normal to palpation.

20th March, 1912.—Suprapubic cystotomy; varicose veins

in mucosa of bladder ruptured. Two veins found—right larger, showing two actively bleeding perforations; left small, showing one perforation plugged with clot. Varicose veins and mucosa excised; mucosa sutured, and drain inserted into bladder.

9th May.—Dismissed well.

This case was admitted to the medical wards of the Western Infirmary, and the hæmorrhage was so severe that Professor Gemmell advised her immediate removal to the surgical side. The amount of bright blood escaping was such as to suggest the necessity of immediate action. The whole presumption being in favour of a bladder origin, and the hæmorrhage so active as to put out of court the use of the cystoscope, I determined to do an immediate suprapubic cystotomy, when we discovered two large tortuous varicose veins extending from the base of the trigone upwards, one on each side of the middle line, and expanding as they reached the dome of the bladder. The area of mucous membrane thus involved was triangular in shape, the apex below and the base above, about an inch and a half in width. The bleeding was principally from the right vein, and when exposed was active, a continuous spray of blood playing upwards into the wound. Two scars were visible on the left vein, evidently the point which had bled while the patient was in hospital at Belfast.

The mucous membrane was incised and the veins removed, following the same principle as in similar operations on the leg; the wounds of the mucous membrane being closed by fine catgut sutures, and a glass drain inserted in the bladder as usual.

The patient made an uninterrupted recovery, and is now well.

Bilharzia hæmatobium.—Apart from the distressing symptoms which this disease gives rise to in Eastern climes, we have occasionally here lesser degrees of the affection causing obscure hæmorrhage, where the bladder lesion is limited and the active propagation of the worm has ceased. The type of bleeding is rather that met with in early tubercle, but without the very serious irritative phenomena found in the advance of that disease.

Thomas K., admitted 18th April, 1910, complaining of attacks of hæmaturia, not specially severe, but consisting of pure blood, the first portion passed being smoky and porter-coloured, the latter portion being pure blood. He had also pain at the point of penis, and sometimes flow of urine was suddenly obstructed. Cystoscope showed no stone or stricture, but there seemed to be something like a tumour on anterior wall. Urine so far free of blood.

This soldier had been affected in Egypt, but from the condition found the affection had been a slight one; though the bilharzia had managed to reach the bladder wall the ova were dead, and the local lesions from which the blood was escaping were no doubt due to the endeavour of the surrounding healthy tissue to get rid of the foreign bodies. I assisted nature by excising five affected areas of the mucous membrane, stitching each wound with the finest catgut and draining above the pubes.

In this connection I would draw attention to the fearlessness with which one may excise large portions of the bladder, especially if the organ be moderately healthy and fairly free from sepsis. With a fairly free abdominal incision, and a lateral notching of the rectus muscle above the pubes, one can, with the patient in the Trendelenburg position, bring the bladder within easy surgical control; occasionally aid may be required by an assistant pressing upwards from the perineum or rectum. I have succeeded in this way in removing cancer of the base of the bladder involving the prostate and the whole of the trigone.

The case was that of an elderly gentleman from Ayr (Mr. C.). He was suffering from the usual symptoms of prostatic enlargement; but blood in his urine, and evidences of ulceration in the trigone, suggested probable malignancy. As there did not seem to be any glandular involvement, however, we decided to operate, and had in the course of our proceedings to remove not only the prostate, but the whole of the trigone, with the ends of the ureters and also a portion of the anterior wall of the bladder. Each ureter was split and stitched to the margin of the wound, the bladder in front drawn together as far as possible, and as hæmorrhage continued troublesome the bladder was packed with natural sponges, which were removed on the third day and the suprapubic drain substituted. There was considerable shock, but healing went on without complication. The patient lived for two years without any evidence of recurrence, and died from, I believe, acute pneumonia. He was able to attend to business and take a moderate amount of exercise, wearing, of course, a permanent suprapubic drain.

In connection with this case, I would like to suggest the use of natural sponges for the arresting of vesical hæmorrhage not controllable by other methods. Sometimes in ulceration of the bladder, a few times in the removal of extensive papilloma, I think we have saved the life of the patient by the elastic pressure which such sponges exert. This they do without harming the mucous membrane, and certainly without interrupting the flow of urine. It seems reasonable to suppose that it must be wise in many cases, particularly delicate patients, to avoid the risk of that prolonged oozing which one meets with in bladder cases—a risk which may not be immediate, but which may lead to secondary consequences in subjects often in a poor condition to begin with.

I was induced to have recourse to this simple line of treatment many years ago when acting in Sir Hector Cameron's wards. A patient was admitted with a fracture of the pelvis and a hæmorrhage, which not only filled the bladder but flooded the peritoneum. We performed an immediate laparotomy, cleared out the peritoneum, found a ·rent in the base of the bladder, and the bladder full of blood-clot. On emptying the bladder through an anterior incision, the hæmorrhage was found to be so copious and persistent that one was glad to stop it by compression; but intermittent pressure, however, failed to arrest it; I therefore determined to sew up the posterior rent and pack the bladder with natural sponges. And this I did, not knowing that the urine would find its way through the porous sponge. Such was, however, the case, and Dr. Eric Wilson, a most excellent house surgeon, devoted himself wholeheartedly to keeping the parts aseptic till three days had elapsed, when the sponges were removed and a suprapubic drain established. The patient made a perfect recovery.

Since then the proceeding has been with me a routine practice in cases of serious hæmorrhage, or where it was deemed inadvisable to have even the ordinary oozing to contend with. Such oozing is not infrequently found after prostatectomy.   As a rule it may be ignored, but some cases, I am confident, will benefit from this method.

Papilloma of the bladder.—This is singularly amenable to surgical interference.   Frequently, however, it becomes malignant, and I therefore make it a rule in all cases to remove an elliptical -portion of the bladder wall, fearlessly removing muscular substance.   Out of three cases of papilloma with malignant change, operated on within recent years, two have remained well.   The third patient, from Dr. Ferguson, of Paisley, had in the scar, two years after the primary operation, a secondary cancer, which I again excised ; and in the meantime the patient is enjoying the best of health and comfort.

Calculus.—In regard to calculus and the various methods of treatment little need be said.   Indeed, the condition has so infrequently come within my notice during the past decade as to lead me to believe that the complaint is becoming less frequent.   Nor can one say much now in regard to stone in the kidney and ureter.   In the latter condition I have no doubt that the transperitoneal method of operation is the right one.   Only five cases, however, have come under my care, but all did well.   The ureter was opened by a longitudinal incision a short distance above the stone, where the dilatation permitted the suturing without unduly stricturing.   In two cases a counter-opening was made and a drainage-tube led through the loin.   The other three were closed, and all made uninterrupted recoveries.

Generally, I believe it will be found advisable to do the great bulk of kidney surgery by an anterior incision, certainly so if there be no sepsis to contend with ; and even if sepsis be present, by suturing the opening in the posterior peritoneal wound to the anterior a cofferdam will be obtained which will enable one to work with impunity.   In some cases where the patient is thin, and with a long abdomen, one may keep the incision so far out as to be able to lift the parietal peritoneum from the flank so as to leave the peritoneal sac intact.   By this method malignant disease of the kidney can be attacked much more accurately than by the lumbar incision.   I would like here to put on record my experience that malignant disease more frequently gives rise to serious hæmaturia than seems to be generally accepted.

It has been the fashion for some years to classify many malignant tumours of the kidney as hypernephroma, and I am more than interested to hear that Dr. Shaw Dunn is now quoted as holding the view that they are not to be considered as such, but merely as carcinoma originating in the epithelial structures of the kidney. The prognosis in malignant disease of the kidney seems not unfavourable.

Chronic capsulitis.—Chronic capsulitis is occasionally met with, and gives rise to most intense suffering, simulating stone, but without any of the other symptoms.

The most striking case of this I have seen was that of a West Highlander. He was admitted to the Western Infirmary suffering from the most intense pain, persistent and unrelieved by anything but opium. The kidney was explored with the expectation of finding a stone; instead of which the capsule was found to be much thickened, a mass of dense fibrous tissue a quarter of an inch thick enveloping the organ, and evidently restricting it, since on making a longitudinal incision the kidney immediately bulged through the gap. The greater portion of the capsule was therefore stripped off and removed, with a most satisfactory result.

I have since occasionally seen the same condition in a lesser degree, but have, unfortunately, not been able to diagnose it prior to an exploratory incision.

Abdominal tubercle.—There can be no doubt that the great bulk of tubercular disease in the abdomen is primarily due to intestinal lesions. These for the greater part will be found in the ileum or cæcum. I have found not infrequently a solitary tuberculous ulcer in the ileum giving rise to localised tenderness and a tendency to slight colic, and a general want of vitality. Usually infection of the corresponding lymphatic glands takes place, and from these, or it may be directly from the primary focus, the germ may enter the peritoneal cavity, giving rise to the numerous manifestations with which we are all familiar. It has been a matter of interest to observe the frequency with which one finds tubercle of the peritoneum without any symptoms.   Thus, in the course of operating for a radical cure of hernia we have in four cases, one a young adult and the others children, found well-marked miliary tubercle.

The amount of good to be derived from laparotomy must still remain *sub judice,* but on the whole I am satisfied that good is obtained where the whole peritoneum can be reached by lavage, particularly so in cases where there is effusion.   Where extensive adhesions exist the efficacy of the treatment is more questionable, though it has been my practice—and I have seen no cause to regret it—to remove all tuberculous foci, freely dissecting away the thickened omentum, and in many cases dissecting out all the tuberculous glands in the mesentery. That this can be done with great advantage was well illustrated in a case which I recorded to the Eastern Medical Society many years ago.   It was that of a child sent to me by the late Dr. Lindsay Steven and Dr. Mathie.   In the opinion of Dr. Steven the case was quite hopeless if allowed to pursue its course, and in consultation we determined to try the effect of laparotomy. The temperature had been ranging nightly to 103°, and the abdomen was much distended.   We found fluid in the peritoneal cavity, and slight tuberculous infection in the peritoneum.   The most striking feature, however, was the extraordinary extent of glandular involvement in the mesentery of the small intestine. These glands were caseated, and a number of them fluctuant. Commencing on the ileo-cæcal valve, we patiently dissected out all the affected glands in the mesentery, amounting in all to about two small bowlfuls.   The numerous holes so created were sutured, and after the operation it was found that the circulation of the intestine had not been appreciably interfered with. The child made a good recovery, and within three months, with an apparently normal abdomen, looked as robust and vigorous as a child could.

Her subsequent history, however, was rather unfortunate, as, about two years afterwards, she had an intestinal obstruction owing to an adhesion.   She was again under my care, and collapsed after her operation, but we had an opportunity of observing that except for a few glands in the gastro-hepatic omentum there were little evidences of tubercle.   Since then I have frequently had occasion to remove masses of tuberculous glands, and I do so without fear of interfering with the circulation. Indeed, comparatively little blood may be lost if one selects the side of the mesentery where the bulk of the gland projects. Thus one gland will come more readily from the posterior, another from the anterior, side. No doubt tuberculous glands in the mesentery may be spontaneously recovered from. Every surgeon is familiar with the frequency with which he finds calcareous glands; on the other hand, it is very certain that such glands may overdose the patient, and determine a general and fatal tuberculosis.

Calcareous glands in the mesentery.—It is also to be borne in mind that calcareous glands themselves not infrequently give rise to marked abdominal discomfort. Sooner or later the gland ulcerates through the peritoneum, acts as a mechanical irritant, and gives rise to reflex disturbance and even to local irritation, which may simulate lesions of other organs. Quite frequently I have seen such a gland giving rise to pains and tenderness in the appendix region, the innocent appendix being removed in the hope of relieving the symptoms. Comparatively recently such a gland simulated in two cases ureteral colic; and our suspicion of a stone appeared to be confirmed by a skiagram, except that two shadows were present. Dr. Riddell, who kindly made the photographs for me, suggested the true origin of the shadow, which we confirmed by operation, dissecting from the surface of the right ureter the calcareous mass, which had become incorporated with the outer wall of the tube. There is no doubt that relief can be obtained from troublesome symptoms by the free removal of such calcareous masses.

Intestinal surgery: A. Stomach.—The anterior wall of the stomach is for the greater part hidden under the ribs, only a portion near the pylorus being in a normal individual palpable, this varying somewhat according to the distension of the organ, and being greater in some individuals in whom a degree of gastroptosis exists.

This hidden condition of the stomach is a most important consideration in the diagnosis of tumours and ulcerations, since many of these are absolutely beyond the reach of palpation, and must be diagnosed by means other than physical signs.

Also, I must remind you that this hollow viscus is furnished with an outlet, the pylorus, a muscular ring with a sphincter action, and that the condition of this muscular ring is of vast significance, as great as that of the other sphincters of the body whose powerful influence in the etiology of disease is frankly and freely recognised.

The pylorus presents many degrees of contraction and many variations in its muscular activity, and like other sphincters may be influenced by causes outwith the organ itself. Just as we have in infancy a spasm of the sphincter of the bladder induced by peripheral irritation, so dilatation of the stomach from undue retention of its contents may be due, not to a rigid organically contracted pyloric ring, but to disordered sphincter action; and, as in one case recently under observation in the Western Infirmary, apparently to a disordered peristaltic wave of the duodenum, since with extreme dilatation of the stomach we found a dilated duodenum and a sphincter so wide that we could with ease introduce three fingers. In that particular case I believe we had to deal with an interesting congenital adhesion, extending from the whole length of the gall-bladder to the duodenum. As you are aware, considerable attention has been recently paid to such adhesions in connection with the colon as a cause of peristaltic disorders, and I venture to suggest that this congenital adhesion band does in some cases cause peristaltic disorder at the pylorus, and, as I know from experience, in the gall-bladder and its ducts. The cardiac orifice is guarded by a sphincter, but this is of less surgical importance than that of the outlet. In development we may have to deal with complete occlusion of the pylorus, and a degree of insufficiency is by no means uncommon. A vomiting baby means not infrequently dyspepsia in later life.

The pancreas lies for the greater part behind the body of the stomach, and is liable therefore to be implicated by perforating ulcer of the posterior wall.

(*To be continued.*)

CASE OF COMPLETE AURICULO–VENTRICULAR HEART–BLOCK.*

By GEO. A. ALLAN, M.B., Ch.B.,

Senior Assistant to the Professor of Medicine, University of Glasgow ;
Dispensary Physician, Western Infirmary.

THIS case was under observation in the Western Infirmary from 27th January till 13th May, 1914, being sent by Dr. Laurie, of Greenock, to be under the care of Professor Monro, who kindly allowed me to investigate and report on the condition. The patient was a man, aged 39 years, a riveter to trade, and gave the following history :—

One forenoon, about seven months previously, when he was at his work, and apparently in his usual health, he fell down in a faint, but quickly regained consciousness, and was able to walk about till dinner time. On reaching home he went to bed, had fainting fits in rapid succession, and remembered nothing till next morning. A few days later he was removed to Greenock Infirmary, where he remained four weeks, and had fainting fits every day. After dismissal he was on holiday for a time, but got worse, and returned to the Infirmary in October, 1913, where he remained till 10th January, 1914. After the second week of this residence he had no fits.

In these fainting fits he lost consciousness for a few seconds, and occasionally his left hand was seen to shake, but he had no general convulsion. Posture did not seem to influence the liability to attacks, as they came on as frequently when he was in bed as when he was moving about.

These attacks, we have reason to believe, were associated with the inception of a new and very slow ventricular rhythm, dependent on a complete auriculo-ventricular heart-block.

During his residence in the Greenock Infirmary, I am informed, his pulse-rate ranged between 24 and 30 per

* Paper read and patient shown at a meeting of the Medico-Chirurgical Society of Glasgow held on 1st May, 1914.

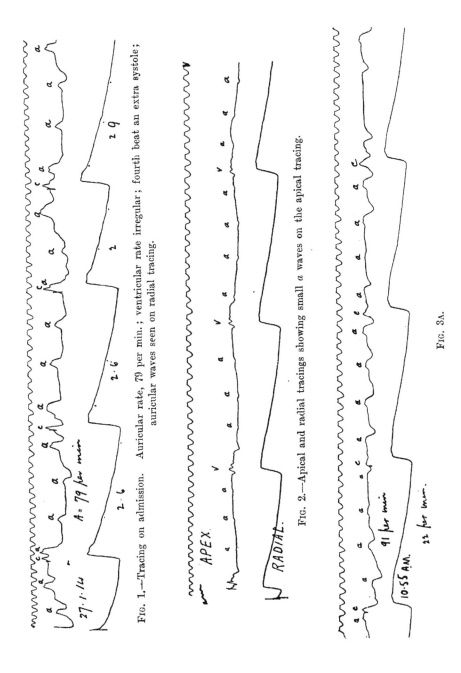

FIG. 1.—Tracing on admission. Auricular rate, 79 per min.; ventricular rate irregular; fourth beat an extra systole; auricular waves seen on radial tracing.

FIG. 2.—Apical and radial tracings showing small *a* waves on the apical tracing.

FIG. 3A.

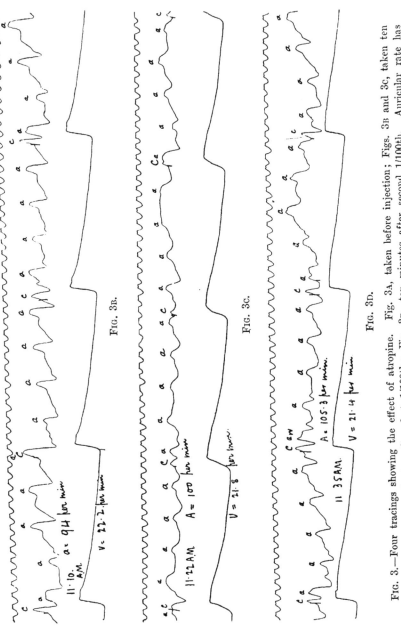

FIG. 3.—Four tracings showing the effect of atropine. Fig. 3A, taken before injection; Figs. 3B and 3C, taken ten and twenty-two minutes after first 1/100th; Fig. 3D, ten minutes after second 1/100th. Auricular rate has increased from 91 to over 105, while ventricular rate is practically unaltered.

FIG. 3B.

FIG. 3C.

FIG. 3D.

minute, and our own records gave a range of 20 to 40. He had been seen by doctors shortly before this illness, and no abnormally slow pulse was noted. While it is probable that there was some auriculo-ventricular dissociation before this time, the block evidently became complete at the time the first fainting fit came on. The fits were quite frequent during the earlier months and quite absent during the later months he was under observation, although there is no essential difference in the pulse records in the two periods. This is most likely to be explained by the gradual, development of compensatory vasomotor control allowing of a more steady supply of blood to the vital centres in the medulla. Had his pulse been much under 20 (although there is no record of it), we might have expected to have had other manifestations of the Stokes-Adams syndrome, such as general convulsions, but these were absent.

His previous health is of importance. He had disease of his occipital bone and of one of his metacarpals when a child, rheumatism at the age of 28, pleurisy at 36, and a venereal sore at the age of 39. This last was followed by secondary symptoms, but he only carried out treatment for five weeks. His blood was examined for the Wassermann reaction, with positive result, and a luetin test, undertaken by Dr. M'Nee, was also distinctly positive. Further, when in hospital he developed an iritis, and Dr. Inglis Pollock, who was asked to see him, diagnosed a corneo-iritis of syphilitic origin, and a week later gummata appeared in the iris. The evidence of syphilis is thus quite clear. During his residence he developed a slight pleural effusion; his urine remained non-albuminous throughout. .

Circulatory system.—His pulse-rate at first averaged about 24 per minute, but latterly kept nearer 30. There was distinct pulsation in the neck and in the suprasternal fossa. In the latter situation it could be counted with fair accuracy, and on admission numbered about 74 per minute. His heart was slightly enlarged to the left, and the apex beat, though usually palpable, was not specially forcible. Feeble impulses could often be felt at the apex following the ordinary cardiac impulse, and were so definite that the student reporting the case thought they were feeble ventricular contractions. The heart's sounds were pure, but the first at the apex was rather soft. The auricular sounds were audible at the apex, being heard as dull, single sounds in the diastolic interval. They became much more evident when the patient received atropine. Systolic blood pressure was 125 mm. of mercury, and the diastolic was 55 mm., estimated by the auscultatory method.

With the polygraph one had no difficulty in getting tracings showing the complete dissociation of auricular and ventricular contractions. Tracing Fig. 1 (p. 184) was taken on the day of admission, and shows ventricular cycles occupying from 2 seconds to 2·9 seconds, corresponding to rates of from 30 to 20·3 per minute, while the auricle is seen to beat fairly regularly at about 79 per minute. On the radial tracing small undulations are visible, corresponding in time to the auricular contractions. Similar waves are seen on the tracing from the apex (Fig. 2, p. 184).

On one occasion I tried the effect of injections of atropine in removing vagal inhibition. Although the patient had been having atropine drops for his eyes for ten days, the effect of the drug is quite striking. The auricular rate was distinctly accelerated, while the ventricle continued to beat at the same slow rate. Before injection the auricular rate was 91, and the ventricular was 22. In twenty-two minutes, after getting $\frac{1}{100}$th of a grain, the auricular rate was 100, and the ventricular was 21·8. Another $\frac{1}{100}$th was then injected, and the auricular rate rose to 105·3, while the ventricular rate was unaltered, or a little less. From the tracings (Fig. 3, pp. 184, 185) it can be easily seen that whereas in the first the apices of four a waves appear between successive c waves, in the last five a waves appear in that space.

The question of the action of atropine in increasing the contractility of the auricles is raised by Ritchie,[1] and it is interesting to note in this connection that after the injections the auricular sounds became much more evident than previously, and, in addition, the waves on the jugular tracing were more prominent than at any other time, though one would not have laid much stress on this latter point alone.

The heart was also examined by the x-rays. The movements were well seen. With the patient in the dorso-ventral position, one could see the ventricle slowly distending in the left lower portion of the shadow. This distension was not continuous, but was interrupted two or three times by additional slight impulses, and was terminated very abruptly by the contraction of the ventricle. These slight impulses correspond no doubt to the small waves seen on the apical tracings, and are to be referred to the additional force exerted on the inflowing blood by the contracting auricle. In the right lower portion of the shadow right auricular pulsation was distinctly visible, but was not so easy to count as the ventricular. It presented more an undulatory movement, three or four times faster than the ventricular contractions. In the left upper region the movement could not be analysed with any degree of accuracy. One was thus able to corroborate the previous observations that the auricle was beating at a rate much more rapid than the ventricle.

In the great majority of cases of heart-block which have been examined *post-mortem*, a definite lesion has been demonstrable in the auriculo-ventricular connecting bundle sufficient to destroy its conductivity, and so cut off the ventricle from stimuli coming from the auricle by way of the auriculo-ventricular node in that muscle. There are, however, a few cases on record in which no lesion has been found, and these await an explanation.

Apart from the acute infections, such as diphtheria and septicæmia, sclerotic processes and gummata occupy a prominent place among the lesions found. This patient had syphilis, and the fact that full doses of iodides produced no effect on his condition does not negative the possibility of a syphilitic process too far advanced, or of a nature not to be influenced by iodides. On the other hand, he also had rheumatism, and although there are no gross endocardial lesions, one must recognise the fact that the myocardium may suffer alone.

Thus, while the clinical condition is easy to recognise, the exact pathological diagnosis is matter for speculation.

REFERENCE.

[1] W. T. Ritchie, *Auricular Flutter*, 1914.

SERIES OF SIX CASES OF LUMBAR NEPHRECTOMY AND ONE CASE OF RESECTION FOR RENAL VARIX.*

By DAVID NEWMAN, M.D.,

Surgeon, Glasgow Royal Infirmary.

I. Three cases of pyonephrosis, two of which were calculous; II. Aneurysm of renal artery occupying the renal pelvis; III. Hypernephroma; IV. Renal carcinoma; V. Renal varix in which resection was performed.

I.—*Three cases of pyonephrosis, two of which were calculous.*

1. *Calculous pyonephrosis of the right kidney—Renal colic —Enlargement of kidney—X-ray shadow—Pus from right ureter—Lumbar nephrectomy—Cure.*

The patient, T. H., aged 29 years, was admitted to the Glasgow Royal Infirmary on 14th November, 1913. He had been in the Edinburgh Royal Infirmary in May, 1907, when the late Professor Annandale opened a large pyonephrosis in the right kidney, and removed a calculus; the pyonephrosis remained open for a considerable time thereafter. The patient was admitted to the Glasgow Royal Infirmary in March, 1912, still suffering from pyuria, and on cystoscopic examination shoots of pus were seen emerging from the right ureter only. The patient was advised to have the kidney removed, but he refused the operation and left the hospital of his own accord. Since then the urine has always contained a considerable amount of pus, and has a strong alkaline reaction, and during the last two years the patient's general health has materially deteriorated. Pain has also been present in the right renal region for the last two years, but it was never very severe until a few days prior to admission. At that time the symptoms became suddenly worse, and the pain

* These cases were demonstrated at a meeting of the Medico-Chirurgical Society of Glasgow, 6th March, 1914. Dr. Newman showed the cases and Dr. J. A. G. Burton exhibited the microscopic sections.

was so bad that the patient sought readmission to the Infirmary, and was anxious to have anything possible done for his relief. On admission both kidneys were easily palpable, but the right kidney was more enlarged than the left, and considerable tenderness existed over the right kidney. On cystoscopic examination pus was observed issuing from the right ureter, while the urine from the left kidney was normal in appearance. On bacteriological examination coliform bacilli and short streptococci were found. The *x*-ray photograph showed a shadow, probably a stone in ,the right kidney.

On 6th November, 1913, the right kidney was removed by lumbar nephrectomy, which showed the whole organ to have been destroyed and replaced by a sac of pus. A large phosphatic stone occupied the pelvis. The patient made a good recovery, and two days after the operation the urine was free from pus.

9th January, 1914.—The patient reported himself to-day. The urine is normal. The patient feels much better in general health, and his appearance is greatly improved. The wound is closed.

2. *Calculous pyonephrosis with discharging sinus—Renal colic, pyuria—No enlargement of kidney—Pus from right ureter—X-ray shadow—Lumbar nephrectomy—Cure.*

E. A., aged 43 years, was admitted to Glasgow Royal Infirmary on 30th October, 1913, suffering from pyonephrosis and calculus. He complained of pain over the region of the right kidney of six years' duration, but about three weeks ago it became very severe. In the Western Infirmary about ten years ago a stone weighing $3\frac{1}{4}$ oz. was removed from the right kidney, and also a part of the kidney itself which was said to be diseased. (This is the patient's statement.) Twelve months ago a vesical calculus was extracted in the Western Infirmary by the suprapubic route, and the patient was advised not to have the kidney removed, though he desired to get rid of it on account of the pain and pyuria. The patient was admitted to the Royal Infirmary complaining of severe pain and of the continual annoyance of a discharging sinus from the right kidney. The urine contained much pus and some blood. At times, he says, the urine is quite clear, and when it is so there is severe pain in the right loin radiating to the front of the abdomen. When the urine becomes turbid, again the pain passes off; when he walks about the quantity of blood is increased, and the urine becomes more turbid. There is also frequent micturition, but there is no rigidity of the abdominal wall, although there is some tenderness on pressure over the right kidney, which, however, being diminished in size, is not palpable.

6th November, 1913.—The patient had very severe pain over the right kidney, which demanded the administration of morphia. A cystoscopic examination showed the pus to be coming from the right kidney only, and there was a distinct x-ray shadow. On pressure over the right kidney pus could be made to escape from the right ureter, while the urine escaping from the left was normal.

9th November.—The right kidney was removed through a lumbar incision, and the organ found almost completely destroyed. It was cystic, and contained a number of phosphatic stones, and a considerable quantity of pus.

9th December.—The wound was now practically healed, there was no discharge, and the patient was considerably improved in general health.

6th February, 1914.—The patient reported himself to-day. The wound is perfectly healed and he is about to resume his work.

3. *Pyonephrosis of the left kidney—Great enlargement of kidney—Nephrotomy and drainage—Pyuria and hæmaturia—Pus from left ureter only—Lumbar nephrectomy—Cure.*

D. M'I., aged 28 years, was admitted to the Glasgow Royal Infirmary on 18th October, 1913, complaining of a swelling in the abdomen, which she first noticed a week before admission, but it must have been present long before. On examination a large swelling occupied the left side and front of the abdomen, extending from the left lumbar region to $3\frac{1}{2}$ inches to the right of the umbilicus, and in the middle line from $5\frac{3}{4}$ inches above to $3\frac{1}{2}$ inches below the umbilicus. The swelling was fluctuant, tense, elastic and movable, dull on percussion, but with an area giving a tympanitic note between the swelling and the pubes. Uterus was normal. The left ovary enlarged. Abundant pyuria and slight hæmaturia. Right ureteral opening very small, but the shoots coming from it were clear. The left ureteral opening was large, the lips thickened, and large shoots of pus were seen to escape slowly from it.

On 26th October, 1913, nephrotomy was performed, evacuating 80 oz. of pus, and drainage was continued until the patient was readmitted on 13th January, 1914. The general condition of the patient was so poor at the time of the first operation that it was not considered advisable to remove the kidney. After drainage for two and a half months patient was readmitted, and the left kidney was cut down on by a lumbar incision and the large pyonephrotic sac was removed.

31st January, 1914.—The large cavity from which the kidney was removed has not yet closed, but the discharge has steadily become less, so that now the patient is able to be out of bed and is looking well.

24th February.—Wound is closing up well, and the patient has gained in weight, but still there is some little discharge from the sinus.

27th February.—Dismissed well.

II.—*Aneurysm of renal artery occupying the renal pelvis— Hæmaturia at first slight, afterwards severe—Little pain— Plugging of left ureter with clot—Severe hæmorrhage—Lumbar nephrectomy—Cure.*

A. M., aged 52 years, was admitted to the Glasgow Royal Infirmary on 7th January, 1914. When first seen on 31st July, 1913, he complained of hæmaturia of four days' duration. He had suffered from frequency of micturition for some years previously, but no difficulty or pain in passing urine. Four days ago the urine became very red in colour, and he passed clots of blood at every act. He had pain at times, caused by obstruction, but this soon passed off when the clot of blood had escaped. At all other times he had no pain. His frequency became more and more marked, and he passed a very little urine at a time. He had no difficulty and no pain except when a clot passed into the urethra, but there has been some discomfort in the lumbar region. The patient was admitted for a few days in October, 1913, but beyond a slight hyperæmia of the floor of the bladder the cystoscope failed to discover anything abnormal. There was some enlargement of the prostate, but no hæmaturia was noticed while the cystoscopic examination was being made.

7th January, 1914.—Since October last the patient has had no bleeding until 2nd January, 1914, when he noticed the urine slightly red. Then it became redder, and that night some clots came away. He had very little pain when these clots were being passed—only discomfort in the abdomen immediately above the symphysis pubis. This was present only occasionally, and preceded the hæmaturia. For the first few days after admission the urine was quite red, but on 9th January it was again clear. On 11th January the urine was clear, but contained blood on the 12th, and this was preceded by pain over the pubes. On two occasions attempts were made to use the cystoscope, but a good view could not be obtained on account of the bleeding, and only masses of clot occupying the floor of the bladder were seen.

On 9th January another attempt was made at cystoscopic examination, a large quantity of blood being washed out, also many clots. Ultimately the fluid coming away was quite clear, and, on examination, the opening of the left ureter was seen to be plugged with a considerable blood clot.

On 16th January the bladder was again washed out without difficulty, and a good view was obtained. The opening of the left ureter was dilated, and on an assistant pressing the left kidney between the hands shoots of blood were observed entering the bladder. If much pressure was exercised the quantity of blood escaping became very copious, and was in direct proportion to the amount of pressure employed.

17th January.—Last night, just after passing urine, which was highly coloured with blood, the patient felt that his bladder was again full, and he passed about two pints of what looked to the house surgeon like pure blood. On account of the extent of the hæmorrhage the kidney was at once exposed and removed, and, on examination, the pelvis was found to be occupied by an aneurysm of the renal artery completely filling the cavity.

After the operation the patient was very collapsed, and saline had to be administered intravenously, and later on *per rectum.* At the operation very little blood was lost, but the severe hæmorrhage preceding it greatly exhausted the patient.

18th January.—Ninety oz. of urine passed. On the 19th January, 66 oz., and it was clear, containing no blood.

Patient made an uninterrupted recovery. The Wassermann reaction was negative.

It is interesting to note that this aneurysm of the artery involves a portion of the vessel after it has entered the kidney. The pelvis of the organ was found completely filled by the aneurysm, the walls of which pressed upon and were adherent to the mucous membrane of the pelvis. In most cases of aneurysm of the renal artery the sac is outside of the kidney, and, of course, in such instances hæmaturia is not a necessary accompaniment of the disease.

III.—*Hypernephroma of the left kidney—Hœmaturia from left kidney for five weeks, soon followed by great enlargement of kidney—Lumbar nephrectomy—Good recovery.*

J. A., aged 42 years, was admitted to the Glasgow Royal Infirmary on 13th November, 1913, suffering from a large hypernephroma. He complained of pain in the left flank and back for about six weeks prior to admission. He had pain at the beginning and end of micturition, and had difficulty in starting the flow of urine. Five weeks ago he noticed blood in his urine, and this condition has prevailed until within six days. Since then he has not noticed any blood. There is marked tenderness over the left flank, but no distinct swelling can be detected. The urine is acid; specific gravity, 1012; clear and transparent; contains no deposit and no blood. Cystoscopic examination showed some hyperæmia of the bladder; there is a curious scoop-shaped area of whitish colour just below the right ureter orifice, and there are slight papilliform projections at the neck of the bladder.

21st November, 1913.—Guinea-pig inoculated; killed, and found normal.

1st December.—Patient was readmitted to-day. A distinct enlargement of the left kidney was discovered for the first time. Hæmaturia is now present, but on cystoscopic examination nothing can be discovered in the bladder to account for it.

12th December.—Hæmaturia this morning was very slight. The bladder was washed out without difficulty. At the base of the bladder, attached to the area around the orifice of the left ureter, there was a mass of material, which may be discoloured blood-clot, or may be a tumour.——It extends from the left margin of the trigone across the middle line almost to the orifice of the right ureter. The left part of this mass appears like a miniature coil of intestine which has become deeply congested, whereas the right aspect of the swelling is rounded like the upper surface of a mushroom. Through the centre of this mushroom-shaped swelling there is a deep cleft as if it had been torn. It is difficult to say at the present examination whether this is a blood clot or a tumour. The patient is to be examined again in a few days. The patient states that he has a slight pain prior to the onset of hæmaturia, but as soon as blood appears the discomfort in the left renal region subsides. The difficulty of diagnosis in this case is between a tumour of the bladder obstructing the exit from the left ureter and a tumour of the left kidney with clot adhering to the base of the bladder, a portion of which has become discoloured.

13th December.—Another cystoscopic examination made to-day; the mass which was described yesterday is found to have disappeared, showing that it was simply an adherent blood clot.

15th December.—The left kidney, which was now much enlarged, was removed by lumbar nephrectomy. A large nodulated tumour involving the cortex, but not the part round the pelvis, was found occupying the kidney. On account of the shortness of the renal vessels it was considered advisable to clamp them rather than to trust to a ligature. The forceps was removed ten days later.

16th January, 1914.—The patient was dismissed well. The tumour, on microscopic examination, proved to be hyper-nephroma.

IV.—*Renal carcinoma—Severe hæmaturia from left kidney —No x-ray shadow—Little pain—Lumbar nephrectomy.*

The history was that of severe renal hæmaturia for ten days, with several less severe attacks during the previous six months. The patient was admitted to the Regent Home on 5th November, 1913, suffering from very profuse hæmaturia and some pain over the left kidney, and there was a distinct increase in the size of the organ.

The patient was poorly nourished, pale, and looked thoroughly ill, though he complained very little of bad health. A cysto- scopic examination showed the blood to be flowing from the left ureter only. There was no shadow in the *x*-ray plate and no pyuria. Temperature febrile, pulse rapid, patient weak on account of loss of blood. It was therefore decided to operate as early as possible, and on 12th November the left kidney was explored through a lumbar incision and was found to be occupied by a large carcinoma. The kidney was removed, and for some time the patient made a very satisfactory recovery.

The wound healed and his general condition improved, but about three weeks after the operation his temperature again became febrile, although there was no discharge from the wound and nothing local to indicate the cause of the tempera- ture. A careful examination made by Dr. George S. Middleton failed to discover anything in the chest or abdomen, but still the temperature continued to oscillate—normal in the mornings and febrile in the afternoons. The patient took his food moderately well, but while in the Home seemed to remain very much at a standstill. The wound was practically healed, and he returned home on 22nd December.

V.—*Renal varix — Hæmaturia — Kidney enlarged and movable—No x-ray shadow—Shoots of blood from left ureter —Nephrorrhaphy without improvement—Resection—Cure.*

The patient was admitted to the Glasgow Royal Infirmary on 13th October, 1913, complaining of hæmaturia of three weeks' duration. The hæmaturia began while the patient was at work. It began painlessly, and continued so, except upon two occasions when he felt considerable discomfort in the left kidney and passing across to the right lumbar region.

The first attack of this pain was two days after the onset of the hæmaturia, and the second attack two weeks later. When lying in bed the patient's abdominal muscles appeared rigid, so that palpation failed to reveal any enlargement of the kidneys, and an *x*-ray plate did not give a shadow either over the renal region or the bladder. The urine was dark red, and blood was intimately mixed with it. Reaction acid, and specific gravity 1018. No pus, and no organisms present.

13th October, 1913.—Cystoscopic examination shows the line of the left ureter to be marked by a very distinct ridge, and about the centre of this ridge the mouth of the ureter appears as a wide oval opening with pouting lips. While watching for a few seconds, a large shoot of almost pure blood was thrown from the ureter into the bladder. This was repeated time after time. The orifice of the right ureter is normal. Under the anæsthetic the left kidney is easily palpable, and found to be slightly enlarged and unduly mobile.

27th October.—Lumbar exploration was performed, and the left kidney found to be very dark red in colour from congestion. There was very little enlargement, but the range of movement was greater than normal, and it was thought that the hæmaturia was the result of obstruction of the renal vessels, caused by the displaced kidney. Nephrorrhaphy was therefore performed, the kidney being fixed by sutures at the lower pole, and the wound was packed with gauze.

28th October.—Hæmaturia still continues as before; no diminution in the amount.

2nd November.—Hæmaturia being undiminished, the nephrorrhaphy wound was opened up and the kidney exposed in the loin. On account of the traction on the vessels, the artery probably being twisted while the vein was free, the parenchyma of the kidney was very anæmic, so that when an incision was made from pole to pole to expose the whole cavity of the pelvis, very little bleeding occurred. The kidney was enlarged, but at the lower pole two pyramids (the second and third from the lower pole) were found to be of a dark purple-red colour, and this colouration extended from the apex of the pyramid to within a quarter of an inch of the capsule. The mucous membrane at this point was very deeply congested, and while the epithelium appeared to be intact, it was studded over by innumerable "granulations," giving the surface the appearance of a raspberry, except that the individual "seeds" were extremely small, none being larger than half the size of a mustard seed. The kidney measured $5\frac{3}{4}$ inches from pole to pole. Of that $1\frac{1}{4}$ inch was removed from the lower pole, including the varix, the diseased mucous membrane, and a large adventitious artery which supplied the lower portion of the kidney. The cut surfaces of the kidney were united by mattress sutures, three being introduced to keep the longitudinal section together. The lower incision, namely, that by which the varix was removed, was sutured both by mattress sutures and continuous superficial sutures. All the sutures were loosely tied so as not to exert undue pressure on the renal substance, and so avoid cutting. The muscular edges were brought together by a row of interrupted sutures, and the skin united by continuous sutures.

4th November (evening).—Since last operation the quantity of blood present has been increased; but later to-day it suddenly diminished, and now is very small in amount.

Three days after the operation blood disappeared from the urine, and the patient was dismissed on the 21st November, 1913, and has remained well.

Obituary.

JAMES DUNCAN FARQUHARSON, M.B., C.M. Glasg.,
NEWCASTLE.

WE regret to announce the death of Dr. J. D. Farquharson, which took place in Newcastle on 27th July. Dr. Farquharson, who was born at Perth in 1858, studied medicine at Glasgow University, and in 1884 took the degrees of M.B., C.M., with commendation. Though thus distinguished in his professional curriculum, he also found time to distinguish himself both in athletics and in journalistic work. After his graduation he built up a large practice in the West End of Newcastle, and also became a conspicuous figure in the public life of the town, being in 1897 elected a member of its Council. He was a keen Volunteer, and afterwards a keen Territorial officer, and at the time of his death was Major in the Royal Army Medical Corps (Territorial Force). He was a Fellow of the Edinburgh Obstetrical Society, and among other appointments he held those of Commissioner on the Immigration Board for the Tyne ports, and joint secretary of the Northumberland and Durham Medical Society. His death, at the comparatively early age of fifty-six, will be widely regretted both by the laity and by his professional colleagues.

DAVID YOUNG, M.D. Glasg.,
PARKHEAD.

WE regret to announce the death of Dr. David Young, which occurred at his residence on 3rd August. Dr. Young, who studied medicine at the University of Glasgow, took the degrees of M.B., C.M., in 1872, and that of M.D. three years later. Settling in the East End of Glasgow he rapidly acquired an extensive practice there, and became one of the best known of its practitioners. His death, which took place in his sixty-seventh year, will be mourned by many who were both his patients and his friends.

CURRENT TOPICS.

UNIVERSITY OF GLASGOW: GRADUATION IN MEDICINE.—A special final examination in medicine for those who had completed their course of study, and desired to volunteer for active service, was held in the University on 12th August and the following days. Twenty-two candidates offered themselves, and of these, nineteen were successful. The results were announced on the afternoon of the 15th, and thereafter the degrees of M.B., Ch.B., were conferred on the successful candidates by the Vice-Chancellor, Principal Sir Donald MacAlister. The graduation took place in the Senate Room, in the presence of a small company consisting of the examiners and a few friends of the graduands. At the close of the ceremony, the Vice-Chancellor addressed those on whom degrees had been conferred in the following terms :—

"The University, recognising the national emergency which has unhappily come upon us, has sought by every means in its power to make it easier for you to serve your country, as you propose to do, in the medical profession. We wish you god-speed whatever enterprise you may have to undertake for the good of your fellow-countrymen. We hope and believe that as doctors you will never forget that the honour of the University is in your hands, and that you will not only maintain it but advance it. I would remind those of you who are about to serve your country in the field, that your work extends not only to the wounded of your own side but to those of the other side also. It is incumbent upon you as physicians and surgeons to do all you can to alleviate suffering, and to preserve the life of friend or of foe. I speak with feeling on this subject, because only to-day I have returned from the seat of war. I passed through the ranks of thousands of soldiers, and personally as a physician, but largely because I am Principal of this University, I met with nothing but kindness, courtesy, and helpfulness at a time of very great difficulty and stress. As members of the medical profession you are non-combatants and helpers of all your fellowmen, though some may meantime be technically your foes. The Senate, small in numbers, but representing, I am perfectly sure, the feeling of all members of the University, sends you forth to your work with prayers that all may be well with you."

The following gentlemen received the degrees of M.B., Ch.B. :—

With honours.—Archibald Munn M'Cutcheon.

With commendation.—Andrew Picken (distinction in midwifery), William Semple Wallace (distinction in surgery and clinical surgery), Joseph Bannister Williamson, B.Sc.

Ordinary degree.—Edmund Tytler Burke, John Eglinton Cameron, Thomas Ingram Dun, James Jackson Findlay, Allan Dumbreck Fraser, M.A., B.Sc., Robert Masson Greig, Fergus Leslie Henderson, Alastair Caulfield Jebb, Douglas Reid King, George M'Callum, Joseph M'Culloch, David Mackie, John Percival Moir, John Stuart Prentice, James Vallance.

THE ROYAL COLLEGES OF PHYSICIANS AND SURGEONS : DIPLOMA IN PUBLIC HEALTH.— After passing the required examinations, the following, amongst other gentlemen, received, on 30th July, Diplomas in Public Health from the Royal Colleges of Physicians and of Surgeons of England:—William Henry M'Kinstry, M.B., C.M.Glasg. (1887); Hyacinth Bernard Wenceslaus Morgan, M.B., Ch.B. Glasg. (1909); and William David Henderson Stevenson (Capt., I.M.S.), M.B., Ch.B. Glasg. (1903).

Diplomas of L.R.C.P. and M.R.C.S. were conferred upon 97 candidates, among whom was John Bowman Hunter, B.A. Cantab., of Ayr.

THE TRIPLE QUALIFICATION.—At the quarterly examination of the Royal College of Physicians of Edinburgh, Royal College of Surgeons of Edinburgh, and Royal Faculty of Physicians and Surgeons of Glasgow, held in Glasgow, and concluded on 25th July, the following candidates, having passed the final examination, were admitted L.R.C.P.E., L.R.C.S.E., and L.R.F.P. & S.G. :—

Laurence Fraser, Shetland; Richard Bridge Lilly, Tynemouth; George Loudon Neil, Lesmahagow; Rona Lockhart, Nitshill; Sengarapillai Ponniah, Ceylon; Andrew Crawford, Glasgow; John William Cowie, Tillicoultry; John Gilchrist, Glasgow; George Frederick Walker, Southport; John Rennie Carrie Gordon, Whiteinch; Andrew Wilson Cochrane, Glasgow; Abraham Isaac Clarke, Belfast; Babu Singh Thakur, India; Cyril Armand Bernard, Liverpool; Cyril Gray, County Durham; David Winthrop Woodruff, Glasgow.

At the quarterly examination held in Edinburgh, and concluded on 17th July, the following candidates were admitted to the same degrees :—

Joseph Kendrick Venables, Christchurch, New Zealand; Kenneth Grant Fraser, Scotland; Thomas Ebenezer Lawson, Coventry; David Charteris Graham, Darjeeling, India; Robert M'Cheyne Paterson, Punjab; Reginald Ernest Illingworth, Edinburgh; John Miller Chrystie, Dumfries; Edward Claude Brooks, Karachi, India; Robert Ryland Whitaker, Edinburgh; William Millerick, Co. Cork; Jan Martinus Beyers, South Africa; Walter Chapman, British Guiana; Theunis Botha Trutor, Cape Colony; and Joseph Vincent Duffy, Hebburn.

APPOINTMENT.—The following appointment has recently been made :—

William Wright, M.D.Glasg., to be Interim Medical Officer of Health for Glasgow, in the absence of Dr. A. K. Chalmers on active service.

GLASGOW ROYAL MATERNITY HOSPITAL.—A recent number of *The Nursing Times* gives great praise to the Glasgow Royal Maternity and Women's Hospital, which it says may be well described as the finest hospital in Great Britain. It considers that while it must be exceedingly encouraging to the directors to be able to record the fact that at a recent bazaar no less a sum than £16,000 was raised for the institution, there is another side to the picture, namely, that the whole of that large sum has had to be devoted towards wiping off the debt, and that there is still not enough money in hand to enable the directors to reopen the gynæcological wards. The necessity for doing this as soon as possible, as it points out, was emphasised by Lord Strathclyde and by Dr. Jardine at the recent annual meeting. For this purpose £1,000 annually is required. The hospital was built after visits had been paid to a number of British and Continental hospitals by a committee of doctors, who gave careful preliminary study to all the aspects of the question before building was begun. The result is a magnificent erection, with large, sunny, light, and airy labour wards, and an isolation block for septic cases and all necessary equipment. Patients are admitted from all over the West of Scotland. Last year 21,000 visits were paid to patients in their own homes by nurses and students. Nearly 1,500 cases were treated in the wards at the same time. The number of abnormal cases dealt with is very remarkable.

SUPPLY OF RADIUM: GLASGOW AND WEST OF SCOTLAND SCHEME.—In connection with the recent appeal for funds for the purchase of a central supply of radium for Glasgow and the West of Scotland, the committee, of which Sir John Stirling-Maxwell, Bart., is chairman, has to date received subscriptions amounting to over £7,300. In addition to this sum the Bellahouston Trustees have made a grant to the committee of £500 per annum for three years to secure the expense of custody and administration and afford a proper trial for the scheme, provided the future progress, in the Trustees' opinion, justifies the continuation of the grant. Arrangements have been made for the purchase of 600 milligrammes of radium, which will be ample for the committee's requirements in the meantime, and the University authorities have kindly placed a room in the University at the disposal of the committee. This room is in course of being fitted up as a radiometric laboratory under the supervision of Professor Frederick Soddy, F.R.S., and on his recommendation a very capable physical chemist has been appointed. Arrangements are in course of being completed with certain infirmaries and hospitals in the city for the treatment of patients with radium.

BRITISH MEDICAL ASSOCIATION.—The annual meeting of the British Medical Association, held this year at Aberdeen, will long be memorable to those who attended it, not only for its scientific value or for its social attractions, but for the contrast between the auspices under which it opened and those which attended its close. It began in sunshine; its last days were overshadowed by the imminent threat of European war. Events have moved so quickly since then, and future consequences of such magnitude now occupy our minds, that even to the participants the meeting must seem a distant yet a pleasant memory. This is not the place to dwell upon its scientific work, distinguished though it was; its record will be found in the *Journal* of the Association. It is, however, a duty and a pleasure to express to the profession, to the University, and to the city of Aberdeen the grateful thanks of those who were their guests, and in whose service and entertainment they spared themselves no trouble, and reaped every possible success. The arrangements must have been unusually difficult; Aberdeen was full of summer visitors, and it was the season of the annual holiday. Yet the reception committee triumphed over all difficulties, and many members have reason to be grateful to the private hospitality which was so liberally offered. Alike in indoor and outdoor entertainments, in receptions, garden parties, excursions, and sports, and in the weather which shone upon it, the meeting was brilliantly successful, and the fortunate members of the Association who were present will long look back upon it with pleasure that they were there, and with regret that it is not still to come.

CALEDONIAN MEDICAL SOCIETY.—The Caledonian Medical Society held their annual meeting on Friday, 24th July, in the rooms of the Royal Faculty of Physicians and Surgeons, Glasgow. Dr. J. T. Maclachlan was elected President for the current year; Dr. S. Rutherford Macphail, of Derby, was elected President-elect; Dr. W. A. Macnaughton and Dr. D. Rorie were re-elected Editors of the *Journal*.

Dr. Maclachlan, in his presidential address, dealt with the subject of the parasitic causation of disease. He stated that once the parasite or parasites of any given disease were discovered, and their habits ascertained, they could be destroyed with as much certainty as the wild beasts of the forest. It was only a question of money, and the appointment of expert men to devote their entire attention to such investigation. He advised men over 60 years of age, possessed of wealth, to subscribe £100,000 as their best insurance policy to the investigation of the parasite or parasites concerned in the causation of pneumonia, which was so fatal to elderly people. In his opinion, cancer would sooner or later disclose a parasitic origin. He appealed to the large cities to appoint at least one expert to devote his entire time to the elucidation of the cause of any single infectious disease, and predicted the final annihilation of all infectious diseases that afflict humanity.

PUBLIC HEALTH CONGRESS.—The congress of the Royal Institute of Public Health which sat in Edinburgh from 15th to 20th July, under the presidency of the Marquis of Linlithgow, was very largely attended by medical men and sanitary authorities from all parts of the kingdom. The subjects for discussion were divided into six sections — state medicine, bacteriology and comparative pathology, child welfare, industrial hygiene; naval, military, and colonial hygiene; and tuberculosis; and in most of these the opinion of the West of Scotland was well represented. The inaugural address of the Marquis of Linlithgow dealt with the means of spreading a sound knowledge of the operation of natural laws in the causation of disease, while Dr. Leslie Mackenzie's presidential address in the state medicine section discussed the problem of the control of tuberculosis, which, he said, was essentially the problem how to dissociate the tuberculous patient from the unfitted home. Among the contributions of special interest to Glasgow and the West of Scotland were papers by Professor Glaister, on the conservation of Scottish watershed areas, in which he dealt with Glasgow's water supply; by Dr. A. K. Chalmers, on the prevalence of diphtheria in Scotland in recent years; by Dr. Alexander Scott, on deformity as a cause of industrial disablement, in which he referred to Glasgow's bad eminence in the matter of rickets; by Dr. John C. M'Vail, on the relation of the National Insurance Act to public health administration; by Dr. Arbuckle Brown, on the nutrition of Glasgow children; by Dr. Trotter, on co-ordination in administrative method in dealing with infection and infant mortality; by Dr. J. T. Wilson, on the administrative control of tuberculosis in Lanarkshire; by Dr. A. S. M. Macgregor, on features in the

city incidence of tuberculosis; and by Mr. Harry J. Wilson, on physical deterioration in its relation to the industrial classes. Papers of outstanding interest were those of Sir Thomas Oliver, on the declining birth-rate; and of Professor von Pirquet, on bronchogenous,. placentogenous, and enterogenous infection with tuberculosis in infancy. The dinner of the congress, held on 17th July, was attended by a large number of distinguished members and guests.

HOUSING IN SCOTLAND.—The sixth annual conference of the National Association for the Prevention of Consumption and other forms of Tuberculosis, held at Leeds University in July, was particularly noteworthy to Scottish readers for its denunciation of the system of housing prevalent in the large towns of Scotland. The addresses of Sir William Younger, a member of the Royal Commission on Housing in Scotland, and of Sir Robert Philip, M.D., were unsparing in their condemnation of the conditions existing in Glasgow and Edinburgh. Sir William Younger said that the back lands of Glasgow had a widespread and sinister reputation. He had seen in Glasgow single-roomed or two-roomed ticketed houses, with defective ventilation, so dark that you could hardly see to read a paper at the back of the room, opening into a common lobby 20 ft. to 27 ft. long, itself without light or ventilation, and consequently foul and dirty. Let them imagine a consumptive patient sleeping in a dark enclosed bed, living in this "home" with several other members of the family, and they would realise something of the problem which confronted them. An inquiry was made into 2,500 actual cases of phthisis, and it was found that there were over 10,000 persons living in direct and intimate contact with them, not of course from choice, but from dire necessity. One and two apartment houses were responsible for 2,438 children and 4,813 adults being brought into direct and constant contact with 1,870 sufferers from phthisis. In the case of 1,166 patients the only bed available, in most cases the recess bed, an ideal breeding-ground for the tubercle bacillus, had to be shared with other members of the family. This resulted in over 1,600 persons actually occupying the same bed with their consumptive brother, or sister, or parent, or child, as the case might be. They must attack the abominable slum if they were ever to realise the hope which he had heard expressed that phthisis would one day be relegated to the list of maladies conquered and obliterated by the march of science.

Sir Robert Philip, dealing with the records and statistics accumulated by the Royal Victoria Hospital of Edinburgh during the past twenty-six years, said that time after time it had been found that tuberculosis had appeared in different families occupying successively the same house. He had notes of four such houses. In one street in Edinburgh every one of twenty-two rather ancient houses had yielded one or more cases of tuberculosis, and one house of four flats showed a record of thirty-six cases in eighteen families. A short street of nineteen modern houses yielded seventy-five cases, one house giving no fewer than eighteen cases. It was no uncommon thing to have ten or twelve cases from one particular house. He urged the importance of the training of fathers and mothers to rear healthy children, and persistent and well-directed efforts on the part of intelligent doctors and well-trained nurses who have the *entrée* into the houses where cases exist. Great possibilities attached to a well-directed system of skilled domiciliary visitation. The insanitary house must be condemned ruthlessly. It should constitute an offence to offer insanitary dwellings for occupation no less than to expose tainted milk or meat for human consumption.

THE " BRITISH PHARMACOPŒIA."—We have received an intimation from the Medical Council that in view of the outbreak of war, and possible changes arising out of it, the publication of the new edition of the *British Pharmacopœia* is indefinitely postponed.

THE WELLCOME RESEARCH LABORATORIES.—We have received from Messrs. Burroughs Wellcome & Co. descriptive catalogues of the exhibits shown by the Wellcome chemical and physiological research laboratories at the Anglo-American Exposition now open in London. The catalogues show how much valuable research work has already been done in these laboratories, and will greatly add to the value of an inspection of the exhibits themselves.

THE RIBERI PRIZE.—The Royal Academy of Medicine of Turin announces for competition the thirteenth Riberi Prize of 20,000 francs, to be awarded for research work in the medical sciences. Those who desire to send in researches in competition for the prize are requested to enrol their names by 31st December, 1916. Forms of enrolment may be had from the secretary of the Royal Academy of Medicine, 18 Via Po, Turin.

THE MEDICAL PROFESSION AND THE WAR.—The declaration of war was immediately followed by the embodiment of those members of the medical profession who were liable to be called up for active service. The Royal Army Medical Corps Officers of Field Ambulances and those attached to regiments embodied on Wednesday, 5th August, and before the week was well out all had gone on field service. Those members of the profession whose services were available on mobilisation were next sworn in, and will act as physicians and surgeons to the 3rd and 4th Scottish General Hospitals.

The medical arrangements for the Lowland Division are in the hands of the Assistant Director of Medical Services, Colonel D. J. Mackintosh, M.V.O., M.B., LL.D., with Lieut.-Colonel A. K. Chalmers, M.D., as Sanitary Officer, and Major G. St. C. Thom, M.B., R.A.M.C., as Staff Officer.

The following is a list of the officers of Field Ambulances and of those attached to regiments who are now on field service:—

Lowland Mounted Brigade Field Ambulance. — Lieut.-Colonel H. Wright Thomson, M.D., commanding; Major James Bruce, M.B.; Captains R. Yuill Anderson, M.B., Farquhar Gracie, M.B., Hugh Forrest, M.B., Andrew Ross Muir, M.B.

First Lowland Field Ambulance. — Lieut.-Colonel G. H. Edington, M.D., F.R.F.P.S., commanding; Captains W. Bryce, M.D., W. Cochrane Murray, M.B., and J. W. Leitch, M.B.; Lieutenants W. Ferguson Mackenzie, M.B., F.R.F.P.S., Neil M'Innes, M.B., A. D. Downer, M.B., W. C. Gunn, M.D., R. S. Taylor, M.B.; Quartermaster and Honorary Major James Kenny.

2nd Lowland Field Ambulance.—Lieut.-Colonel A. D. Moffat, M.D., commanding; Majors J. M'Kie, M.B., M. Dunning, M.B.; Captains W. Adam Burns, M.B., J. A. H. Aitken, M.B., D. Shannon, M.B., A. M. Watson, M.B.; Lieutenants W. H. Manson,

M.D., D. H. MacPhail, M.B.; Lieutenant and Quartermaster J. Macdonald.

R.A.M.C. Officers attached to Regiments:—

Lanarkshire Yeomanry.—Major H. Kelly, M.D.

3rd Lowland Brigade Royal Field Artillery.—Captain R. Bruce, M.B.

Scottish Rifles.—*5th Battalion,* Major F. V. Adams, F.R.F.P.S.; *6th Battalion,* Major J. L. Loudon, M.D.; *7th Battalion,* Major T. Forrest, M.B.; *8th Battalion,* Captain A. B. Sloan, M.D.

Highland Light Infantry.—*5th Battalion,* Lieutenant A. D. Kennedy, M.D.; *6th Battalion,* Lieutenant J. H. Martin, M.D.; *7th Battalion,* Captain P. M. Dewar, L.R.F.P.S.; *9th Battalion,* Captain T. Douglas Brown, M.D.

By a far-seeing arrangement, the military authorities have secured that when the Territorial Force is mobilised the services of civilian physicians and surgeons shall be available for performing the work of the "General Hospitals" at the base. This arrangement was easily made, because it allowed those physicians and surgeons to carry on their private work almost as freely as before, and did not necessitate their leaving home.

The 3rd and 4th Scottish General Hospitals are accommodated at Stobhill, where 1,040 beds are now available. At the time of writing some thirty cases are in hospital. The 3rd Hospital is under the charge of Lieut.-Colonel A. G. Hay, M.D., commanding, with Major B. Riddell, M.D., as Registrar, these officers residing at the hospital; while Lieut.-Colonel T. K. Dalziel, M.B., and Major W. K. Hunter, M.D., are at present on duty as visiting surgeon and physician, with, in addition, an orderly officer on duty daily. The 4th Hospital is under the charge of Lieut.-Colonel A. Napier, M.D., commanding, with Major J. Grant Andrew, M.B., as Registrar, these officers residing at the hospital; while Lieut.-Colonels J. C. Renton, M.D., and G. S. Middleton, M.D., are at present on duty as visiting surgeon and physician, with, in addition, an orderly officer on duty daily.

Volunteers for service abroad have been numerous. It is obviously impossible to obtain a complete list of those who have thus offered their services in Glasgow and the West of Scotland, but it may be mentioned that from the Glasgow Royal Infirmary Drs. A. J. Gibson, T. Gilchrist, M. White, W. E. Elliot, D. A. M'Alpine, W. E. Maitland, J. MacInnes, and J. M. Grier, and from the Western Infirmary Drs. D. K. Adams, D. P. Brown, R. Barlow, R. W. Brander, J. C. Walker, S. Robertson, W. Meikle, and A. M. Russell have sent in their applications.

DOCTORS ON ACTIVE SERVICE.—At a meeting held in Edinburgh on 12th August a committee was formed consisting of the Deans of the Faculties of Medicine in the four Scottish Universities, the Presidents of the Royal College of Physicians, of the Royal College of Surgeons, and of the Royal Faculty of Physicians and Surgeons of Glasgow, with Dr. John Playfair, Dr. John Steven, and Dr. J. C. M'Vail, Edinburgh; Dr. John Adams, Glasgow; Dr. John Gordon, Aberdeen; Dr. J. R. Hamilton, Hawick; Dr. J. C. Anderson, Methil; and Dr. Norman Walker, Edinburgh (convener), to take steps to meet the emergencies arising owing to so many medical practitioners having been called up or liable to be called up for active service.

FREE MEDICAL ATTENDANCE DURING THE WAR.—At a joint meeting of the Local Medical and Panel Committees for the Burgh of Glasgow it was unanimously agreed to recommend to medical practitioners in the city that free medical attendance be given to the necessitous dependants of all persons called up for active service with any of the Imperial Forces during the present war. It was also resolved unanimously to take such steps as may be necessary to safeguard the interests of all members of the medical profession called up for service, and to make arrangements for carrying on the practices of colleagues during absence. Four District Committees were formed to give effect to these recommendations.

THE WAR AND THE SUPPLY OF DRUGS.—Through the courtesy of Mr. J. Reid Douglas, managing director of Messrs. Frazer & Green, Limited, we are enabled to lay before our readers a statement with regard to the effect of the war upon the supply and the prices of drugs. That effect has already been that business has practically been brought to a standstill, so far as wholesale drug markets are concerned. International events have moved so fast that there was no time to enable importers to lay in extra stocks of articles coming from abroad;

and the bought contracts on their books, in many cases, are of no value, since sellers cannot deliver. Supplies of German chemicals have entirely ceased, and, if it were possible, it would be illegal to obtain them. Supplies of other products are limited, uncertain, or available only at greatly advanced prices. Manufacturers and wholesalers have been swamped with orders, and in many instances stocks are already depleted. Some articles, such as citric and tartaric acids and cream of tartar, are almost unobtainable, and fancy prices are being paid for them. In regard to supplies of goods of foreign origin, the following statements are applicable :—

It is impossible to obtain goods from Germany, and therefore impossible to obtain supplies of salicylates, aspirin, chloral hydrate, potassium permanganate, and many other chemicals in respect to which it is common knowledge that the goods come only from Germany.

Other countries, with which England is not at war, have made it illegal to export their products, *e.g.*, Russia (affecting ergot, Russian petroleum, cantharides, &c.).

In other cases, where the goods come only from a certain country not at war, but closed to us for the present on account of the war (*e.g.*, Norwegian cod liver oil from Norway; lemon and bergamot oils from Sicily; olive oil from Italy, &c.), it is impossible to obtain supplies from the country of origin.

In many cases the chief portion of the total output of the article comes from Germany, Austria, or other closed countries (*e.g.*, sugar), so that the war has entailed a great rise in value. Confections, pulv. glycyrrhizæ co., and all syrups have therefore risen in price. Some goods which are made or could be made in England or elsewhere contain as an essential ingredient or raw material a product falling within the above categories, *e.g.*, bismuth salts from bismuth metal (German controlled); hexamythylene-tetramine from formaldehyde (obtained from Germany); bromides from bromine (German controlled).

At the time of writing (15th August) bismuth has advanced enormously in price, potassium bromide is quoted at 10s. per lb., and cod liver oil is unobtainable. Retailers are being supplied by the wholesale trade with only portions of their orders, in order to protect the stocks.

The following is a list of the articles which have advanced in price since the beginning of the war, and some of these are rapidly becoming unobtainable :—

Acetic acid and acetates, acetylsalicylic acid and salicylates, carbolic acid and its preparations, citric acid and citrates, lactic acid and lactates, salicylic acid and salicylates, tartaric acid and tartrates; bismuth and its salts; lard, lanolin, paraffin, and ointments; synthetic benzoic acid and benzoates; all bromides; all starches, arrowroot, and foodstuffs, including children's and invalid foods; acetanilid, aspirin, and all German synthetic preparations; belladonna and atropine; glycerophosphates; cantharides; chloral hydrate; cocaine and its salts; opium, its preparations and alkaloids; ergot and its preparations; formaldehyde; mercurials; linseed; magnesii sulphas; all honeys, syrups, and preparations containing sugar; many essential oils; cod liver oil, castor oil, and olive oil; potassium bicarbonate, carbonate, nitrate, and permanganate; quinine and its salts; saccharin; sodium hyposulphite; strychnine and its salts; thymol; zinc and its salts; all effervescent preparations; iodine and iodine preparations, including iodoform. Cotton wool, wood wool, and bandages have also considerably increased in price. Salvarsan is unobtainable.

It is evident that in some of the cases mentioned the stringency will be only temporary, and that with the reopening of trade routes supplies will reappear; but in the case of preparations coming from a hostile country the difficulty must last till the end of the war. Even here, however, those goods which have been hitherto manufactured in Germany from raw material derived from other countries will now in all likelihood be manufactured in Great Britain, although necessarily at the outset at higher prices. It would thus seem to be possible that the war may bring among other unexpected consequences a great opportunity to British manufacturing chemists.

HEALTH OF THE ARMY.—The inaugural address of the Earl of Derby, president of the twentieth annual congress of the Royal Sanitary Institute, was delivered on 6th July at the opening of the congress in Blackpool. Its subject makes it of vital interest at a time when all our naval and military forces are engaged to the last man in a war against military despotism.

Lord Derby, who said that the army had been his profession, referred to the value of even the brief training of the Territorial Force in the improvement of physique, and the inculcation of habits that made for human welfare. The training of the Ulster Volunteers had resulted in a reduction of crime and drunkenness in Ulster. The figures which he submitted for the British Army, given him by Sir Lancelot Gubbins, Chief of the Royal Army Medical Corps, showed, with regard to the incidence of all diseases in the British Army in the United Kingdom, that the number of admissions, which in 1892 was 761·3 per 1,000 of the strength, had dropped in 1912 to 364. The deaths, which were 4·38 in 1892, had dropped in twenty years to 2·34, while the average number of constantly sick, which in 1892 was 42·75, had dropped in the same period to 19·50. For the Colonies, the admissions in a similar ratio were 865·4 in 1892; in 1912 they had dropped in twenty years to 425. The deaths had dropped from 8 to 3; and the average number constantly sick had fallen from 45 to 24. The figures for India were, in 1892—admissions per 1,000, 1,514; deaths, 17; and average constantly sick, 83; in 1912—admissions, 547; deaths, 4; average constantly sick, 28. These were all very startling figures, illustrating the advance of medical science in the army. He proceeded to give statistics relating to enteric fever in India. In 1903 there were 1,366 cases; nine years later there were only 118. The number of deaths had fallen in the interval from 292 to 26, and the average number constantly sick from 203 to 20. The number of cases of malaria in 1903 was 17,037; in 1912 there were 5,847; and the number of deaths had dropped from 35 to 12, the latter figure being an increase on the records for 1910 and 1911, when there were only 7 and 6 respectively. The average number constantly sick was down from 371 to 210. Lancashire had, through the Liverpool School of Tropical Medicine, played a prominent part in the cure of Mediterranean or Malta fever. In 1904 there were 320 cases of this disease, and 12 deaths; in 1910 and 1911 there was not a single case; and in 1912 there were 3 cases. Referring to malarial fever in Mauritius, Lord Derby mentioned that the average number constantly sick, which at one time was as high as 34·75, had fallen as low as 2·35. As regards venereal disease, the average number constantly sick had fallen in twenty years, in Britain, from 16·46 to 5·51; in the Colonies, from 16 to 9; and in India, from 29 to 7. The figures he had given proved the enormous advance in the work of the Royal Army Medical Corps for the army which it served, and for the country which the army served. He gave further details as to the effect on recruits of six months' service with the gymnastic class. The figures were taken in the year ending 30th September, 1904. The average height of recruits on enlistment was 5 ft. 5 in.; after six months training they averaged 5 ft. 6 in. In the old days the soldier was too often looked upon as a sort of outcast, who, when he came back from the army, was a worthless creature. That was no longer the case. The social status of the soldier had improved, and he ventured to think that the army was now a powerful missionary for health.

NEW PREPARATIONS, &c.

From Messrs. Allen & Hanburys, Ltd.

"*Byno*" *Phosphates.*—This deals with a preparation of which the formula is stated to be as follows:—Ferri phosph., 1 grain; calcii phosph., 1½ grain; potassii phosph., ⅛ grain; sodii phosph., ⅛ grain; "bynin," 1 oz. "Bynin," of course, is a liquid malt.

Infant Feeding during Summer.—A pamphlet dealing with the use of various foods, rusks, &c., supplied by the firm.

Leaflets are also sent us dealing with "*Azoule*," *sterilised Catgut and Sutures, Pituitarin, Pituitarin-Adrenin, Quinine-Urea-Hydrochloride* as a local anæsthetic, and "*Iodolysin*," which is stated to be an improved preparation of thiosinamin and organically combined iodine.

From Messrs. Casein, Ltd.

A pamphlet containing tables for split proteid percentage, and the method of calculating "*Secwa*" powder mixtures. "*Secwa*," of course, is a dry whey powder which we have already favourably dealt with in these pages.

MEETINGS OF SOCIETIES.

MEDICO-CHIRURGICAL SOCIETY OF GLASGOW.

SESSION 1913-1914.

MEETING XIII.—1ST MAY, 1914.

The President, MR. A. ERNEST MAYLARD, *in the Chair.*

I.—CASE OF COMPLETE AURICULO-VENTRICULAR HEART-BLOCK.

BY DR. GEO. A. ALLAN.

Dr. Allan's communication is published as an original article in this issue at p. 183.

II.—MALIGNANT GANGLIO-NEUROMA OF LEFT SUPRARENAL.

BY PROFESSOR T. K. MONRO AND DR. J. SHAW DUNN.

This communication was published as an original article in our issue for August, 1914, at p. 81.

III.—MALIGNANT TUMOUR OF THE NECK, INVOLVING THE SPINE AND CERVICAL AND BRACHIAL PLEXUSES.

BY PROFESSOR T. K. MONRO AND DR. G. HASWELL WILSON.

Clinical report by Professor Monro.—Fanny K., aged 56, unmarried, was admitted to the Western Infirmary on 17th October, 1913, on the recommendation of Dr. Marion Gilchrist. Her complaint was of pain in the right shoulder and arm of six months' duration, and of a swelling in the neck which began two months earlier than the pain.

In February, 1913, patient noticed swellings on the right side of the neck, and these gradually increased in size. In April she began to have pain in the right shoulder, near the tip of the acromion process. Then the glands on the left side of the neck became enlarged. The pain afterwards became less in the right shoulder, but it involved the outer wall of the axilla, and at the time of admission it was most severe at the right elbow. The pain was worst when she was lying down, and it interfered with sleep.

Past health.—Always good.

Family history.—Good.

Social condition.—Patient kept a vegetable shop, and had to be constantly using her arms, and had to stand for long periods.

Condition on admission.—Patient was well-nourished and of good colour. The glands on the right side of the neck were much enlarged, hard, and fixed, and were more or less matted together. Those on the left side were not so large or hard, and were discrete. The thyroid gland was slightly enlarged. The temperature was normal, the pulse somewhat accelerated. The tongue was dirty, and the teeth were very defective in number. Patient was a total abstainer, and was moderate in her use of tea. The organs of circulation and of respiration were healthy, and the urine also was normal. There was slight loss of tone in the muscles of the right arm. Sensation was unimpaired. The knee-jerks and plantar reflexes were normal. There had been slight difficulty in swallowing solids for three weeks before admission.

While patient was in the infirmary it was ascertained that both the Wassermann and the luetin tests gave negative results.

On 3rd November patient was transferred to Dr. Edington's wards, in order that one of the enlarged glands might be excised for histological investigation. When she returned to the medical wards on 26th November, a decided change in her condition was observable. The left arm had now become the seat of pain, and she required an opiate at night to procure sleep. It was noted about this time that the head was carried far forwards, as if from disease of the cervical spine, and that rotation of the head was restricted, if not actually prevented. The right arm was cold and livid, and apt to sweat.

7th December.—The condition of the left arm is now similar to that of the right. Pain is constant and severe.

The backward projection of the spine in the cervical region is becoming greater.

15th January, 1914.—The pain has become worse.

1st February.—The weakness and numbness of the arms are constantly becoming worse.

26th February.—There is a severe curvature of the cervical spine, the head being thrown far forwards. There is discolouration at the back of the neck, with thickening of the soft tissues. There is great loss of power in the upper limbs, and the muscles of the hand are wasted. There is partial loss of, control over both sphincters. On both sides the knee-jerk is exaggerated, ankle-clonus is present, and the plantar reflex is of extensor type. There is slight wasting of the right lower limb. Morphine has to be given every six hours.

15th March.—A large bedsore is present over the sacrum. Just above this, a sinus has formed, which discharges great quantities of foul-smelling pus.

17th March.—The bedsore is growing larger. A slough of four inches square is gradually separating.

28th March.—Patient is cyanosed and at times unconscious.

31st March.—Patient was unconscious all morning and died in the afternoon. In the last few weeks of life, the temperature had been febrile, as might have been expected in view of the suppuration in the lower part of the back.

Pathological report by Dr. G. Haswell Wilson.—*External appearances:* A hard mass is palpable on the right side of the neck, and the head is slightly inclined towards the right shoulder. A very large bedsore over the sacrum exposes the sacral spinous processes. Smaller bedsores are present over the scapulæ and on the calves of the legs.

On reflecting the skin from the right side of the neck a considerable tumour mass is found which, in places, is closely adherent to the skin. The sterno-mastoid muscle is extremely atrophied; it is tightly stretched over the tumour, and is partly invaded by it. On further dissection the tumour is found to weld all the structures on this side of the neck into one firm mass, and on removing the clavicle it is seen to extend downwards into the axilla, surrounding the brachial nerve plexus and axillary vessels. The tumour is closely adherent to the first rib and has invaded its substance. It also adheres to the trachea and œsophagus, and binds them firmly to the vertebral column. A small process extends into the posterior triangle on the left side of the neck. On opening the trachea a small rounded patch of tumour is found under the mucous membrane in the upper part. The bodies of the cervical vertebræ are extensively invaded, and can readily be cut with a knife. To such an extent is the bone destroyed that, on removal of the tumour mass from the neck, the vertebral column is unable to support the weight of the head and snaps across through the body of the fourth cervical vertebra. The dura mater at this level is closely adherent to the bone, and, on separating it, a nodule of tumour is seen inside the spinal canal. The dura is greatly thickened, and is found on section to be invaded by tumour. The spinal cord itself shows a slight constriction at this level. Well marked purulent meningitis is present over the cauda equina and the lower part of the cord, and this is found to be due to a gangrenous condition of the sacrum in relation to the bedsore. The sacrum is completely necrosed, crumbling readily on pressure, and on section much pus of extremely foul odour exudes. The suppuration has opened into the spinal canal and both sacro-iliac synchondroses. The retro-peritoneal tissues in the pelvis are in a gangrenous condition, and a large pocket of pus is found on the right side, communicating with the sacral bedsore. All the pelvic veins, both femoral and iliac veins, and the inferior vena cava are filled with firm thrombus, which, in places, is undergoing suppurative softening.

The tumour tissue is pinkish-white in colour and somewhat translucent, with areas of necrotic softening. It infiltrates the various structures diffusely, and no clear margin can be distinguished. Histologically it is a sarcoma. The cells vary in size in different parts, and the amount of stroma also varies. Much of it is necrotic. It has apparently originated in the cervical lymph glands, probably from the gland stroma rather than the lymphoid tissue.

The tumour was shown and its relationship to the structures in the neck demonstrated. Microscopic sections from different parts were also shown.

IV.—LACERATION OF KIDNEY: NEPHRECTOMY.

By Mr. G. H. EDINGTON.

· The patient whom I now show you, John D., aged 16
years, sheet-iron worker, was admitted to the Western
Infirmary on the evening of 16th October last. At 11 A.M.
on that day he fell while on the deck of a torpedo boat, and
struck his back against a fixed ring projecting from the
deck. On admission to the infirmary ten and a half hours
later he was very pallid, complained of pain and tenderness
in the right side below the costal margin, and had not passed
water since the accident. No pain was elicited in the side
by pressure on the sternum. At 11·50 P.M. 25 oz. of bloody
urine withdrawn by catheter.

The following morning 20 oz. of urine, normal in appearance, were drawn off by catheter; there was great tenderness
in flank, and some swelling. Under $CHCl_3$ a mass the size of
a cocoanut was felt in the flank. Transverse laparotomy,
immediately above the umbilicus, from middle line to mid-
axillary line, showed the cæcum and ascending colon with
subperitoneal extravasation of blood, and floated forwards by
retroperitoneal swelling in renal region. The left kidney,
apparently normal, was present in its usual situation.
Vertical incision through posterior parietal peritoneum,
external to ascending colon, allowed of quantity of clot being
turned out of cavity in which lay right kidney in two pieces,
the lower of which quite loose and picked out by fingers.
The larger upper piece was attached by pedicle, which was
ligated and kidney removed. Drainage-tube through stab
wound in loin; peritoneal incision closed; abdominal wound
closed by through-and-through silkworm-gut stitches. Recovery was uneventful. He has reported himself monthly
since. Took up light work on 23rd January, and resumed
ordinary work on 7th April. The scar is sound, and he
feels quite well and none the worse for his accident.

Examination of the kidney after removal showed that it
measured 13 cm. in length and 4·5 to 5 cm. transversely.
It had been completely torn across at the level of the lower
end of the hilum, 5 cm. from the lower pole, the tear being

directed upwards and forwards. The surface of the kidney showed white areas, extending well into the cortex. The lower fragment was very hard, swollen, and dark coloured.

Dr. Shaw Dunn reported that the kidney tissue was normal, the pale areas showing " early autolytic changes."

The severe results of what did not look like a serious accident, and the ¯good scar resulting from transverse laparotomy, are worthy of note.

V.—PARTIALLY PYONEPHROTIC KIDNEY, WITH DOUBLE URETER
AND PELVIS: SPECIMEN OBTAINED BY NEPHRECTOMY.

By Mr. G. H. Edington.

The specimen was removed from a married woman, Mrs. A., aged 33 years, who was sent to see me by her doctor in May of last year. Six years previously, when allowed up after the birth of her third child, she felt a pain in the right side. The pain was accompanied by an attack of bilious vomiting, lasting 24 hours, and was followed by swelling of the body and face. She was ordered back to bed, and the temporary diminution of urine which had been noted was succeeded by the passage of a large quantity, which was muddy. Attacks of pain occurred every three months, when she was up and exerting herself; but during successive pregnancies—there have been four since first onset—they were absent, except during the last, when the pain was only mitigated. The attacks became more frequent, latterly weekly, and during the five weeks preceding her visit to me pain had been constant. Her child was at this time 8 weeks old. A swelling which had formed in the right flank used to disappear coincidently with free flow of muddy urine, but not so during this prolonged attack. Of late she had become white and thin, and sweated profusely at night.

On examination the right flank was seen to be occupied by a swelling which extended down as far as the cæcum. Its surface was smooth and lobar, percussion dull, with tympanitic area between it and the liver dulness. The swelling was hard near the umbilicus, and more fluctuant further out. Impulse was communicated from the loin. The urine contained copious pus, but no tubercle bacilli in the deposit. There was little hesitation in diagnosing pyonephrosis, and she was admitted into the infirmary early in August to undergo operation. Before operation the urinary sediment yielded a growth of coliform bacilli, but no tubercle bacilli were found. Nephrectomy was performed on 1st September. The kidney was removed transperitoneally through a transverse incision in anterior abdominal wall. The ureter, which was thickened, was ligated well below the level of the kidney. On cutting it across it was seen to be double. The left kidney was in its usual situation and apparently normal. The abdominal wound was stitched in layers, and drainage was made through a slit in the loin.

She made a good recovery and was discharged well on 23rd September. During convalescence, examination of the urine yielded a Gram-positive diplococcus on culture; also large Gram-positive bacilli and bacillus coli communis.

After removal of the organ it was observed that there was double ureter and pelvis, and that the pyonephrosis affected the lower pelvis. The upper ureter led up to a normal pelvis and kidney perched on the upper surface of the cyst. The appearance was strongly suggestive of a sigmoid kidney, and if there had not been proof of the presence of a kidney on the left side would have caused us grave anxiety.

A cystoscopic examination could not be made prior to operation, but during her convalescence the cystoscope showed a single ureteral orifice on each side of the trigone.

Pathological report by Dr. Shaw Dunn.—The kidney, on examination, is found to possess two separate pelves and ureters: of these the upper are of normal appearance and take origin from the upper half of the kidney, which, on section, exhibits quite normal characters. The upper ureter passes from its origin over the front of a large smooth sac attached to the lower half of the kidney. On dissection it is found that this sac represents a second pelvis, which has drained the lower half of the organ. It is much distended, and filled with foul-smelling purulent material: the part of the kidney to which it belongs is stretched out, and the renal substance· is greatly thinned and atrophied. The ureter of this lower pelvis makes its exit by a distinctly valved orifice, and it would appear that the main obstruction to the outflow of urine from this cavity took place at this point: the lower ureter beyond its origin contains some pus, but it is not dilated. There is nothing to indicate the original cause of development of obstruction. No calculi are present in pelves or ureters.

VI.—MR. HENRY RUTHERFURD showed—

1. A colon with ulceration and perforation at root of volvulus of sigmoid, after operation for reduction.

2. The parts concerned in a fracture of the femur by direct violence, where gangrene resulted from pressure, by the lower fragment, on the femoral artery and vein at the lower end of Hunter's canal.

3. Water-colour drawing of a case of gangrene of the penis from causes so far unexplained.

REVIEWS.

—

Practical Bacteriology, Blood Work, and Animal Parasitology, including Bacteriological Keys, Zoological Tables, and Explanatory Clinical Notes. By E. R. STITT, M.D. Third Edition. London: H. K. Lewis. 1913.

WHERE a book "overflows" on every available particle of space, including the pages of the covers themselves, it is evident that the author wishes to give the maximum information, while keeping the size of the book within handy limits, and Dr. Stitt has succeeded in this endeavour to a very marked degree.

Of course, Dr. Stitt's book on these subjects has become well known through the medium of former editions, but in the present edition the author has compressed a most extraordinary amount of information into what seems at first sight an impossibly small bulk. Careful perusal, however, will show that there is no scrimping of any essential point throughout, and altogether the present work of handy pocket size may safely be consulted as authoritative in any of the branches included.

The general arrangement is the same as in the previous editions, but the new material added is by no means inconsiderable, and this has been made possible, without unduly increasing the size of the book, by employing smaller type for the paragraphs which are supplementary to the text proper.

In Chapter I, on apparatus, the description of the technique for dark ground illumination with the oil immersion objective is too scanty, and this method of investigation has now become of such importance that it seems desirable that very full instructions should be given in a book of this kind, as good results depend very largely upon little *minutiæ*, which require careful and full description.

The chapter on general staining methods is full, and yet put in remarkably small compass.

The author's remark (page 82) that Pappenheim's method of staining the bacillus of tubercle does not appear to have an advantage over the older method is not supported by other observers; the results obtained by Pappenheim's method are at least as good, and the saving of time is often a point of very great importance indeed.

The chapters dealing with the study and identification of bacteria in general are excellent. The relations of the various lactic acid bacilli are given, and in this connection the Boas-Oppler bacillus is given due attention.

Moulds and fungi generally are given a short chapter, and although the matter is shortly put, the low pathogenicity of this group may be held as justifying this treatment in a book like the one under review.

The chapter on the bacteriology of water, air, milk, &c., is certainly far too limited in its scope, and perhaps it might be well to leave this now quite special department of bacteriology for separate treatment elsewhere.

In the description of Wassermann's test no mention is made of the Hecht-Fleming modification, although the latter is as satisfactory in practice as many of the other modifications, and has further advantages of its own.

There is a short but excellent description of the condition of anaphylaxis.

Part II, on the study of the blood, is exceptionally full and accurate. It seems strange, however, that no mention is made of Jenner's stain here. Many workers prefer this stain for all routine blood-staining of films. Further, no mention is made of Simon's counting chamber; for leucocytes especially this has many advantages over the Thoma or its modifications.

Naturally, malaria gets a very full description, and nothing but praise can be given in the treatment of this section.

Parasites of all kinds receive due consideration, and, indeed, the section on animal parasitology is perhaps not only the best in this book, but better than many in much more ambitious cognate works.

Part IV, on clinical bacteriology and animal parasitology of the various body fluids and organs, is excellent. It is to this part that the ordinary medical practitioner will most often refer for information as to securing proper and adequate specimens for bacteriological investigation.

. The illustrations are excellent throughout, and are not unduly numerous, a point of importance in a small book, where space is a consideration.

There is a very useful appendix and a rather contracted index.

The tables, factors, &c., on the covers will be found of considerable value.

Altogether, Dr. Stitt's book should be one of the most frequently consulted works in the library of every medical practitioner.

Diseases of the Heart. By JAMES MACKENZIE, M.D., F.R.C.P. Third Edition. London: Henry Frowde and Hodder & Stoughton. 1913.

THE third edition of this excellent work on the diseases of the heart has appeared within five years of the publication of the first. This in itself is sufficient indication of the popularity of the book. Dr. Mackenzie has not been content merely to correct minor mistakes and to make small alterations, but to a large extent has re-written the book. The recent advances in the study of the diseases of the heart have necessitated this. Whilst the first edition was largely based on his own investigations, in this edition the author has availed himself of the results obtained by many other workers in this field; and he has not hesitated to abandon views which the more recent researches have shown to be erroneous.

In the first four chapters the pathology of heart failure is discussed. The author considers that it is defects in the heart muscle rather than in the valves that bring about failure. He attributes heart failure to exhaustion of the reserve force of the cardiac muscle. The production and significance of the symptoms of heart failure are then carefully considered; and their consideration is of special value, as Dr. Mackenzie is recognised as an authority on symptoms and their interpretation.

The myogenic theory of the heart's action and the anatomy and development of the heart are then described. While the author admits that it would be beyond his province to enter into a discussion as to the relative merits of the myogenic and neurogenic theories of cardiac action, he considers that the myogenic theory is a useful working hypothesis. The relation between heart affections and sensory and vaso-motor disturbances is carefully worked out. In many cases the pain produced by cardiac affections is thought to be a reflex protective phenomenon.

The description and application of instrumental methods in the investigation of heart affections is gone into fully, and it is in this part of the book that Dr. Mackenzie avails himself largely not only of his own investigations, but also of the opinions of many of his co-workers in this field. As examples of this we would mention the chapters on auricular fibrillation and auricular flutter, which show clearly the immense strides that have been made in cardiology since the publication of the first edition of this work.

It may seem strange to some that only twenty-two pages are devoted to the sounds, murmurs, and valvular defects of the heart, and for this reason the book might appropriately be called "The diseases of the myocardium;" but we agree with the author that in the older writings too much stress has been laid on the affections of the valves and too little on those of the myocardium.

The chapters on treatment are written with the same sound commonsense that illuminates the other parts of the book. Dr. Mackenzie is in agreement with most authorities in considering rest as a most important factor in the treatment of the failing heart. We agree that to a large extent the virtues of spa treatment lie rather in the mental and physical rest so readily obtained in such resorts than in the healing properties of the waters. As regards drugs, digitalis is considered to be almost a specific for auricular fibrillation. Many of the so-called cardiac tonics, such as camphor and strychnine, are considered to be of little or no value.

The concluding pages are devoted to an appendix, in which

ninety-two cases, illustrative of conditions referred to in the text, are carefully described. This is not the least valuable part of an excellent book.

––––––

Report of the Proceedings of the English-speaking Conference on Infant Mortality. London: National Association for the Prevention of Infant Mortality and for the Welfare of Infancy. 1913.

THIS conference was held at Caxton Hall, Westminster, on 4th and 5th August, 1913, and this volume of 456 pages reports fully the business of the meetings. The papers read are printed apparently in full, and the discussion on each paper seems very fully given. Needless to say, the papers and discussions teem with interest for all thoughtful people. This year's conference was distinguished from those of 1906 and 1908 in embracing representatives from every English-speaking country, and twenty-two English-speaking Governments were represented by specially appointed delegates. A large proportion of the work of the conference was contributed by the representatives from oversea.

There were two main sections, viz., administrative and medical. These are divided respectively into subsections on *A*, the responsibility of central and local administration; *B*, the administrative control of the milk supply; and *A*, the necessity for special education in infant hygiene; *B*, medical milk problems; *C*, antenatal hygiene.

Following the work of these sections was a joint meeting of the two main sections, at which resolutions were passed to the following effect:—

1. That maternity benefit belong to the mother.

2. That in the education of girls attention should be paid to establishing good bodily health and development, and complete fitness for maternity and the practical care of the home.

3. That stillbirths should be registered.

4. That certification of death be more complete, and that certificates be confidential.

5. That midwives be better trained.

6. That infant hygiene be given a more important place in the medical curriculum.

7. That the respective governments of the countries represented appoint commissions on venereal diseases.

8. That the grant earned by "recognised" infant welfare centres depend in future on their efficiency.

9. That steps be taken that a negative result on microscopical examination of milk for tubercle bacilli be not accepted without confirmation by inoculation tests.

10. That the Milk Bill be passed with as little delay as possible.

This is most interesting reading, and the impression left on the mind is that there is plenty of work along these lines for the future, but that already very much has been done in certain places, and by no means least in Glasgow, towards lessening the present unsatisfactory infant mortality.

The joint honorary secretaries who sign the preface are Dr. A. K. Chalmers and Dr. Eric Pritchard, and they are to be congratulated on the excellence of this report.

The conference covered a wide scope, and this report of its labours is recommended to the notice of all practitioners.

A Guide to the Mental Deficiency Act, 1913. By JOHN WORMALD and SAMUEL WORMALD. With a Preface by T. EDMUND HARVEY, M.P. London : P. S. King & Son.

IN the appendix to this volume the text of the Act is given, and this is followed by a very good index. The body of the book extends to 95 pages, and in the first section or introduction is discussed the history of the movement preceding the introduction of the Bill, beginning with the Royal Commission of 1904. The operation of the Act, with its definitions of defectives, the circumstances rendering defectives subject to be dealt with, and the Act in its relation to the Local Education Authority, are expounded in Section II. The authorities under the Act, how these are appointed and related to the Lunacy Commissioners, the staffing of the Board of Control, the administration of the property of lunatics and defectives, the local authorities and the duties of these bodies, are all set forth in plain language in the third section. The succeeding section discusses the administration of the Act, *e.g.*, how defectives are to be dealt with by boarding out, in colonies, in private homes, or in State institutions for the criminal classes, how patients are to be employed and classified, the procedure under the Act, and numerous other points of administration. Offences against the mentally defective are next discussed, and the financial and statistical matters are explained. Finally under the heading "Conclusions," it is pointed out that the Act is founded on popular control, and its success will largely depend upon co-operation between the parents of defectives and the local authority. It is claimed as a charter of real liberty to a large number of chronic mentally defectives who in the past were the Ishmaelites of society.

The book is clearly and well written, and should prove useful to all who may have occasion to utilise the Act, or who may be called upon to help in its working. It deals with the Act as confined to England.

The Trial and Acquittal of Professor Carlo Ruata, Professor of Materia Medica at the University of Perugia, Italy.

THIS is a translation from the *Vita e Malattie*, and is published by the National Anti-Vaccination League.

Professor Ruata was indicted on a charge of having instigated the people of Italy to evade the vaccination laws. Briefly, Professor Ruata holds that isolation should be substituted for vaccination, and his acquittal may or may not be held as to some degree exonerating him from the indictment proper. On the whole, the magistrate seems to have been greatly impressed by the fact that Professor Ruata acted in a *bonâ fide* manner throughout, and did not attack the vaccination laws *per se*, but signified his belief that the matter was one in which legitimate difference of opinion might prevail among the members of the medical profession itself.

The statistics in Professor Ruata's defence are by no means free from obvious fallacy, but this abuse of figures is one which is not altogether confined to the anti-vaccinators, and thus it would serve no useful purpose to go into the sources of possible error in the figures as given here.

Official Year-Book of the Scientific and Learned Societies of Great Britain and Ireland. Thirtieth Annual Issue. London: Charles Griffin & Co. 1913.

A COPY of the twenty-eighth annual issue was reviewed in our pages in 1911, and the present issue is on the same general lines.

In addition to the list of the various societies there is in each case a short record of the work done during the year, including the published papers, although the bracketed remark "No Return" appears more frequently than it should. By the medical profession special interest will be taken in the extended returns of the papers read at the annual meeting of the British Medical Association in 1913, also the long list (almost seventeen pages) of papers read before the Royal Society of Medicine during the same year.

As a book of reference this supplies information, officially compiled, in a compact form.

E. Merck's Annual Report, 1913. Darmstadt: E. Merck.

THIS *Annual Report* is arranged as usual. There is first an exhaustive monograph on a particular drug which is of present interest to the profession, and then follow shorter monographs arranged alphabetically under the names of the drugs dealt with. This year the principal monograph is on lecithin, and this drug is discussed in the fullest possible way; a copious bibliography is appended to the article. The succeeding monographs are stated to be compiled from the publications of the authors referred to in each, and deal not only with the specialities of the firm of E. Merck, but also with a very large number of other drugs. The book is a mine of information, and should prove as useful as its predecessors to practitioners of medicine.

———

Natural Therapy: A Manual of Physiotherapeutics and Climatology. By Thomas D. Luke, M.D., F.R.C.S.Edin., and Norman Hay Forbes, F.R.C.S.Edin., F.R.S.Edin. Bristol: John Wright & Sons, Limited. 1913.

It is stated that this is the second issue of a previous work, to which a chapter on climatology has been added.

Water, heat and light, massage, electricity, and diet in the treatment of disease are dealt with in successive chapters, and then follow chapters on the modern "cure" and on climatology. There are 30 plates and 125 smaller illustrations in the text; there is a bibliography and an index.

The size of the book prevents a very full discussion of the various subjects dealt with, but as a manual or introduction to the subject it is well enough. The explanations of the methods employed are, as a rule, concise and clear; but in the theoretical portions dogmatic assertion is rather in evidence, and occasionally the sentences are somewhat obscure in meaning.

On the whole, however, the book forms a safe and satisfactory manual on the subject. It is easily read, the illustrations are apt and good, and, in spite of its comparatively small size and large subject, one may say that it fulfils the object of its authors. May we venture to suggest, however, that treatment by means of drugs is not quite out of date, even in the case of *B.P.* drugs?

ABSTRACTS FROM CURRENT MEDICAL LITERATURE.

EDITED BY ROY F. YOUNG, M.B., B.C.

MEDICINE.

The Blood Picture in Hodgkin's Disease. By C. H. Bunting, M.D. (*Johns Hopkins Hospital Bulletin*, June, 1914).—The author has studied the blood of fourteen cases of Hodgkin's disease, in which the diagnosis had been established by histological examination of a test gland. The study of the blood in those cases has shown that there is a deviation from the normal leucocytic picture in all cases, but that there is not a single constant picture found in them. The blood findings are summarised as follows:—Throughout the disease there are two constant features—an increase in blood plates, and an absolute increase in the transitional leucocytes. In regard to the other elements, in early cases there is a transitory increase in lymphocytes and basophiles and a deficiency in eosinophiles, with a normal or low neutrophile count, followed by a gradual decrease in lymphocytes and a moderate eosinophilia. In late cases there is a marked neutrophile leucocytosis, and a diminution in percentage of all other elements, except the transitional leucocyte.—ARCHD. W. HARRINGTON.

DENTAL SCIENCE.

Iodine. By Wesley Barritt, Ph.C., L.D.S.Eng. (*British Dental Journal*, 2nd March, 1914).—Iodine is an element which has been experimented with in every disease known, and it is remarkable with what success it has met, new applications for its use being continually brought forward.

Coindet, a native of Geneva and a student of medicine at Edinburgh University, appears to have been the first to discover that the therapeutic value of various substances was due to iodine.

The author classes iodine as a powerful antiseptic, bactericide, disinfectant, counter-irritant, and resolvent. As an antiseptic it is largely used in general surgery, and Owen points out its value as a household remedy as a valuable first-aid adjunct, and that as such it should be used in preference to all other antiseptics.

In a solution of 3 grm. to a litre, its bactericidal properties are equal to 1 in 1,000 sublimate solution, streptococci having been completely destroyed in broth in eight minutes. Its antiseptic properties are due to both its local and diffused action, as much by its sterilising influence as by its antitoxic action on the products of cellular elaboration.

As an antiseptic mouth wash a few drops of tincture of iodine in a small tumbler of warm water is excellent in mouths where caries are prevalent. Iodine readily stains the skin and linen, and its volatile nature is a factor which we are obliged to heed.

When extracting septic teeth a solution applied to the gum both before and after operating is a good precautionary measure against infection of the sockets, and also these properties may be taken advantage of for sterilising the gum before inserting a hypodermic needle.

In pyorrhœa alveolaris it may be advantageously applied to the gum pockets after thorough cleansing and instrumentation.

As a counter-irritant iodine relieves pulpitis and periodontitis, and reduces all inflammatory conditions ; its action in such cases is probably due to diapedesis of the leucocytes being brought about, and ultimate resolution taking place. Its property as a counter-irritant, resolvent, and vasomotor stimulant favours this diapedesis, augments the activity of the tissues, and promotes the absorption of exudations and the disappearances of pathological conditions.

The intensity of its action appears to be due to the quantity of albuminates present, the greater their amount the less the effect to be obtained, as iodine quickly combines with them to form organic compounds. Hence its action on the mucous membrane is much more intense than on any other part.

A colourless tincture of iodine is made which is worthless as an application to the skin. Colourless tinctures are made by the addition of ammonia or hyposulphite of soda, the iodine forming with them double salts which are colourless ; salts of iodine are practically unabsorbed by the skin when their solutions are applied as paints. If the colour is an objection, the official compound liniment of potassium iodide and soap is to be recommended. This is in the form of a white cream, and should be rubbed into the part until absorbed. During the process of friction the acid contained in the secretion of the sebaceous glands frees the iodine, and in this way does it act.

Rabuteau proved the liberation of iodine by the blueing of his shirt after rubbing a cream on his body. Iodine is liberated from its salts by acids, oxygen, paraldehyde, and most metallic salts.

The author mentions the liability to iodism during internal administration, and draws attention to the fact that potassium iodide is quickly absorbed by the stomach, is decomposed, and may be detected in the saliva five minutes after administration. In the decomposition which takes place, part of the potassium iodide forms sodium iodide and part is freed into iodine, which combines with the albuminates of the body and remains longer in the system.

This affinity of iodine for organic bodies is taken advantage of in the preparation of numerous organically combined iodides. These remain inert until they reach the small intestine. Decomposition is slower than that of alkaline iodides, and elimination is prolonged, iodism being rare. The elimination of the sodium iodide in the mouth is by means of small submucous glands of the gum, so that the iodide is liberated in the mouth in the neighbourhood of the teeth, and right at the seat of the peridontal disease where it is difficult to gain access.

The author mentions the method of liberating iodine in the mouth where the patient is taking iodide internally by use of hydrogen peroxide or the electric current. He uses iodipin by Merck, and gives a tablet representing $\frac{3}{4}$ gr. iodine thrice daily after food.—J. Forbes Webster.

Certain Affections of the Nose and Throat which cause Deformities in and about the Mouth, and the Earliest Treatment of the Same. By David Rankin, M.S.Lond., B.S.Durh., F.R.C.S. Eng. (*British Dental Journal*, 1st April, 1914).—The presence or absence of deformities of the maxillary and mandibular arches, as also irregularities in the teeth and about the mouth, depend very largely upon the perfect equalising pressure of the lips, tongue, cheeks, and palate, together with efficient mastication. Any alterations in these factors causes and augments irregularities. It follows, therefore, that when nasal breathing is not fully performed, and the mouth is constantly kept open, deformities occur, and of these the most important is contraction of the arches and narrowing of the palate due to inefficient pressure of the tongue.

Obstruction to the passage of air through the nasal channels and naso-pharynx may be due either to conditions arising in these passages themselves, or to conditions of the surrounding parts which interfere with nasal respiration. The most important of the first class are—adenoids, deviated septum, hypertrophy of the turbinated bodies, polypi, and other new growths. Among the latter causes are diseases of the antrum, such as empyema, mucocele, osteoma, sarcoma, and carcinoma. Of all these adenoids is the most frequent.

The symptoms of adenoids are subjective, objective, and collateral. Of the subjective symptoms the most important are the impairment of the mental faculties, difficulty in attention on the part of the child, and, secondly, epipharyngeal catarrh, which catarrh has a great tendency to extend up the eustachian tubes to the middle ear and cause aural complications. Among the objective symptoms one finds the typical expressionless face, open mouth, protruding incisor teeth, and snoring at night. Adenoid masses may be both seen and felt. A better idea of the amount of adenoid tissue to be removed may be obtained by inspecting the masses through the anterior nares, cocainising if necessary. This is a better way in small children than inserting the finger into the naso-pharynx, hurting and terrorising the child. *When tonsils are hypertrophied adenoids are usually present.* Certain changes in the hard palate and in the teeth are characteristic of adenoids. The palate is usually abnormally arched, especially in the anterior portion, and apparently higher than normal. This apparent heightening is due to the fact that the upper jaw contracts laterally, while the height of the arch remains the same. This same fact also causes the central incisors to protrude and to be twisted upon their axis so as to cause their posterior surfaces to face one another; the teeth are also often irregular.

The treatment of adenoids resolves itself into their removal. If the tonsils are hypertrophied they should also be removed at the same time. The author employs for the removal of adenoids the curette of St. Clair Thomson, and for the tonsils the Ballenger modification of the Sluder guillotine.

The shaft is inserted into the mouth, and the edge of the ring is inserted between the tonsil and the posterior pillar of the fauces on the same side; the anterior is pressed upon by means of the finger or thumb so that the tonsil is thrust through the ring, counter pressure being exerted by the shaft against the lower jaw, and the handle is then pressed, the tonsil being thus enucleated in its capsule.

The improvement in the mental growth of the child after removal of the adenoids is often marvellous, provided the operation is performed during infancy and childhood.—J. FORBES WEBSTER.

Case of Congenital Absence of Teeth.

By F. N. Doubleday, M.R.C.S., L.D.S. (*British Journal of Dental Science*, 15th June, 1914).—The patient, a youth, aged 17 years, is believed to have had all his temporary teeth present. When he came under observation nine months ago he had present the following teeth only :—

$$\frac{M_2 - M_1 - T_3}{M - 3} \quad \bigg| \quad \frac{T_3 - M_1 - M_2}{3 - M}$$

No other permanent teeth appear to have been erupted, and the skiagrams do not indicate that there has been any sign of their development within the jaws.

Another case, that of a solicitor, was found on examination to have the following teeth only :—

$$\frac{M - T_3}{M - T_3 - T_2} \quad \bigg| \quad \frac{- T_3 - M}{T_3 - M}$$

He stated that no other teeth had ever been erupted. According to him he could thoroughly enjoy good dinners, and never suffered from indigestion. In both cases the jaws seemed well developed.

Mr. Doubleday mentioned that although both of these patients were members of large families, no history of any member of them having had a deficient number of teeth could be found.—J. FORBES WEBSTER.

X-RAY, &c.

Twelfth Report from the Cancer Research Laboratories

(*The Archives of the Middlesex Hospital*, vol. xxx).—Dr. W. B. Lazarus Barlow and Dr. T. J. B. Dunbar report experiments with the radiations of radium on muscle-nerve preparations of the frog. Experiments are given in detail. The conclusions are to the effect that under the conditions the radiations act beneficially. This is shown by the facts that—

1. The preparation responds to a smaller electrical stimulus than does the control preparation.

2. The preparation has a longer life than the control.

The action is due to the alpha radiations, there being no evidence that the beta or gamma rays take part in producing the effects.

Drs. Barlow and H. Beckton contribute an article on "Radium as a stimulus to cell division." The experiments were made on the ova of *Ascaris megalo-cephala*. Varying doses were administered from very small ones, which produced no recognisable change in the rate of development, up to doses so large that definite interference with growth was observed. Reference is made to previous work on the same lines published in the Eighth Cancer Report, 1909. The conclusion then arrived at was that small doses, or doses of short duration, cause cell division to proceed at a faster rate than normal; larger doses have an inhibitory action. From these later experiments they conclude—

1. If radium act on ova of *Ascaris megalocephala* in the resting stage in a given small quantity, and for a continuous period of about thirty hours at 0° C, cellular division subsequently proceeds at an accelerated rate.

2. Greater quantities than the above, or more prolonged exposures, pro-gressively retard the rate of division.

3. These effects are brought about by the action of alpha, beta, and gamma rays acting together.

4. Beta and gamma rays alone (alpha rays being excluded) act similarly.

5. The action of alpha rays appears to be about one hundred times as great as the action of beta rays.

Upon the whole, the results of using large amounts of radium for short periods are similar to the results of using smaller amounts of radium for longer periods. In other words, the retarding or accelerating effect of radium upon cell-division is governed by the "radium dose," the product of quantity of radium and length of exposure, while to produce a given effect either of these factors may vary within wide limits, provided that the other factor varies correspondingly in the inverse direction.

The fact that, clinically, this relationship of time and amount of radium is only recognisable within narrow limits is probably to be explained by the greater complexity of the cell and tissue layers upon which the radium is acting.

As a result of the action of the beta plus gamma rays from a few milligrammes of radium there occurs a disturbance of normal growth. This has been found to obtain both in the case of an animal cell (ova of *Ascaris megalocephala*) and vegetable.

This disturbance of growth is more marked if the cells, during irradiation, be in active division.

Dividing ova of *Ascaris* are at least eight times as vulnerable as resting ova.

The most vulnerable stage in division is the metaphase.

Beta and gamma irradiation is followed by profound nuclear changes affecting the chromatin; and such changes, though present, are less marked if the cells have been irradiated in a resting condition.

From the point of view of treatment of new growths by radium, this research indicates that satisfactory results may be expected in proportion to the percentage of neoplastic cells in active division during the period of irradiation, and, conversely, may explain the general experience of radiologists that rapidly growing tumours are more amenable to radium treatment than slow growing tumours. Further, since the vulnerability of a tissue must vary directly with the number of dividing cells present, it follows that a radium treatment may be so directed as to act upon rapidly dividing neoplastic cells, while it leaves the surrounding tissues relatively untouched. In order to affect the maximum number of neoplastic cells while in the dividing stage, the period of irradiation must be as prolonged as possible, consistent with lack of injury to the cells of the surrounding normal tissues.

N. Greenwood, jun., contributes "statistical notes" on the paper on "Radium as a stimulus of cell division." He concludes—"The evidence adduced by the authors in support of their contention that the effect of exposure to small quantities of radium is to increase the proportion of dividing cells, cannot be dismissed as vitiated by errors of sampling. Looked at from the statistical standpoint, there is a substantial probability in favour of their belief."

—JAS. R. RIDDELL.

"Focussing" X-Rays.—The rays from the *x*-ray tube are generated on a small area. They diverge as they pass on towards the part to be treated.

The result is that when the area lies deeply, as in the case in a fibroid or other tumour with sound skin over it, the skin receives a dose greatly in excess of that reaching the tumour. To obviate this Dr. Freiherr Von Wiéser, in conjunction with the Veifa Merke, Frankfurt, has devised a special tube. In it the target on which the *x*-rays are generated is of large size, and in front of the tube is placed a lead screen intercepting the path of the rays. Through this screen are a series of holes converging towards a predetermined point. From each point on the target *x*-rays arise and travel in all directions, but all are absorbed by the lead screen excepting those which converge towards the predetermined point. These pass through the holes in the screen. Photographs taken with this tube show that there is an actual increase of energy at the focal point, as compared with any other point nearer the tube. For deep-seated therapy the immense advantage of this is apparent.—JAS. R. RIDDELL.

The Control of the Quality and Quantity of the X-Rays issuing from the Tube.—Perhaps the greatest difficulty which confronts the radiologist in his work is the control of the quality and quantity of the *x*-rays issuing from the tube. Dr. W. D. Coolridge, from Schenectady, N.Y., has invented a tube which is described in the *Physical Review of the American Physical Society*, December, 1913. The peculiarities are : the vacuum is very high—several hundred times greater than that of the ordinary tube. The cathode is spiral in form, the two ends of the spiral being attached to two wires separated from each other, which pass out of the tube and are connected through a rheostat to a low tension battery ; this circuit has got an ammeter in it. When the cathode is cold no current can be forced through the tube at all, but when the current from the batteries is sent through the spiral it heats the spiral. The heated cathode is a source of the electrons which form the cathode stream by means of which the *x*-rays are generated. If the temperature of the spiral is low only a small number of the electrons escape from it, consequently only a small discharge current can be sent through the tube. As the temperature of the spiral is raised the discharge current through the tube increases, and with a given temperature the discharge current is always the same ; the current thus being constant the penetration of the rays is increased by simply increasing the voltage in the high tension circuit. As the tube is capable of giving an immense output as compared with the ordinary tubes in use at present, it is highly dangerous and must be used with the greatest caution.

" This new and very powerful Roentgen-ray tube differs in principle from the ordinary type in that the discharge current is purely thermionic in character, the tube and the electrodes being freed from gas as thoroughly as possible, so that the positive ions play no appreciable role in the discharge.

" The tube rectifies its own current, so that it can be driven by either direct or alternating current.

" Both the intensity and the penetration of the *x*-rays produced are under the complete control of the operator, and either can be instantly increased or diminished independently of the other, enabling us to obtain an intense homo. geneous beam of primary *x*-rays of any desired penetration.

" The tube can be driven continuously for hours, with either high or low discharge current, without showing an appreciable change in the intensity or penetrating power of the radiations.

" The tube shows no fluorescence and no local heating of the anterior hemis. phere."—JAS. R. RIDDELL.

Reyn's Electrolysis and its Application in Tuberculous Rhino-Laryngological Diseases. By Dr. Ove Strandberg (*Archives of the Roentgen Ray*, May, 1914).—The object of this method is the production of free iodine in the diseased area. The patient is given a large dose of sodium iodide ; in the case of an adult 5 grammes. An hour and a quarter after taking the drug the application is made. The electrode consists of a number of fine platinum-iridium needles placed side by side, and attached to a metal handle. The needles are made to pierce the mucous membrane at the diseased area. The electrode is attached to the positive pole of a battery or other source of galvanic current, and a current of from 3 to 5 milliamperes is made to flow for three or four minutes. Experimental work is recorded by which it was established that, an hour and a quarter after taking the dose mentioned, iodine actually is liberated in the tissues by the current named. To quote from Dr. Standberg's paper—

"1. In the human organism it is possible to set free nascent iodine electrolytically from sodium iodide given internally.

"2. For an adult the dose must be at least 3 grammes in a single dose.

"3. The maximum effect of the electrolysis is obtainable from one to two hours after the administration of the sodium iodide.

"4. In this reaction the positive is the active pole.

"5. The current must be at least 2 milliamperes at 65 volts."

Details are given of the classes of cases treated, and three cases are reported in full ; in all 217 patients have been treated.

"Reyn's electrolysis offers many advantages ; one of these is the comparatively short duration of the treatment which has nevertheless proved effective even in inveterate cases."—JAS. R. RIDDELL.

Ionisation and Electrolysis in Affections of the Nose and Ear. By A. R. Friel, M.D. (*Archives of the Roentgen Ray*, November, 1913).— The agent used is the zinc ion derived from a 1 per cent solution of the sulphate. Various forms of electrodes are described. For example, for the maxillary antrum a Eustachian catheter covered with a piece of rubber tubing is used ; for the frontal sinus a frontal sinus cannula painted externally with celloidin to insulate it where it touches the tissues ; for the nose a vulcanic speculum is placed in the nostril, and inside this is a wire dipping into the solution filling the nose. Before filling the nose with the solution the patient lies down, and a small balloon attached to the end of a catheter is passed down one of the nostrils into the naso-pharynx ; it is then blown up so as to block posterior nares. The current used is 2 or 3 milliamperes, and the length of application ten minutes. The writer says, "My experience is if ionisation is going to do good it does so straight away." The treatment should be repeated about once a week.

JAS. R. RIDDELL.

Books, Pamphlets, &c., Received.

The Child's Diet, by J. Sadler Curgenven, M.R.C.S., L.R.C.P. Second edition. London: H. K. Lewis. 1914. (2s. 6d. net.)

A Handbook of Fevers, by J. Campbell M'Clure, M.D.Glasg. London: Shaw & Sons. 1914.

Diseases of the Stomach and their Relation to other Diseases, by Charles G. Stockton, M.D. With 5 plates, 22 radiograms, and 65 illustrations in the text. London: D. Appleton & Co. 1914. (25s. net.)

Anæmia and Resuscitation: An Experimental and Clinical Research, by George W. Crile. London: D. Appleton & Co. 1914. (21s. net.)

The Occupational Diseases: Their Causation, Symptoms, Treatment, and Prevention, by W. Gilman Thompson, M.D. Illustrated. London: D. Appleton & Co. 1914. (25s. net.)

The Newer Physiology in Surgical and General Practice, by A. Rendle Short, M.D., B.S., B.Sc.Lond., F.R.C.S.Eng. Third edition, revised and enlarged. Bristol: John Wright & Sons, Limited. 1914. (5s. net.)

Examination of the Urine and other Clinical Side-room Methods (late Husband's), by Andrew Fergus Hewat, M.B., Ch.B., M.R.C.P.Ed. Fifth edition. Edinburgh: E. & S. Livingstone. 1914. (1s. 6d. net.)

The Practical Medicine Series, under the general editorial charge of Charles L. Mix, A.M., M.D., and Rodger T. Vaughan, Ph.B., M.D. Series 1914. Chicago: The Year Book Publishers. (Price of the series of ten volumes, $10·00.)

Vol. I.—General Medicine, edited by Frank Billings, M.S., M.D., and J. H. Salisbury, A.M., M.D. ($1·50.)

Vol. II.—General Surgery, edited by John B. Murphy, A.M., M.D., LL.D. ($2·00.)

Vol. III.—The Eye, Ear, Throat and Nose, edited by Casey A. Wood, C.M., M.D., D.C.L., Albert H. Andrews, M.D., and William L. Ballinger, M.D. ($1·50.)

Gonorrhœa and its Complications in the Male and Female, by David Watson, M.B., C.M. With 72 illustrations and 12 plates, 9 of which are in colours. London: Henry Kimpton. 1914. (15s. net.)

A Surgical Handbook for the Use of Students, Practitioners, House Surgeons, and Dressers, by Francis M. Caird, M.B., F.R.C.S.Ed., and Charles W. Cathcart, M.B., F.R.C.S.Eng. & Ed. With 208 illustrations. Sixteenth edition, revised and enlarged. London: Charles Griffin & Co., Limited. 1914. (8s. 6d.)

The Brain in Health and Disease, by Joseph Shaw Bolton, M.D., D.Sc.Lond., F.R.C.P.Lond. London: Edward Arnold. 1914. (18s. net.)

Mechano-Therapeutics in General Practice, by G. de Swietochowski, M.D., M.R.C.S. With 31 illustrations. London: H. K. Lewis. (4s. net.)

GLASGOW.—METEOROLOGICAL AND VITAL STATISTICS FOR THE FIVE WEEKS ENDED 15TH AUGUST, 1914.

	WEEK ENDING				
	July 18.	July 25.	Aug. 1.	Aug. 8.	Aug. 15.
Mean temperature, . .	57·2°	60·8°	57·0°	57·1°	60·0°
Mean range of temperature between highest and lowest,	24·2°	13·3°	17·8°	12·5°	16·2°
Number of days on which rain fell, ...	1	1	1	7	1
Amount of rainfall, . ins.	0·043	0·010	0·03	1·52	0·05
Deaths (corrected), . .	256	287	238	238	293
Death-rates, ...	12·8	14·3	11·9	11·9	14·6
Zymotic death-rates, . .	0·8	0·9	0·4	0·9	0·9
Pulmonary death-rates, .	2·1	2·4	2·3	2·0	2·9
DEATHS—					
Under 1 year, . . .	64	53	45	52	63
60 years and upwards, .	55	70	66	63	72
DEATHS FROM—					
Small-pox, ...	...	...	...	...	...
Measles, ...	2	3	3	1	...
Scarlet fever, . . .	1	3	...	2	2
Diphtheria, . . .	2	..	...	2	1
Whooping-cough, . .	11	7	5	11	12
Enteric fever, . . .	1	2	...	3	2
Cerebro-spinal fever, . .	1	3	...	...	...
Diarrhœa (under 2 years of age),	11	11	15	19	18
Bronchitis, pneumonia, and pleurisy, . . .	26	30	33	32	38
CASES REPORTED—					
Small-pox, ...	...	...	...	...	...
Cerebro-spinal meningitis, .	...	2	...	1	5
Diphtheria and membranous croup, ...	23	18	16	17	18
Erysipelas, . . .	21	21	24	37	29
Scarlet fever, . . .	48	70	64	88	62
Typhus fever, . . .	1	...	...	...	...
Enteric fever, . . .	7	8	9	5	23
Phthisis, ...	26	41	35	62	28
Puerperal fever, . .	2	1	1	8	3
Measles,* . . .	35	17	30	11	10

* Measles not notifiable.

SANITARY CHAMBERS,
GLASGOW, 25th August, 1914.

THE

GLASGOW MEDICAL JOURNAL.

No. IV. OCTOBER, 1914.

ORIGINAL ARTICLES.

THE USE OF NEO–SALVARSAN IN MENTAL DEFICIENCY.*

BY LEONARD FINDLAY, M.D., D.Sc.,
Physician, Royal Hospital for Sick Children, Glasgow.

OUR opinion regarding the frequency or infrequency with which mental deficiency is a consequence of syphilis depends on the reliance which we place in the Wassermann test. Before the introduction of this reaction it is true that some authors, e.g., Ziehen,[1] had found evidence of syphilis in as many as 17 per cent of the cases, but Shuttleworth,[2] on the other hand, concluded that only 1 per cent of cases of idiocy were due to this malady. With the advent of the serological test, however, some of us have come to look upon syphilis as a very serious element in the production of mental weakness. With the help of this test Fraser and Watson[3] found evidence of lues in 60 per cent of 205 mentally defective and epileptic children, and Robertson and I, working with the same technique, obtained a positive Wassermann reaction in 59 per cent of 15 mentally defective children. Dean[4] concluded that at least 15 per cent

* The Wassermann tests were in part done by Drs. C. H. Browning, Madge Robertson, and H. F. Watson.

of cases of idiocy were due to syphilis, and Krober[5] puts the figure at 21 per cent.

Undoubtedly the highest percentages have been obtained by workers in the West of Scotland using the Browning, Cruikshank, and M'Kenzie method, and these same figures have caused some authorities to question the diagnostic value of the test. If anything, in the absence of both a history of lues and specific stigmata, were required to confirm our opinion that the spirochæta pallida is a frequent cause of idiocy, and also that salvarsan is exceedingly efficacious in the treatment of syphilitic manifestations, the following experience in the treatment of mental deficiency would suffice. It must be admitted that my experience is limited, and I await with interest the reports of other workers.

M'Kenzie,[6] one of the strongest supporters of the syphilitic basis of much mental deficiency, remarks that the condition is peculiarly unsuitable for treatment by salvarsan. This, to my mind, is purely a theoretical objection, for we really do not know the nature of the lesion in such cases, and there is no à priori reason why a syphilitic affection of the brain, just as similar lesions elsewhere, should not be relieved by such a potent antispecific remedy. It is quite true that nervous tissue has practically no power of regeneration, but certainly any such capacity in this direction that it may possess will be met with during early life. In view of the fact, too, that it is the vessels of the cerebrum which suffer earliest and most frequently in congenital syphilis, one need not be surprised if antisyphilitic treatment should prove of some service in syphilitic brain lesions.

In all probability the effect of salvarsan in this condition would have been thoroughly tested before this had it not been for the fear of inducing encephalitis. So far as one can judge from the records in the literature of the treatment of nervous diseases by salvarsan, such a fear is well founded, but as the condition of mental deficiency, if left alone, is such a hopeless one, even a modicum of success would, in my opinion, far outbalance an occasional accident.

Stimulated by good results in the treatment of old-standing congenital syphilitic lesions, and fortified by the experience that the drug and its administration are almost, if not absolutely, safe, I determined to use it in some cases of mental deficiency. I felt, too, that were my efforts successful the results would go far to substantiate the true syphilitic nature of cases of idiocy, which reacted positively to Wassermann's test, and yet which did not present specific stigmata.

CASE I.—E. H., female, æt. 8 years. First seen 14th November, 1912. Father and mother alive and well. Patient is one of a family of five, all of whom are living. The other children are normal, and there is no specific history in the family.

Patient began to walk at 15 months, and to talk at 18 months, but she has never talked well. She commenced to get teeth at 18 months; the upper incisors have never appeared. She was always a backward child, has never been to school, and is subject to nervous attacks, during which shaking of the hands and feet occurs. She would never associate with other children, could not be sent messages, was not able to dress herself, and frequently soiled her clothes. Shortly before coming under observation she had been looked upon as a cretin, and was treated with thyroid gland without any benefit.

She is pale, nervous, mentally deficient to an extreme degree, and undersized. There are no specific stigmata.

Patient, her mother, and four brothers and sisters all give a positive Wassermann reaction.

She was treated with potass. iodid. and hydrarg. perchlor. for four months, but with no improvement. Between 8th April, 1913, and 12th May, 1913, she received in addition four intra-muscular injections of neo-salvarsan in doses varying between 0·4 and 0·6 grm., in all 1·8 grms. By the conclusion of the series of injections she had distinctly improved, and was brighter mentally, but the pain and induration consequent on the treatment had been so severe that it was decided to administer the drug intravenously. From 19th May to 2nd June, 1913, she received three intravenous injections in doses varying between 0·3 and 0·4 grm. at weekly intervals, *i.e.*, in all 1·05 grms. The child by this time had still further improved; she was brighter, was beginning to play with other children, and could be trusted to go messages. From 9th September till 23rd September, 1913, she received other four intravenous injections, the doses varying between 0·35 and 0·25 grm. These last four injections were administered under an anæsthetic, as the child had hitherto been very much afraid at the time of the operation. In all, she received 4 grms. of neo-salvarsan.

At the termination of the salvarsan therapy she was greatly improved. She was anxious to play with other children, could be trusted to go messages, could dress herself, and had ceased to soil her clothes. She would now enter into conversation, and at home was desirous of making herself useful by washing dishes and helping with the baby. Her mother remarked that she was becoming " very wild,' like her younger sister, and when outside could hold her own with other children.

The child was last seen on 9th June, 1914, when the Wassermann and luetin reactions were definitely negative. She had not received any mercury since November, 1913. The improvement in both her mental and physical states has continued. Her mother says that she is very different to what she was before the injections were commenced. She wants now to go to school, and from her sister has learned many letters of the alphabet, and also figures.

CASE II.—W. G., male, æt. 8½ years. First seen on 9th May, 1913, on account of not making progress at school, which he had attended for three years. He is one of a family of three, the other members of which are healthy and intelligent. There is no specific history in the family (father is a soldier) nor of mental disease, nor are the parents related to one another.

Patient never goes out to play with other boys, nor can he defend himself against them. He cannot go messages nor make the slightest attempt at reading, and is only able to recognise pictures of very few common objects.

He is moderately well developed physically, has a somewhat small head and a dull apathetic expression. There are no specific stigmata. Wassermann reaction is definitely positive. From 16th May till 23rd June, 1913, *i.e.*, during a period of 5½ weeks, he received five intramuscular injections of neo-salvarsan in doses varying between 0·3 and 0·45 grm., in all 1·9 grms. At the same time he was given potass. iodid. and hydrarg. perchlor. per os.

After four injections his mother stated that he was distinctly brighter, and for the first time cried on entering the dispensary, apparently recognising that he was going to receive an injection, which always caused considerable pain. He could now go messages, and was able to read such small words as "cat" and "dog," which he could not do previously. Four months after the last injection he was still progressing, had been put into a higher class at school, and was playing with other boys, but still allowed them to "knock him about." Six months after the last injection the Wassermann reaction was still positive but weak. Potass. iodid. and hydrarg. perchlor. were still being continued.

Seen on 25th April, 1914, ten months after last injection. Had not received potass. iodid. or hydrarg. perchlor. for six weeks. He had lost the dull apathetic look, and for the first time conversed freely with me. He is in the same class as his brother, who is 2½ years younger, but is learning just as quickly. His school teacher admits he is only slow, but this same teacher one year ago said that it was impossible to do anything at all with him at school. He can go messages, plays with other children, and is now able to defend himself against boys of his own age.

CASE III.—G. G., male, æt. 7½ years. First seen on 24th February, 1913, because he had been dismissed from school on account of his inability to learn.

Father and mother alive and well. He is one of a family of three, all of whom are living. There is no history of mis-carriages or still-births or of syphilis in parents or family. The other two children are quite normal.

Patient was a healthy baby at birth, walked at twelve months, and talked at eighteen months. Until he was sent to school he seemed quite a normal child. At school he is well behaved but is making no progress, and his mother states that he is gradually getting duller. He used to go out to play and could be sent messages, but now he simply sits about the house taking no interest in anything. If thwarted at home he is subject to severe fits of passion, which will last for one or two hours and during which he will tear his clothes and break any dishes that may be within his reach. He has also not been thriving of late.

He is an undersized child (2 st. 5½ lb.), but does not present any specific stigmata. He cannot recognise pictures of common objects or even the objects themselves, cannot tell where he lives, or if he has any brothers or sisters, and any conversation that he has consists of one or two words. The Wassermann reaction is strongly positive in both the patient and his mother.

On 25th March, 1913, he received an intramuscular injection of 0·45 grm. neo-salvarsan, which caused great induration and tenderness, and in consequence it was decided to administer the drug intravenously. From 8th April till 6th May, *i.e.*, a period of four weeks, he received five intravenous injections of neo-salvarsan in doses varying between 0·3 and 0·45 grm., in all 1·75 grms. At the same time he was treated with mercurial inunctions.

As a result of the treatment he improved considerably. On 7th September he had been back at school and seemed more interested. He could again be trusted to go messages, and always brought back the correct change, whereas before he invariably spent on sweets any change that he received. He had ceased to take the violent fits of temper, and his general health had also improved, but he was still very backward mentally. After this he was lost sight of, but recently it was learned that about Christmas, 1913, *i.e.*, seven and a half months after the last injection of neo-salvarsan, he commenced to take convulsions and suffered from severe headaches. This state of matters persisted until the middle of March, 1914, when he developed blindness. Soon afterwards the convulsions and headaches became more violent and head retraction appeared. He died three weeks later.

CASE IV.—W. B., male, æt. 8½ years. First seen on 22nd January, 1913, in East Park Home for Infirm Children.

Father and mother are alive and well. Mother has had six pregnancies. Patient is the first and the second was still-born. There have been no miscarriages. The other children are alive and well. Patient learned to walk at 2 years, and to talk at 3 years, but he has never been bright. He had never been to school.

When first seen he was an undersized mentally deficient child. He spent most of his time by himself sitting in a chair with his head rolling from side to side. He could walk but very unsteadily, the slightest push causing him to fall. His head was large and square, with prominent forehead, and of a definite hot-cross bun shape. Round the mouth were linear cicatrices and an eczematous condition implicating the mucous membrane of the lips. Both upper central incisors were notched, and interstitial keratitis was also present.

Between 16th October and 8th November, *i.e.*, a period of three and a half weeks, he received four intravenous injections of neo-salvarsan in doses varying between 0·3 and 0·4 grm.; in all 1·3 grm. neo-salvarsan was administered. At the same time mercury was prescribed. After the injections he seemed more interested in things, and commenced to run about and play, but on account of his eyesight getting worse he could not be sent to school.

On 13th December, one month after the last injection, the Wassermann reaction was still strongly positive. In his general health he was, however, much improved, was brighter mentally, and could go messages. His eyesight was, on the other hand, not so good, and seemed to be getting rapidly worse.

Seen again on 18th June, 1914, when the following note was made:—General health has still continued good, and he is mentally brighter than formerly, but is now completely blind. In the right eye there is a slight degree of optic atrophy with disseminated choroiditis, and in the left an extensive cataract. To-day he visited East Park Home, and the sisters and assistant matron are quite emphatic that both mentally and physically he is very much better than when he left the institution one year ago.

Each of these cases, it will be admitted, was a very marked example of mental deficiency, three of them being frankly idiots. The treatment in all had a most salutary effect, and although it did not bring them up to a normal level, it made it possible for two of them to be educated, and to look after themselves. In milder cases, and especially if the treatment were commenced earlier, it might be possible to obtain complete cures. Unfortunately one of the children died, but so long after the cessation of the salvarsan administration that I do not think the issue can be ascribed in any way to the drug.

It is more likely that the mischief, which had been progressive before the child came under observation, was arrested by the treatment, and that it had several months later relapsed with the development of a gumma. Unfortunately no *post-mortem* examination was performed, and thus our opinion can only remain conjectural.

Conclusions.—1. Syphilis is a frequent cause of idiocy.

2. In syphilitic idiocy there may be no luetic stigmata.

3. Neo-salvarsan when introduced intravenously or intra-muscularly has a very marked effect in improving the mental condition.

LITERATURE.

[1] Ziehen, *Psychiatrie*, Leipzig, 1908, p. 613.

[2] Shuttleworth, *Amer. Jour. of Insanity*, 1888, lxiv, p. 381.

[3] Fraser and Watson, *Jour. of Mental Science*, October, 1913.

[4] Dean, *Proceed. Royal Soc. of Medicine*, July, 1910.

[5] Krober, *Med. klin. Wien*, 1911, vol. vii, p. 1239.

[6] M'Kenzie, *Fourth Annual Report of the Scottish Western Asylums' Institute*, 1913, p. 7.

PRACTICAL POINTS IN ABDOMINAL SURGERY, BEING THE "JAMES WATSON LECTURES" DELIVERED BEFORE THE ROYAL FACULTY OF PHYSICIANS AND SURGEONS, 11th and 14th MARCH, 1913.

By T. KENNEDY DALZIEL, M.B., F.R.F.P.S.,
Surgeon to the Western Infirmary, Glasgow.

(*Continued from* p. 182.)

Deformities.—In regard to deformities, that condition of pylorus we have already described may be taken first, as the one which we first see in life.

The pyloric ring may be so thick as to form a tumour, easily palpable, especially if, as is usual, a few weeks have elapsed since birth; during which time progressive emaciation has rendered the subject worthy of an advertisement for meat juice. In some cases the stomach is dilated, in others the ease with which the food can be regurgitated permits the organ to retain its normal size, or even, when irritation sets in, to become somewhat contracted. Such an infant takes food readily for a week or so, retains it some time, and subsequently vomits immediately milk is taken. The child necessarily wastes, the bowels act very slowly, and unless an operation is performed to permit the onward flow of nourishment, the child dies in the course of seven or eight weeks or earlier, usually with a dilated stomach.

Here the deformity is entirely one of the muscular coats. As a rule the mucous membrane is sufficiently well developed readily to expand if a pyloroplasty be performed.

In infants a longitudinal incision is made down to, but not injuring, the mucous membrane. The peritoneum is then drawn from each end of the incision into the gap, while the sides of the wound are pulled transversely and several stitches placed to cover in the surface of the cut muscle. The line of sutures then represents a transverse incision instead of a longitudinal one. No blood need be lost in such an operation, and little anæsthetic is required, and the bowel not being opened there is little fear of sepsis. For additional security to the wound a fold of omentum may be tacked over it. In spite of the fact that some physicians have given an opinion very adverse to this operation, I have been more than satisfied with the results.

I had two in one week recently in the Children's Hospital, so fragile and so wasted—the one after five, and the other after seven, weeks' semi-starvation—that one hardly dare touch them; yet both immediately revived, till now, within a few months after the operation, they may be recognised as fairly well-nourished infants.

CASE 1 (sent by Dr. Murray Young, Hamilton).—Baby H., æt. 2½ months. Admitted with a history of persistent vomiting since 3 weeks old. At first the vomiting was occasional, and not very severe; but it gradually became more severe and more persistent, until at last the child vomited up everything taken. It did not occur immediately on taking nourishment, but usually between one and two hours after taking a drink. The vomited material was white in colour, and contained usually some curds of various sizes up to the area of a threepenny piece; latterly, it was of a light brown colour at times, and of a very watery consistence. In the first three weeks of life the bowels moved quite normally, but since the onset of the vomiting described there was at first some sluggishness, which developed later into complete constipation, the bowels never moving unless after an enema, and the result consisting of small scybala. Simultaneously with the onset of these symptoms the child began to lose flesh, and to get generally out of condition. The child was fed at first on the breast, and, later, on various peptogenic foods; but in spite of these he did not thrive, but continued as described. Medical advice was obtained, but in spite of treatment the symptoms persisted, and the child continued to lose flesh.

He was admitted to the Sick Children's Hospital on 7th October, 1912, and when seen presented the typical appearance of marasmus. The abdomen was normal in appearance, but peristalsis was visible very distinctly in the upper part. It began in the left hypochondrium, was seen to pass downwards and to the right, and was very distinctly intensified by giving the child a bottle to suck. On admission the weight was 6 lb. 7½ oz.; the temperature was 100°, with a pulse of 120, and respirations 32 per minute.

The child was operated on shortly after admission, and pyloroplasty performed. The muscular coats of the pylorus were about a quarter of an inch in thickness, and this thickening was about an inch and a half in length.

After operation a saline (3 oz. with brandy min. 10) was administered, and repeated four-hourly. Peptogenic milk (1 oz.) was given orally, alternately with Valentine's Meat-Juice ($\frac{1}{2}$ oz.) in hot water. The child stood the operation quite well, and was only slightly sick afterwards.

On 9th October—two days after operation—there was some recurrence of vomiting, and so only sterile water was given by mouth, the rest of the nourishment being given rectally.

11th October.—The salines were stopped on this date, and the patient put on Sister Laura's Food ($\frac{1}{2}$ oz.), with boiled water ($\frac{1}{2}$ oz.) hourly. The child was generally greatly better, and vomiting had ceased entirely.

By 13th October the amount of the food given was 1 oz. hourly, and by the 18th 3 oz. three-hourly were taken by mouth, and no inconvenience followed. On this date the weight was 7 lb. $\frac{1}{2}$ oz.

21st October.—Weight, 7 lb. 9 oz. On the 24th the amount of food taken was 2 oz. two-hourly.

On dismissal (31st October) the weight was 8 lb. 1$\frac{1}{2}$ oz., and the child was looking better in every way. The bowels had also improved, and whilst at first laxative medicine was required, latterly the bowels moved normally of their own accord.

Nothing further was heard until 3rd January, 1913, when the child was brought back to report. It was a healthy-looking child in every way, and was taking its food quite well. The weight was 14 lb. 12 oz., a difference of 8 lb. 4$\frac{1}{2}$ oz. from its weight on admission.

CASE 2 (sent in by Dr. Brown, of Dennistoun, and Dr. Findlay).—Alex. M'C., æt. 9 weeks. Admitted on 26th October, 1912, with a history of persistent vomiting since birth until about two weeks before admission. As in the previous case, he had been weaned, and various peptogenic foods of all strengths tried, and even whey alone, but still the vomiting continued, and with it the patient began to lose flesh.

Diarrhœa came on a few days after birth, and continued until about one week before admission. The stools were loose and very frequent, but they did not contain any evident excess of mucus, and there was never any melæna. For the fortnight previous to admission the symptoms were not so clamant, and small quantities of peptonised milk (1 part in sterile water, 3 parts) were often kept down; but the child did not seem to improve any in general health, and was still losing flesh.

When seen on admission the child was pale and very thin, so that the ribs could be seen distinctly under the skin. The abdomen was not so distended as usual, and peristalsis from left to right was seen in the region of the stomach. It was not nearly so evident as in the previous case, and at times was not seen at all. The weight was 6 lb. 10 oz., with a normal temperature, a pulse of 132, and respirations of 28 per minute.

On the following day (27th October) pyloroplasty was performed. Three hours after operation saline (2 oz. with brandy min. 10) was given rectally. The child was somewhat collapsed during the course of the operation, but the saline, which was retained, seemed to have a distinctly beneficial effect. Rectal feeding was instituted, peptonised milk ($\frac{1}{2}$ oz. with brandy min. 10) being given two-hourly. The bowel was washed out once every twenty-four hours.

On 31st October oral feeding was started. Peptonised milk (1 oz. with brandy min. 10) was given two-hourly, while the rectal feeds were now given every four hours.

1st November.—The patient was put on to peptonised milk ($1\frac{1}{2}$ oz. with brandy min. 10) four-hourly, and rectal feeds six-hourly. The bowels moved regularly once every twenty-four hours, and since the operation there had been no sign of sickness. Weight, 7 lb. $\frac{1}{2}$ oz.

By 3rd November rectal feeding was stopped entirely, and the child put on to hourly feeds of the same food as Case 1, with brandy min. 10 in each feed.

Things went on quite well after this. By 6th November the stitches were removed and all was found well, and by 11th November brandy was left out of the feeds. On the 6th the weight was 6 lb. 15 oz.; on the 11th, 7 lb. $4\frac{1}{2}$ oz.

Between 12th and 17th November gastro-enteritis was

present, as shown by vomiting; some diarrhœa, with green stools; fretfulness, and failure to increase weight, although none was lost. The usual weight was about 7 lb. 4 oz. The peptogenic food was stopped, and peptonised milk given, but it was replaced again by albumen water (1 oz.) two-hourly. Stimulant was again called into use. Castor oil min. 10 was given as required.

After 18th November things improved very quickly, and the symptoms noted disappeared. Stimulant was omitted, and peptogenic food again used, with quite satisfactory results.

25th November.—The child went home, weighing 7 lb. 5 oz.

On enquiry we found that by 2nd January, 1913, the child was well in every way, and weighed 11 lb. 1 oz.—an increase of 4 lb. 7 oz. from its weight on admission.

The oldest case on whom I have done this operation is now 10 years of age, and though occasionally troubled with gastric disorder is, on the whole, a good average child.

. I think it more than likely, however, that, as in lesser degrees of pyloric obstruction, such cases will, as age advances, require a gastro-enterostomy. It seems likely that the scar left by operation, plus the rigidity which is likely to follow the presence of the mass of fibrous muscular tissue, will lead to a degree of pyloric insufficiency. It is, however, too early yet to arrive at a definite conclusion.

While in infants this operation seems to be a simple, safe, and effective proceeding, it has not, in my experience, been of the same value in later life. So much so, that after considerable experience of pyloroplasty in adults I have practically given it up. The cases seem to do well for a time—a year or two years or more—but in about 50 per cent of the cases symptoms recur, and in many a gastro-enterostomy has been required.

The relaxation of the sphincter and its powerlessness for a time enables the stomach to empty itself, but as the wound heals cicatrisation advances, the muscle again becomes active, and the old train of symptoms is re-established. In a lesser degree of contraction I believe good may be obtained, but, on the whole, it is an operation which I have come to view rather with disfavour.

A word is necessary regarding the exact operation performed.

After opening the abdomen the pylorus was isolated and incised longitudinally for as far as hypertrophy and stenosis existed; but in depth the incision extended only down to, but not through, the mucous membrane.   The median points of the incision were then drawn apart, and a vertically stitched wound made as usual.   Thus, the lumen of the bowel was never opened into, and hence no gastro-intestinal contents could get into the peritoneum.   Again only one layer of stitches was required in stitching the pyloric wound.

These points indicate safety and simplicity with attendant speed for this operation, as compared with the operation, usually described, of puncturing the stomach, passing a probe or director through stomach puncture and through pylorus, and cutting down on it through all the coats of the pylorus.

Hour-glass stomach.—This is, as a rule, an acquired malformation, the result of cicatrisation following a somewhat extensive ulceration.   Some cases may be suspected from the organic dilatation, from the behaviour of the stomach during lavage, and the appearances presented by a radiography after a bismuth meal.   The symptoms are, indeed, largely those of a combination of chronic ulceration and pyloric obstruction; and, indeed, not infrequently we have, in addition to the hour-glass contraction, pyloric obstruction as well.   It is an interesting fact that in Glasgow we seem to see comparatively little of the hour-glass stomach.   Though surgeons, especially in the midlands of England, are constantly seeing it, yet after some extensive experience I have only had to deal with three cases, in one of which, the pylorus seeming normal, I contented myself with establishing a drain between the proximal dilated portion of the stomach and the jejunum.   In another I felt it right to excise the diseased portion of the stomach, and in a third I felt justified in restoring the shape of the stomach by an incision similar to that practised in pyloroplasty.

The infrequency of hour-glass stomach in Glasgow, if my experience corresponds with that of other surgeons, is interesting as illustrating the fact that different types of diseases are met with in different parts of the country, probably determined by the habits of the people.

Congenital dilatation of the stomach occurs, and a similar

dilatation may result from over-eating; while dilatation from atony, though frequently spoken of in text-books, has been in my experience extremely rare, and probably occurs in a general asthenia. It has been proposed in such cases to distinguish the .size of the stomach by plication, but of this I have no experience.

There is, however, a form of atonic stomach which demands a surgeon's careful consideration, as not infrequently a troublesome complication after operations, not necessarily of the abdomen. This acute dilatation can hardly be described as atony, in so far as there can be no great change in the muscular fibre of the stomach during the short time it exists. One must suppose that it is due to an altered innervation, whether toxic in origin or as a part of the general loss of nerve force which one associates with shock. The symptoms are great epigastric discomfort, amounting to actual pain in some cases; visible distension of the organ; vomiting, which soon becomes offensive and generally dark from the presence of blood. The vomiting is not urgent, but tends to come up in mouthfuls, as if expressed by the muscles of the abdominal wall. Unless active measures be taken this condition may determine the death of the patient.

The worst case I have seen was that of a gentleman from whom a large pedunculated lipoma had been removed from the abdominal wall, an operation which only lasted a few minutes. In about eight hours some dark vomit occurred, when it was amply evident his stomach had become extremely distended. The vomit became black, and he looked as if he might die at any minute. The vomiting continued for nearly a week, and ultimately with lavage, &c., the patient made a good recovery. In every surgical clinic such cases will occur, and the lesser degrees make a spontaneous recovery, but the more serious cases call for active interference. Lavage probably affords the best means of treatment, though I recently had a patient from whose gall-bladder I had removed a collection of stones, and whose pylorus was surrounded with numerous adhesions, in whom I had after the lapse of days to perform a gastro-enterostomy, without which we were satisfied the patient would have died.

In this case we had not only the chronic and acute dilatation to contend with, but a narrow pylorus, anchored by adhesions in such a way as to render spontaneous recovery almost hopeless. Medicinal tonics, such as strychnine, ergot, and pituitary extract are no doubt useful aids.

Chronic dilatation.—Chronic dilatation, a type of gastric disease with which every physician is amply familiar, is characterised by loss of motor power, disordered digestion, and arrested absorption; and the symptoms will be found referable to these conditions, and also to those causing the dilatation.

The clinical picture of a case of chronic dilatation of the stomach you are probably more or less familiar ' with. As Douglas puts it, "such a person may be ravenously hungry at times, and complains of great thirst, though the heavy cutting characteristic of gastritis may be present. His breath is offensive, he eructates foul-smelling gas constantly in a long noisy effort. This belching is due to the fermentation of the stagnating stomach contents. Constipation is obstinate, the stools are dry masses, the urine is scanty, malaise is marked, and headache a constant accompaniment. Vertigo is a frequent symptom. If the distension is great the patient complains of cardiac embarrassment, and has palpitation, feeble irregular pulse, and often precordial pain, which may be mistaken for angina. The peripheral circulation becomes depressed, shown by moist and cold extremities. Occasionally there is a slight toxic temperature."

In some cases there is tetany, which manifests itself by painful spasms of the flexor muscles of the arms and legs. This is probably due to auto-intoxication; it is attended frequently by a rise of temperature, and must always be looked upon as a serious symptom, such patients not infrequently dying during an attack. Nervous depression of a profound type is frequently present; not infrequently unreasoning fears disturb the patient. Indeed, so profound may the nervous disturbance be that coma may terminate the case.

The diagnosis of dilated stomach, however, must rest on the size of the organ. It is not necessary for me to dwell on the numerous methods of estimating the position and size of the stomach. Inspection, palpation, and auscultatory percussion no doubt assist, but unless the stomach be previously washed out and dilated with gas these may be misleading. I have seen a dilated colon mistaken for a stomach for the want of this simple and obvious method of detection.

The surgical treatment of dilatation of the stomach must be familiar to most of you, and while it is true that almost all forms of dilatation can be relieved, and the atonic, especially the acute variety, cured by lavage and medicinal measures, it is also true that in a large percentage of cases of dilatation operative interference is called for, and this resolves itself into pyloroplasty or gastro-enterostomy.

Pyloroplasty.—This we have already discussed in relation to the congenital deformity of the pylorus, and a similar operation has been practised by many surgeons, and by myself for the relief of dilatation when due to the simpler forms of pyloric stenosis.

Gastro-enterostomy.—Gastro-enterostomy, however, holds the field as a more suitable method of draining the stomach. There have been numerous varieties of this operation—connecting the duodenum with the pyloric funnel, the jejunum with the anterior or the posterior wall of the stomach, and in the earlier days with a by-pass to prevent the bile reaching the new aperture. But it seems to me now sure that the best operation is the posterior.gastro-jejunostomy, arranging the parts that the opening in the stomach will lie over the descending jejunum, so that there may be no kinking or undue distortion of parts. This is no easy matter, since the stomach will certainly alter in shape after the operation, and may distort and displace what seems to be an admirable arrangement during operation. It is, I believe, a matter of experience to determine just where the opening should be made in the stomach.

The only complications after this operation which might cause anxiety are the occurrence of ulceration at the margin of the opening, and that of bilious regurgitation. At one time this was supposed to be unavoidable through the new opening, but experience shows that in the majority of cases it really takes place through the pylorus, and is probably determined by a disordered peristalsis of the duodenum. Usually it can be cured by permanently occluding the pyloric orifice, and, indeed, it is rarely found in cases where nature has already accomplished that end by cicatrisation. As I have long taught, we have least trouble from this complication in the worst cases of pyloric obstruction.

Ulceration of the stomach.—As elsewhere, ulcers may be divided into two groups, simple and malignant, the latter of which are sadly common, and for the most part cancerous. The non-malignant ulcers may be tuberculous. According to Professor Sutherland, of Dundee, tuberculous affection of the gastric mucosa is not at all uncommon, but fortunately it rarely advances, the growth being checked by the destruction of the tubercle bacillus by the gastric juices. In tuberculous persons swallowing affected material such superficial tuberculous ulcers are often found. Only occasionally, and especially about the pylorus, does the tuberculous process break away, passing beyond the reach of acid secretions, and becoming a chronic ulcer of a somewhat vicious type. I have seen such ulcers in infants, and not infrequently one finds evidence in the lymphatic glands that an infected atrium must have existed in the stomach or pylorus sometime in early life. Such diseased lymphatic glands may press upon the bile-ducts, and probably interfere with the solar plexus. Superficial ulcers, akin to those met with within the lips, which one associates with a disordered stomach, also occur within the stomach itself, and if in the pyloric ring may give rise to very severe gastric spasm, so intense as to simulate gall-stone colic, occasionally also giving rise to local tenderness. While these ulcers generally heal in a few days with the light diet which nature calls for, it is not improbable that they may start a more chronic process of ulceration, especially if within the sphincter, where the constant unrest may, as in the sphincter ani, establish a vicious circle, the pain causing a powerful contraction of the sphincter, injuring the ulcer and tending to prevent healing. Lastly, we have to deal with the commonest of all—chronic perforating ulcers of the stomach, pylorus, and duodenum. The first portion of the duodenum as far down as the gall-ducts is no doubt under the same influences, so far as contents are concerned, as the stomach, suggesting that the acidity of the stomach contents plays a not unimportant part in perpetuating, if not in creating those chronic ulcers. The neutralisation of the acid contents by the bile and pancreatic juices seems to remove these influences which act higher up.

One rarely sees ulceration in the small intestine; indeed, I have only known of two cases of tuberculous ulcer of the jejunum, and two cases of malignant ulcer. The primary cause of perforating ulcer is a matter of speculation. The theories of arteriospasm, septic infection of veins, hæmorrhage from degenerated arterioles, and so on, are but theories, and are not supported by any actual observations. I sometimes wonder if it be necessary with our knowledge of ulcerative processes elsewhere to search for such abstruse theories. It seems not unreasonable to suppose that such chronic ulcers may develop from small blisters, determined by an abnormal condition of the stomach contents, aided perhaps by constitutional weakness, such as anæmia.

It is an undoubted fact that in almost all cases of ulceration excessive acidity of the stomach contents will be found, and medically most relief will be obtained by a dietary which will diminish such acidity, or by medicines which will neutralise it. The surgical treatment of such chronic perforating ulcers, whose conical shape, hardened margins, and terraced sides you are all familiar with, will depend for the most part on the effects produced, and the surgeon is rarely asked to see such cases unless the ulcer happens to be a painful one; and here, in the stomach, as on the leg, you may have an ulcer absolutely callous and painless, or it may give rise to the most intense agony. Surgical interference may be called for on account of the ulcer penetrating a large blood-vessel. Thirdly, the ulcer may perforate the stomach wall, and give rise to a septic peritonitis; or may penetrate into one of the adjoining organs —the pancreas, liver, or spleen; or eat its way into the anterior abdominal wall; or through the diaphragm into the thorax.

And lastly, and perhaps more important than all, such an ulcer situated on the outlet of the stomach wall will in all its stages prevent proper emptying of the organ, and so induce dilatation—in the early stage by causing spasm of the sphincter, later by inducing disordered peristalsis, and ultimately by cicatrising and organically and mechanically blocking the outlet.

For long it has been taught that the ˉcardinal symptoms of ulceration of the stomach were pain after taking food and during the process of digestion, vomiting, local tenderness, and hæmorrhage, with the addition of secondary symptoms according to the situation of the ulcer, and the effect produced from malnutrition.

After a considerable experience of operations for gastric ulcers, it has been amply evident to me that these clinical symptoms are absent in the majority of cases.

That a person may have a chronic perforating ulcer of the stomach for years without any pain, vomiting, or tenderness is undoubted.   My attention was forcibly drawn to this many years ago by the history of a patient, a daughter of a deceased colleague, whom I saw with that most distinguished physician, Dr. R. S. Thomson.

A young lady of 26 years developed acute abdominal symptoms pointing to perforation of the stomach.   On opening the abdomen we found an ulcer in the middle of the anterior wall, from which the stomach contents were escaping.   This lady had at no time suffered from pain, sickness, or vomiting.   During conversations we had I tried hard to obtain any suggestion of suffering, but her only complaint was hunger.

And here I may state that in my experience hunger pain, by which I understand a hunger so intense as to amount to suffering, is very frequently met with in ulceration of the stomach, and only occasionally does it occur in ulceration of the duodenum. In this I am aware I differ from the views of others who have had even greater opportunities for observation than I have had ; and yet I am so definitely clear on the point that I do not hesitate to express the view quite frankly, nor do I see any physiological reason why an ulcer of the stomach should not be more likely than that of the duodenum to give rise to hunger.

That in cases of ulcer of the duodenum hunger has been complained of may well be accounted for by the fact that a person may have more than one ulcer.   In duodenal ulcer pain may no doubt be accounted for when the stomach contents scald it, and the taking of food, by arresting the stomach evacuation, may relieve the pain.   But this pain has, to my mind, been entirely different from the pain I have observed in gastric ulceration, where the discomfort is one of true hunger, and where the taking of food by diluting the stomach contents, or introducing alkalinity, will for a time arrest the gnawing hunger.

The lady I speak of found it necessary to resort to the pantry every two hours or so, and at night furnished herself with a supply of bread and butter, in this way making life more comfortable. She had not, however, actual pain—only intense hunger.

Whether local tenderness might have been detected or not is an open question, as she had had no medical advice until perforation occurred.

Pain from gastric ulcer may be very intense when the pancreas is invaded, and in the seven cases I have seen of gastric ulcer invading the pancreas, pain, especially referred to the back in the neighbourhood of the tenth and eleventh dorsal vertebræ, has been a marked feature. Localisation of pain not infrequently enables one to form a shrewd guess as to where the ulcer may be found. If at the cardiac orifice pain is generally referred up the œsophagus, patient complaining of pain behind the middle of the sternum. On the anterior wall referred pain in the left shoulder or under the shoulder blade may be noted. Posterior wall, apart from pancreatic perforation, gives rise to pain in the right shoulder. Ulcer of the lesser curvature may involve the disturbance of both pneumogastric and splanchnic nerves, and so give rise to pain in both shoulders. Ulceration in the duodenum and pylorus not infrequently implicates the hepatic plexus, and this refers the pain to the right shoulder. In such cases, however, we have a possibility of local tenderness to guide us. The tender area to the left of the eleventh and twelfth dorsal vertebræ, which has been noted by many observers, has not in my experience been much of a guide.

After this general *résumé* of pain in relation to ulceration of the stomach, one may state that the pain due to the involvement of the pancreatic or other organs may demand surgical interference, our objects being so to alter the condition of the stomach contents as to prevent extension of the ulceration; secondly, to save the organ which is involved.

Ulceration into the pancreas is extremely fatal. In the first three cases which came under my observation I contented myself with performing a gastro-enterostomy, hoping that by draining the stomach the ulcer might heal; but in one, paralysis of the whole intestine and stomach ensued, the distension becoming so extreme that the silkworm stitches which I had used in the abdominal wound broke, and some intestine protruded.   This was quickly rectified, but paralysis persisted, and the patient died in a couple of days, there being no evidence, *post-mortem*, of any peritonitis or cause for death. The second case died-from hæmorrhage from perforation of a large artery in the pancreas; and the third died some months after the operation from abscess in the neighbourhood of the pancreas.

The penetration of the ulcer into the pancreas presents peculiar features, the secreting lobes persisting while the fibrous matrix disappears.   It may be that the alkalinity of the pancreatic juice neutralises the effect of the acid secretions of the stomach.   Latterly, I have in every case deliberately separated the stomach from the pancreas, using the hole in the stomach, after refreshing its edges, to anastomose with the intestine, or closing it and making an ordinary gastroenterostomy.   I then carry down to the ulcer in the pancreas a funnel of parietal peritoneum, down which an antiseptic dressing can be introduced into the ulcer of the pancreas.   Of the four. cases so treated one died, apparently from shock; the rest did well.

When situated on the lesser curvature near the cardiac orifice the ulcer may perforate the diaphragm.   Two such cases I have seen, and both proved fatal from septic pleurisy. The anterior abdominal wall may be attacked.   Such a case was recently in my wards, the history being one merely of slight dyspepsia, and, when seen, what appeared to be an abscess was found below the left costal margin.   The contents of the abscess indicated its origin.   The stomach was separated from the abdominal wall and sutured, and the patient ultimately made a good recovery.

Ulcers in the neighbourhood of the pylorus present often extremely difficult problems, causing, as they do, great matting of the parts.

(To be concluded.)

NEW MEDICAL ELECTRICAL DEPARTMENT OF THE GLASGOW ROYAL INFIRMARY.

By JOHN MACINTYRE, M.B., C.M.,

Surgeon for Diseases of Throat and Nose, Glasgow Royal Infirmary ;
Consulting Medical Electrician to the Hospital.

In the year 1897 an Electrical Department was instituted in the Royal Infirmary, and at the request of the managers I was asked to take charge of it.

It was a very modest installation, but, probably for the first time in any hospital, arrangements were made for carrying the current from the centre room to the different parts of the hospital by means of wires carried through the building.

In 1894, owing to the kindness and generosity of a few citizens, a considerable addition was made to the apparatus, consisting of gas engine, secondary cells, medical and surgical switchboards, and apparatus generally in use for the treatment of disease.

In the early part of 1896, shortly after the historical discovery of Roentgen, an *x*-ray laboratory, which was the first of its kind in the world, was installed in the Royal Infirmary, and, from that time onwards, the Infirmary, as the science advanced, has been provided with the best apparatus in every department of medical and electrical work.

Glasgow is noted for its generosity and liberality wherever money is necessary to assist the less fortunate of its citizens, and, thanks to a few members of the community, something like £10,000 have been spent in connection with the medical and electrical department, so that nothing has been taken from the funds of the Infirmary for this purpose.

Since the foundation of the electrical department, the managers have given it every encouragement and support. While it is true that the money for the apparatus was got from outside sources, still the chairman and managers of the hospital have provided the building and staff, and have done whatever was possible to give the patients of the hospital the benefit of the most recent advances in science.

It should also be recorded that the apparatus has been very largely used both by the visiting and dispensary staffs, and thousands of patients in the hospital and also under the care of the outside medical profession have benefited by the department.

No one could have predicted in 1896 that within a short period of time such advances could be made. The ever memorable discovery of Roentgen has opened a new chapter in physical, chemical and medical history, and the results recorded in diagnosis and treatment have surpassed all anticipation.

The following notes will show to some extent in what direction medical science has been advancing.

In designing the new installation it was necessary to keep two things clearly in view—the danger, firstly, to the patients, and, secondly, to the doctor and nurses. With regard to the former, the apparatus has been so arranged that it is impossible that the high currents of 500 or 250 volts supplied by the Glasgow Corporation can ever reach the patient. In some transformers this would be quite possible, but Glasgow Royal Infirmary utilises the main only to drive the motors, which in turn work the dynamos, so that there is a complete break between the force outside and that supplied to the patient.

With regard to the second difficulty, and it is a serious one, because nearly all the members of the staff have more or less been injured by the x-rays, and some of them are very sensitive to them, the cubicles have been lined with thick lead, 10 lb. to the square foot, so that the most dangerous or burning rays cannot get outside. The doctor and nurses go inside, and after putting the patient in the proper position come outside, and they can control the apparatus from the switchboard there. Lead glass windows are provided, so that if anything should go wrong the operator can stop the current at once and re-enter the cubicle when the current is switched off.

The electro-cardiograph.—In healthy individuals the contraction of the heart commences at the great veins and then spreads downwards through the auricles to the ventricles, in this way forwarding the blood from the veins into the arteries. Any alteration in the normal sequence of events necessarily interferes greatly with the proper circulation of the blood.

At the end of the nineteenth century, our clinical knowledge of the action of the heart was derived from examination of the pulsations on the chest-wall and in the arteries, which only

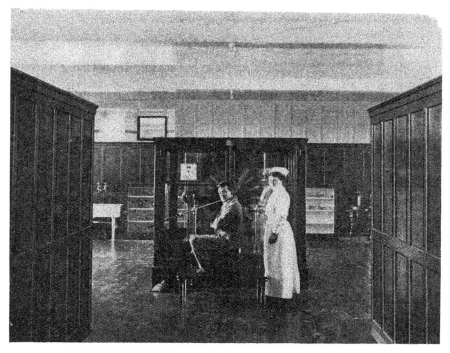

FIG. 1.
Entrance to the main wards.

afforded information as to the action of the ventricles, and gave none as to that of the auricles. In the first years of this century, however, James Mackenzie's ingenuity devised an instrument, the clinical polygraph, by means of which the pulsations in the veins of the neck were recorded on strips of paper side by side with the arterial pulse; and, as the venous pulsations showed the contractions of the auricles, and the arterial pulse the contractions of the ventricles, it became possible for the first time to appreciate alterations in the action of the auricles, and to correlate their activity and that of the ventricles.

During the next ten years a great advance occurred in our knowledge of cardiac diseases from analysis of the data which were thus obtained. It was already known from the researches which had been conducted by W. H. Gaskell at Cambridge, that disturbances of the auricular action might occur, and that the ventricles might or might not share in these disturbances, and it was now possible to examine critically the disorders of the cardiac action which occurred in disease, and to discover the character and the site of origin of the abnormality.

The polygraph, however, has several disadvantages, the most important of which is that it cannot be utilised in patients where breathing is embarrassed, as the respiratory movements interfere with its application. The technique, too, is sometimes difficult.

It has been known for long that muscular contraction produced electrical currents, and that these occur when the heart beats, but the currents in the latter case were so minute and of such short duration that they could not be recorded with the apparatus then available. The first advance was obtained by means of the capillary electrometer (Waller), which achieved a record of the cardiac currents, but this apparatus was too delicate to be used in clinical work ; and it was not till Einthoven, of Leyden, devised the string galvanometer, that the electrical method of examination became available at the bedside. The electro-cardiograph at the Royal Infirmary is the latest and most complete instrument of this kind, and has been designed and manufactured by the Cambridge Scientific Instrument Company.

Electrodes are attached to the limbs of the patient, and the electrical currents produced by the cardiac beats are conveyed to the galvanometer, in which they pass through a very fine fibre suitably mounted in a magnetic field. The movements of this fibre, which are very small, are magnified by means of a microscope, and the shadow of the moving fibre is projected by an arc lamp on to a moving photographic plate or film, the whole of which is exposed save the portion hidden by the shadow. The resulting record is the electro-cardiogram, the curves of which indicate the contractions of both the auricles and the ventricles.

The ordinary methods of examination by palpation, percussion, and auscultation, in the large majority of cases of cardiac disease, indicate truly and accurately the nature of the lesion, and electro-cardiographic examination is therefore superfluous and unnecessary. But in a considerable minority of cases the rhythm of the heart is disturbed, and the polygraph

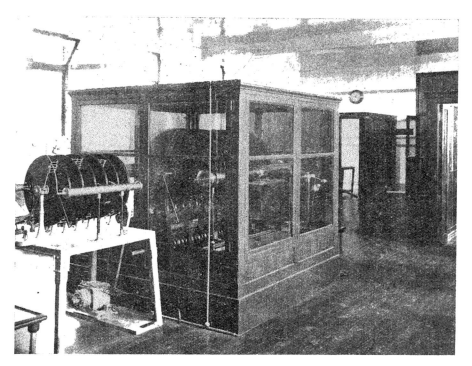

Fig. 2.
Gaiffe and Blythswood static machines.

or electro-cardiograph can alone supply information as to the nature of the disturbance. In some cases polygraphic examination is impossible or insufficient, and an electrical examination is urgently required.

Many of these latter patients are too seriously ill to permit even the minimal exertion of being conveyed to the electrical department, and the difficulty has been surmounted by connecting the electro-cardiograph with all the wards in the medical block, so that records can be obtained in the room on the basement set apart for this work from patients who are lying quietly in their own beds long distances away.

By means of these methods our knowledge of the disturbances of the cardiac rhythm is very rapidly increasing, and three problems now lie in front of us:—To discover all the disturbances of function which may affect the heart, to elucidate their causes, and to learn their appropriate treatment. I am much indebted to Professor Cowan for this description.

Diathermic treatment.—This method of treatment is comparatively new, but great progress has been made of late in the use of it in cases of gout, rheumatism, diseases of the heart, diabetes, &c.

The healing effect of heat has been known and employed for ages. The old methods were confined to the application of heated media, like the electric light and hot air baths, compresses, thermophors, &c. The heat generated by such means does not influence, however, the *internal temperatures*, as the skin is a very bad conductor of heat. It makes the skin hyperæmic and produces perspiration.

Ordinary electric currents, as supplied by galvanic batteries, accumulators, and electric power stations cannot be sent through the human body. Both the continuous and faradic or alternating currents produce violent painful sensations long before any increase in the internal bodily temperature can be noticed, the former on account of its chemical and the latter in consequence of its muscle-contracting effect.

Some twenty years ago the genius of Nicola Tesla enriched science by the discovery of the high-frequency currents. He found that by using extremely rapid oscillations this new variety of electrical undulation can be sent through the human body without causing any harm, even when using high intensities that would be fatal with ordinary currents. He obtained such rapid oscillations by the discharge of Leyden jars, which he adapted as an interrupter to reverse the direction of currents about 100,000 times per second. These extremely rapid changes in the direction of the current prevent the displacement of the ions on account of their inertia, which explains why such strong currents can be sent into the human body without danger.

All electric currents heat the conductors through which they pass. When sent into the body they have to overwhelm .the resistance offered by the organic tissues, whereby electric energy is transformed into Joule's heat. D'Arsonval recognised that by using the high-frequency currents for diathermic purposes we have at our disposal a valuable means of

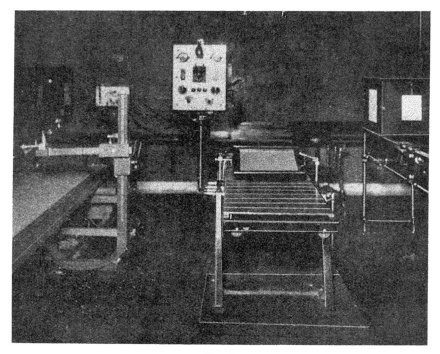

FIG. 3.
X-ray photographic dark room.

treatment. The high-frequency waves as produced by the ordinary high-frequency spark generators have, however, a comparatively low diathermic output, and are not free from faradic subsidiary effects. This explains why for quite a number of years diathermy was employed clinically only on a very small scale.

Just as a steel tuning-fork and a lead tuning-fork produce different sorts of vibration, the former little and slowly damped, the latter few and quickly damped ones, so we may obtain strongly damped, slightly damped, and undamped high-frequency oscillations, according to the construction of the spark-gap employed. Experience has shown in the course of time that the *slightly damped high-frequency oscillations give the best practical results* and permit of *avoiding* the undesired *faradic effect completely.* Such waves are delivered by the so-called *quenched spark-gap.* The construction of this instrument was brought about by the development ˙of wireless telegraphy. Prof. V. Zeynek, of Prague, adopted this new form of high-frequency spark generator in his .diathermic apparatus, and was the first who introduced the new intensive diathermic treatment.

Electro-coagulation.—The same apparatus can be utilised for electric coagulation, and this of late has been used with good effect either as a means of removing diseased tissues altogether, or as a procedure after operation in cancer and other conditions where the disease could not otherwise be removed.

With diathermic currents, coagulating temperatures may be attained in definite sections of the tissues by using special small electrodes. The current can be caused to penetrate into all the corners and cavities, the osseous as well as the soft parts ; thus tumours, otherwise inoperable, can be removed without loss of blood, and tissues are sterilised. There is consequently no danger of spreading germs through the blood canals during the operation.

The cinematograph in medicine.—Eleven years ago I showed the first x-rays film by means of a cinematograph to the Royal Society, London, but, at that time, it could only be used in the study of the lower animals, and many improvements had to be made before we had sufficient power to practise on the body. By process of evolution it is now quite possible to photograph the interior of human bodies by means of the x-rays. In this way all the movements of the heart can be shown on the screen, and also movements of the digestive tract, which will be very valuable in studying all obstructive diseases in the bowel. It will also facilitate the surgeon's work when studying the movements of joints and other conditions.

The apparatus is so powerful that an *x*-ray photograph of the heart in an adult human body can be taken in $\frac{1}{500}$th part of a second, and, by an ingenious mechanical arrangement, twenty-four photographs can be taken in six seconds. When

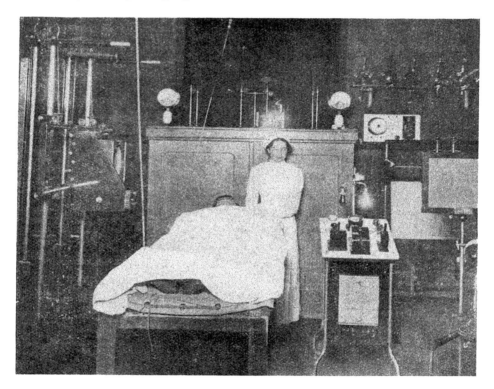

FIG. 4.
Instantaneous and stereoscopic *x*-ray apparatus.

these are reduced to the size of the film of the cinematograph, the complete cycle of the heart's movements can be thrown on the screen.

The cinematograph can also be used in other ways, and the instrument installed in the Royal Infirmary is the latest production. The different movements of the body in cases of paralysis can be shown, and microscopic objects, such as the movements of pathogenic organisms, can also be thrown on the screen. In this way a teacher can show to a class what each student would require to look at through the microscope.

Roentgen-tele-cardiograph.—The perfection of *x*-ray photography is got by instantaneous exposures, which enable us to photograph the heart with one flash of the tube. This has also done much to add to the knowledge of the position of the heart.

These exposures are indispensable, as only such really instantaneous pictures will show sharp and precise details. If such Roentgenograms are taken at a distance of 5 to 7 feet, they will show the actual size of the moving heart far more accurately than the old-fashioned orthodiagrams. The latter are drawn on the flickering picture as it appears on the fluorescent screen, whilst in tele-radiography the dimensions can be measured at ease on the Roentgenogram.

Most heart diseases cause typical changes in the heart's shape. One-flash Roentgenograms allow the study of such pathological alterations even in early stages. For the continuous and exact observation of such changes, in all their various stages, it is of utmost importance to take the different tele-Roentgenograms of the heart at the same time and predetermined phase of the systolic or diastolic curve. Only pictures obtained in this way are comparable. The instrument described takes such predetermined exposures automatically.

Electro-therapeutic apparatus for diagnosis of nerves and muscles.—A very large number of cases of disease of the brain and spinal cord require the electrical examination of muscles and nerves. For long the surgeons have had to use the constant and faradic currents in a more or less imperfect form. The apparatus which has now been got for the Royal Infirmary has been specially devised for what are known as condenser discharges. These discharges have been in use for a number of years for diagnostic purposes, and many men laid the foundation of their practical application. Zanietowski specially devoted much time to the thorough practical development of this new method, but the different opinions regarding the theoretical physiology prevented for a long time their general application. It was, however, more and more recognised that the condenser discharges permit of measurements and stimulation of organic tissues more con-veniently and precisely than any other electric agent. At the Fifth International Congress of Medical Electrology and

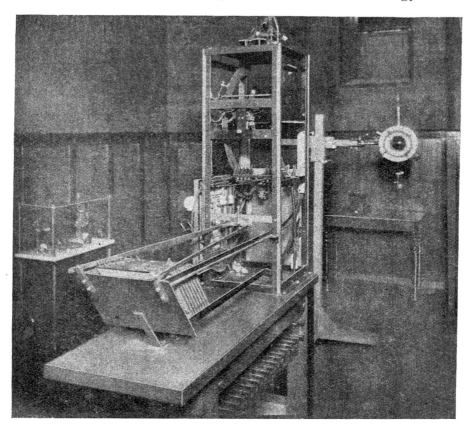

FIG. 5.
X-ray cinematographic apparatus.

Radiology, of Barcelona, 1910, the condenser method was, therefore, unanimously accepted as the electro-diagnostic method that should be exclusively used in future by the medical profession whenever electricity is indicated as a diagnostic medium.

Obesity.—Within the last two years special apparatus has

been designed for causing muscular contraction of the whole body or part of the body. The patient rests on a couch, and the electrodes are placed on any part whence it is desired to remove the deleterious products which are stored up in gout and rheumatism. By a simple arrangement faradic currents are sent to any part, and the muscles are made to contract.

Weights made of sand bags are put on the body up to 50 or 100 lbs., and the interruptions are made a few times more than the number of the beats of the heart per minute.

The result of this treatment is two-fold. If applied frequently it means that the contractions of the muscles in the body or limbs help the stream of blood onwards, and thus give relief after treatment to a patient with a weak heart.

In the same way excessive fat can be reduced in any part of the body or the whole body. It is possible, when a person with a weak heart cannot take exercise, to remove as much as 1 lb. or more per day without any exertion on the part of the patient whatever.

X-ray therapeutics.—X-rays have now been long used with great success in many diseases, but of late special instruments have been constructed so that large quantities may be given. Suitable screens have been designed to prevent the skin of the patient being burned, and by a comparatively simple arrangement the most penetrating of the rays can be sent into any part of the body, and at the required depth. By these means the surgeon hopes that many tumours, such as fibroids, which required operation before, may be helped, and there can be no doubt that in a large number of cases the tumours have disappeared entirely under their influence.

Treatment in the respiratory tract.—The treatment above described has opened a new era in surgical practice, because, by combining this with direct illumination of the throat and chest, the surgeon can look straight into the throat or windpipe and the bronchial tube. This arrangement is of inestimable value in the removal of foreign bodies from the lungs.

In the same way the surgeon can use the instrument in

nose, mouth, or throat, and by means of the electric coagulation (above described), safely destroy tumours in these regions which previously were looked upon as quite inoperable because of the advanced stage of the disease and the risk of hæmorrhage.

Static electricity.—The machine kindly made and presented to the hospital by the late Lord Blythswood is still working, and a smaller instrument has had to be installed to facilitate the work, which is now very heavy.

Baths.—In addition to the above mentioned apparatus, incandescent light baths have been provided for the treatment of the whole body or part of the body, and these have been fitted up in suitable rooms, where the patient can rest afterwards. Some of these light baths are portable, and may be taken to wards in cases where the patient cannot go to the department.

General arrangements.—In addition to the electrical department in the basement of the building, portable instruments have been made that can be taken to the bedside if the physicians wish to use the instruments themselves, or they can be used for treatment in the wards when the patient is too ill to be brought downstairs.

A separate *x*-ray installation has been set up in the surgical side for the use of the surgeons only, and five medical operators have been appointed altogether to carry out the work, which has now become so great that the electrical department requires this assistance and a large staff of nurses as well.

In addition to these new instruments, the whole *x*-ray department has been re-organised and brought up to date. Surgeons requiring a photograph in emergency can have the plates developed at once, and by means of a reducing camera a copy can be sent to the surgeon in a few minutes. The advantages of stereoscopic photography are now universally recognised, and a special instrument has been designed that as soon as the plates have been developed, whatever size they may be, the surgeon may study the stereoscopic effect at once. Specimens of photographs of different diseases have been installed so that the student can not only see what is being done, but for reference and comparison he can see what has been done.

The department, as it stands, has every kind and form of medical and surgical apparatus known, and all of the most recent kind, so that it is quite true to say that the patients in the hospital requiring electrical diagnosis or medical treatment will have even greater advantages than the wealthy.

Obituary.

WILLIAM GILFILLAN, M.B., Ch.B.Glasg., Trinidad.

WE regret to announce the death of Dr. William Gilfillan, which occurred at Falkirk on 30th August. Dr. Gilfillan, who was the son of the late William Gilfillan, schoolmaster, studied medicine at Glasgow University, and took the degrees of M.B., Ch.B., in 1906. After graduation he spent some time in the Glasgow Royal Infirmary in the capacities of resident physician and resident surgeon. He was then appointed Assistant Medical Officer to the Glasgow District Asylum at Woodilee, and after having held that position for some time he went to Trinidad, to take up there the post of Assistant Medical Superintendent to St. Ann's Asylum, Port of Spain. His health failing, he obtained leave of absence in spring and returned to Falkirk, where his death took place after a lingering illness.

CURRENT TOPICS.

THE GLASGOW MEDICAL SCHOOL.

WE publish the following particulars of the medical curriculum in view of the near approach of the winter session, which opens on the 12th inst.:—

UNIVERSITY OF GLASGOW.

The University grants four degrees in medicine. Of these, the M.B. and Ch.B. must be taken together.

The following outlines of the regulations for graduation are in accordance with the New Medical Ordinance, which came into operation on 1st October, 1911:—

Before commencing his medical studies, the student must pass the preliminary examination. This comprises (1) English, (2) Latin, (3) Mathematics, (4) An Additional Language, namely, Greek, French, German, Italian, or such other language as the Senatus may approve. In the case of a candidate whose native language is not English, certain modifications may be made in the preliminary examination.

The certificate of having passed the above examination must, along with satisfactory evidence of the applicant having attained the age of sixteen years, be transmitted to James Robertson, Esq., 54 George Square, Edinburgh, so that the intending student may be registered in the books of the General Medical Council. Certain other examinations, or a degree in Arts or in Science from a recognised University, are accepted as exempting from the preliminary examination.

The degrees of M.B. and Ch.B. will not be conferred unless the candidate has been registered in the books of the General Medical Council for at least five years previously. The academical year commences on the first day of October. In each year there is one medical session of not less than thirty teaching weeks. The session is divided into three terms, two of which are deemed the equivalent of a winter session and one the equivalent of a summer session. Two of the five years of medical study must be spent at the University. There are four professional examinations. Of these, the first comprises Botany, Zoology, Chemistry, and Physics. Candidates are admitted to examination in any of these subjects, after attendance on prescribed course or courses, at times to be determined by the Senatus. Those who have passed the first professional examination may be admitted to the second (Anatomy and Physiology) after the end of the sixth term (*i.e.*, second year). The third examination (Materia Medica and Therapeutics and Pathology) may be taken after the end of the ninth term (*i.e.*, third year). The final examination is open to those who have passed the third examination and completed the fifteenth term (*i.e.*, fifth year). The examination comprises Medical Jurisprudence and Public Health, Medicine, Surgery, and Midwifery, and the Diseases peculiar to Women and to Infants. Every candidate for the final examination must submit a declaration, in his own handwriting, that he has completed his twenty-first year, or that he will have completed it on or before the day of his graduation. The final examination is, like the other three examinations, held twice yearly—at the close of the winter session and of the summer vacation.

Class fees vary; for the majority of classes the fee is £4, 4s.

Clinical courses are taken in the Western and Royal Infirmaries. Attendance on the classes of the physicians and surgeons in both institutions is recognised for purposes of graduation. In addition to clinical courses, the Professors of Medicine, Surgery, and Midwifery at the Royal Infirmary conduct courses of systematic lectures.

Women students are admitted to certain classes in the University buildings. The remainder of the classes are held in Queen Margaret College. The clinical classes are taken in the Royal Infirmary.

The higher degree of M.D. may be taken by anyone who holds the Bachelor's degrees in medicine and surgery, on his complying with certain conditions. These are: That he must be of the age of twenty-four years or upwards; that he produces a certificate of having been engaged subsequent to having received the degrees of M.B. and Ch.B. for at least one year in attendance in the medical wards of an hospital or in scientific work bearing directly on his profession, such as is conducted in the Research Laboratories of the University, or in the military or naval medical services, or for at least two years in practice other than practice restricted to surgery. The candidate must pass an examination in clinical medicine, and must submit a thesis, for the approval of the Faculty of Medicine, on any branch of knowledge comprised in the second, third, or fourth professional examination for M.B. and Ch.B., excepting subjects which are exclusively surgical. Similarly, the degree of Ch.M. may be obtained by examination in clinical surgery and the presentation of a thesis on a subject not exclusively medical.

Full particulars of courses, fees, dates of examination, &c., will be found in the *University Calendar* (Messrs. MacLehose & Sons), or may be obtained from Albert Morrison, Esq., Registrar, the University.

Royal Faculty of Physicians and Surgeons of Glasgow.

(1) *Triple Qualification* (L.R.C.P.E., L.R.C.S.E., & L.R.F.P.S.G.). —In conjunction with the Royal Colleges of Physicians and Surgeons of Edinburgh, the Royal Faculty of Physicians and Surgeons, Glasgow, grants a licence to practise. This Triple Qualification admits to the *Medical Register*, and those possessing it are eligible for the public services. The course of study and the examinations are similar to those for the University degrees, but the class fees are in many cases lower than those payable in the University. Qualifying courses are held in The Anderson College of Medicine and in St. Mungo's College,* and particulars may be obtained from the respective Deans. Regulations for the triple qualification may be had from Walter Hirst, Esq., Secretary to the Royal Faculty of Physicians and Surgeons, 242 St. Vincent Street, Glasgow.

* Many of these courses are recognised by the University as qualifying for graduation. For special regulations, see the respective *Calendars*.

(2) *Fellowship.*—This fellowship is open to registered practitioners of not less than 24 years of age, and of not less than two years' standing. The candidate must pass an examination in medicine or surgery, and in any one of the following subjects which he may select:—Anatomy, Physiology, Pathology, Midwifery, Diseases of Women, Medical Jurisprudence, Ophthalmic Surgery, Aural, Laryngeal and Nasal Surgery; Dental Surgery, State Medicine, Psychological Medicine, Dermatology.

Fee, £50; to one who is already a licentiate of the Faculty, £25. If the candidate does not desire to be eligible to hold office, the fees are £30 and £15 respectively.

EXTRA-MURAL SCHOOLS.

The Anderson College of Medicine.—This school is situated in Dumbarton Road, adjoining the main entrance gate to the Western Infirmary. The classes qualify for the M.B. and the Triple Qualification.

St. Mungo's College.—The school is in the grounds of the Royal Infirmary, Castle Street, and the students, as a rule, attend the clinics in the Infirmary. The classes are recognised by the University. They qualify also for the Triple Qualification.

Western Medical School (University Avenue).—The classes comprise courses upon Anatomy, Surgery, Medicine, Midwifery and Gynæcology, Ophthalmology, and Diseases of the Ear, Throat, and Nose. Some of these qualify for the M.B. and the Triple Qualification; others are conducted as tutorial classes. The students receive their clinical instruction in the Western Infirmary, Eye Infirmary, &c. Usual class fee, £2, 2s.; for the shorter courses, £1, 11s. 6d. or £1, 1s. Further information may be had from the Secretary.

CLINICS.

Royal Infirmary (St. Mungo's College adjoins), 620 beds.— Visit hour, 9 A.M. daily; Outdoor Department, 2 P.M. Fees, including hospital practice, clinical lectures, and dispensary:—

First year, £10, 10s.; second year and perpetual, £10, 10s.; for six months, £6, 6s.; for three months, £4, 4s. Students who have paid fees amounting to not less than £21 to any other hospital in the United Kingdom are admitted on payment of £3, 3s. for six months, or £1, 11s. 6d. for three months. Vaccination, £1, 1s.; pathology, £4, 4s.; or for University graduation, £6, 6s; bacteriology, £2, 2s.; practical pharmacy, £1, 11s. 6d. Fees for the above, as well as for all medical classes connected with St. Mungo's College, are payable to the Superintendent of the Infirmary, Dr. J. Maxtone Thom.

Western Infirmary (adjoining the University), 580 beds.— Visit hour, 9 A.M. daily; Outdoor Department, 2 P.M. Every student shall pay a fee of £10, 10s. for hospital attendance, and, in addition, £3. 3s. for each winter session, and £2, 2s. for each summer session of clinical instruction. Students who have completed their clinical course elsewhere shall be permitted to enter for a six months' course of the *hospital only* on payment of a fee of £2, 2s. The fees should be paid to the Superintendent, Dr. D. J. Mackintosh, M.V.O.

Students who have obtained certificates of attendance during a course or courses of Clinical Medicine extending over not less than nine months, and who have also obtained certificates of attendance during a course or courses of Clinical Surgery extending over not less than nine months, may take courses of instruction on Clinical Medicine and Clinical Surgery on alternate days.

Students "remitted" from the final examination in both Medicine and Surgery can also adopt the alternate day system for their period of further study (which, in the case of candidates "remitted" at the Spring final examination, includes the full term of six months from May till October).

Victoria Infirmary (Langside), 180 beds.—For particulars, apply to the Superintendent, Dr. D. Otto Macgregor.

Royal Hospital for Sick Children (Yorkhill).—The opening of the new Hospital for Sick Children at Yorkhill, with its much enlarged accommodation, will greatly increase the facilities for the study of the diseases of children. Arrangements, however, are not yet complete in every detail, though they will very shortly be completed. Information may be obtained from the secretary, Mr. R. F. Barclay, LL.B., 91 West Regent Street, Glasgow.

Eye Infirmary (174 Berkeley Street, and 80 Charlotte Street).—Hour of visit, 1 P.M. daily. Fee for six months, £1, 1s.; for twelve months, £2, 2s.

Ophthalmic Institution (126 West Regent Street).—Hour of visit, 2 P.M. Fee for a qualifying course, £1, 1s.

Insanity.—During the summer session, a course of lectures is given in the University, and clinical instruction in the Royal Asylum, Gartnavel. Fee for combined course, £2, 2s.

Dr. Oswald conducts, in addition to the above, a clinic on Incipient Mental Disorders in the Out-patient Department of the Western Infirmary.

At Gartloch Asylum, Gartcosh, senior medical students may obtain appointments as resident clinical clerks. The appointments are for six months, and those holding them can attend classes in Glasgow in the earlier part of the day. Applications should be sent to the Medical Superintendent, W. A. Parker, M.B., considerably in advance.

Clinical lectures are given at Hawkhead Asylum by Dr. James H. Macdonald, "Mackintosh" Lecturer on Psychological Medicine in St. Mungo's College. Systematic lectures are given at the College as part of the same course.

Fevers.—Clinical instruction is given in Belvidere and in Ruchill Hospital. Fee, for a course extending over ten weeks (once a week), £1, 1s. Apply to Mr. James D. Borthwick, 285 George Street, Glasgow.

Maternity Hospital.—Clinical instruction in Midwifery is given at the Hospital, and there are exceptional facilities for practical work in the Outdoor Department.

Gynæcology.—Clinical instruction is given in the Gynæcological Departments of the Western and Royal Infirmaries.

Diseases of the Skin, and of the Throat, Nose, and Ear are taught in the special departments of the Royal and

Western Infirmaries. The *Hospital for Diseases of the Throat, Nose, and Ear* (Elmbank Crescent) affords further opportunities for the study of these diseases.

———

APPOINTMENTS.—The following appointments have recently been made:—

A. J. Ballantyne, M.D.Glasg. (M.B., 1898), F.R.F.P.S., to be Lecturer on Ophthalmology at St. Mungo's College.

Walter J. Dilling, M.B., Ch.B.Aberd., to be Robert Pollok Lecturer in Materia Medica and Pharmacology in the University of Glasgow.

Malcolm Hutton, M.B., Ch.B.Glasg. (1903), M.A., B.Sc., to be Medical Officer of the Oldham Union Cottage Homes.

Alexander M'Lean, M.B., Ch.B.Glasg. (1902), D.P.H., to be Acting Medical Officer of Health for Glasgow.

George Richmond, M.B., Ch.B.Glasg. (1903), to be Medical Officer of the Ashton-under-Lyne Union Workhouse.

J. H. N. F. Savy, M.B., Ch.B.Glasg. (1910), to be Medical Superintendent, Crooksby Sanatorium, Farnham.

Alexander Scott, M.D.Glasg. (M.B., 1875), to be Medical Referee under the Workmen's Compensation Act in cases of industrial disease (except nystagmus) arising in the Sheriffdoms of Ayr, Lanarkshire, Renfrewshire, Bute, Stirling, Dumbarton, and Clackmannan, and to take also cases of telegraphists' cramp and writers' cramp arising in the sheriffdoms.

J. A. Stewart, M.B., C.M.Glasg. (1888), M.R.C.S., L.R.C.P., to be District Medical Officer to the Dewsbury Union.

C. R. White, L.R.C.P. & S.G., L.R.F.P.S.G. (1899), to be District Medical Officer to the Hay Union.

Medical Department, Royal Navy: Sir William Macewen, M.D., LL.D., F.R.S., F.R.C.S., F.R.F.P.S., to be Consulting Surgeon.

Royal Army Medical Corps (gazetted 24th August): The following are granted the temporary rank of Lieutenant:— Fred. J. Whitelaw, M.B., Ch.B.Glasg. (1912); F. L. Napier, M.B., Ch.B.Glasg. (1909).

Supplementary to Regular Units (24th August): From the unattached list Officers' Training Corps:—Lieutenant W. C. Mackie, M.B., Ch.B.Glasg. (1908), to be Lieutenant.

Special Reserve of Officers (25th August): W. E. Maitland, M.B., Ch.B.Glasg. (1913), to be Second Lieutenant, 3rd Battalion Seaforth Highlanders.

Royal Army Medical Corps (26th August): Colonel Robert Porter, M.B.Glasg. (1878), is restored to the establishment and is supernumerary; Major G. S. Crawford, M.D., L.R.C.P. and S.E., L.R.F.P.S., to be Lieutenant-Colonel.

The following are granted the temporary rank of Lieutenant:— T. L. Fraser, M.B., Ch.B.Glasg. (1911); Walter Groome, M.B., C.M.Glasg. (1889); H. W. Moir, M.B., Ch.B.Glasg. (1906); W. G. Goudie, M.B., Ch.B.Glasg. (1911); N. M'N. Rankin, M.B., Ch.B.Glasg. (1908); W. L. Scott, M.B., Ch.B.Glasg. (1912); R. H. Jones, L.R.C.P. and S.E., L.R.F.P.S.G. (1912).

28th August: The following are granted the temporary rank of Lieutenant:—J. R. C. Greenlees, M.B.Glasg. (1907), B.C.; E. E. Steele, L.R.C.P. and S.E., L.R.F.P.S.G. (1913).

Canadian Army Medical Corps (28th August): The following are granted the temporary rank of Lieutenant:—A. Turnbull, B.Sc., M.B., Ch.B.Glasg. (1909); A. T. I. Macdonald, M.D.Glasg. (M.B., 1907); Major Thomas Kay, M.B., C.M.Glasg., F.R.F.P.S.

Royal Army Medical Corps (29th August): Granted the temporary rank of Lieutenant:—K. D. Murchison, M.B., Ch.B. Glasg. (1912).

1st September: The following are granted the temporary rank of Lieutenant:—J. S. Buchanan, M.B., Ch.B.Glasg. (1912); W. Dawson, M.B., Ch.B.Glasg. (1908); Douglas M'Alpine, M.B., Ch.B.Glasg. (1913).

The following cadets and ex-cadets of the Officers' Training Corps to be Lieutenants (on probation):—Alex. Glen, M.B., Ch.B.Glasg. (1913); A. L. Robertson, M.B., Ch.B.Glasg. (1912).

3rd September: The following are granted the temporary rank of Lieutenant:—James Fairley, M.D.Glasg. (M.B., 1905); Laurence T. Stewart, M.B., Ch.B.Glasg. (1912); Matthew White, M.B., Ch.B.Glasg. (1914); Alex. Lundie (Cathcart), M.B., Ch.B. Ed. (1903); John F. Barr, B.Sc., M.B., C.M.Glasg. (1891).

3rd September: The undermentioned Lieutenants are confirmed in their rank :—J. W. P. Harkness, A. Picken, M.B., Ch.B.Glasg. (1914).

The undermentioned cadets and ex-cadets of the Officers' Training Corps to be Lieutenants:—O. H. Mavor, M.B., Ch.B. Glasg. (1913); J. H. Magoveny, M.B., Ch.B.Glasg. (1913); Ronald Stewart, M.B., Ch.B.Glasg. (1912).

The undermentioned to be Lieutenant:—Clark Nicholson, M.B., Ch.B.Glasg. (1910).

4th September: Fourth Scottish General Hospital—The undermentioned Lieutenants to be Captains:—A. J. Archibald, M.D. Glasg. (M.B., 1911); W. H. Brown, M.D. Glasg. (M.B., 1901).

Attached to units other than medical units—The undermentioned to be Lieutenant:—W. J. Giblin, M.B., C.M.Glasg. (1888).

First Lowland Field Ambulance:—Lieutenant W. F. Mackenzie, M.B., Ch.B.Glasg. (1906), F.R.F.P.S., to be Captain.

Royal Army Medical Corps (8th September): The undermentioned cadets and ex-cadets of the Officers' Training Corps to be Lieutenants (on probation):—J. R. M'Curdie, M.B., Ch.B. Glasg. (1912); William Fotheringham, M.B., Ch.B.Glasg. (1914); A. W. Russell, M.B., Ch.B.Glasg. (1913).

Territorial Force (8th September): Attached to unit other than medical unit:—Lieutenant James M'Glashan, M.D.Glasg. (M.B., 1892), to be Captain.

Royal Army Medical Corps (15th September): The following have been granted the temporary rank of Lieutenant:—J. C. Dick, M.B., Ch.B.Glasg. (1909); D. M. Hunter, M.B., Ch.B.Glasg. (1913); J. Mowat, M.B., Ch.B.Glasg. (1911); G. D. M'Lean, M.B., Ch.B.Glasg. (1912); D. M'Intyre, M.B., Ch.B.Glasg. (1909); R. C. Robertson, M.B., Ch.B.Glasg. (1914).

17th September: The following gentleman to be Lieutenant on probation :—C. A. M'Guire, M.B., Ch.B.Glasg. (1912).

NATIONAL RELIEF FUND.—We have been asked to give publicity to the following letter, which we regret to state was received too late for insertion in our September issue :—

NATIONAL RELIEF FUND.
Treasurer: H.R.H. The Prince of Wales.

York House,
St. James's Palace, S.W.

To the Editor,

Dear Sir,—We regret to say that the Subscription Sub-Committee of the National Relief Fund has heard of a good many cases in which use has been made of its name, or of the names of those connected with it, with the object of securing support for appeals which are quite unauthorised.

We hope you will be so good as to permit the appearance of this letter, the object of which is to inform your readers that they may be assured that any extravagant or grotesque appeals emanate from persons who have neither the authorisation nor the support of this Committee.—Yours faithfully,

C. Arthur Pearson.
Hedley F. Le Bas.
Frederick Ponsonby.
Joint Secretaries, Subscription Sub-Committee,
National Relief Fund.

24th August, 1914.

It must, we imagine, be entirely unnecessary to commend the objects of the National Relief Fund to the sympathetic attention of any of our readers. There is no medical man so little acquainted with distress, or so poorly equipped with a prophetic imagination, as to be unable to foresee the calamitous results of the absence of the bread-winners at the seat of war. Should that absence be temporary only, it must yet bring privation in its train; and for the dependants of those who do not return there must in too many instances be nothing left but destitution. The medical profession has always been generous in giving work for nothing; it will be no less generous in giving money, not for nothing, not even merely for the relief of suffering, but to strengthen the hands of the nation, as every such movement of relief must do, in its righteous battle against armed oppression. There must be few of us who have not already subscribed to the National Relief Fund. Those of us who have not yet done so will find in our advertisement pages a coupon upon which subscriptions may be intimated; and those who have subscribed may be reminded that such a fund requires not only support at the outset, but steady maintenance as long as the war shall last.

SANITARY SERVICES: CIVIL AND MILITARY CO-OPERATION.—
The Local Government Board for Scotland has issued a circular
to medical officers of health in the following terms :—

It is likely that during the next few months there will be
occasions when the military forces will desire the assistance of
the public health service in various parts of the country, and, after
consultation with the military medical authorities in Scotland, the
Local Government Board invite medical officers of health of
districts in which troops are, or are likely to be, stationed to
place themselves in communication with the local military
medical authorities offering any services that may be useful.
Communications dealing with matters of importance should be
directed to the Deputy Directors of Medical Services of the
Scottish Command, Edinburgh. As medical officer of health
you will be able to give valuable information and assistance to
military sanitary officers in the following, among other,
directions :—

1. In advising as to all local water supplies, and as to their
protection from contamination.

2. In helping to secure satisfactory disposal of garbage and
other refuse.

3. In securing satisfactory drainage or conservancy arrangements.

4. In the control of infectious disease, and in arranging for
hospital provision for the ordinary infectious diseases and for
convalescent cases of enteric fever, and for the carrying out of
disinfection.

In this work the assistance of the sanitary and cleansing
inspector or inspectors in your district will be very valuable,
and their services should be utilised to the fullest extent.

It will be important for each medical officer of health to keep
the medical officer in charge of any local troops informed of any
cases of infectious disease within the area, and it is desirable to
ask this officer to give the medical officer of health information
of cases of these diseases among the troops. It may be useful
to recall the fact that the three diseases for which, under present
circumstances, a constant outlook should be kept are typhus
fever, enteric fever, and small-pox, especially the two last
named.

The War Office state that they propose to arrange for each

medical officer of health to have notified to him any soldiers convalescent from enteric fever coming into a sanitary area. These convalescents should be kept specially under supervision. For safeguarding the health of nurses and other attendants on the sick, and of populations exposed to the infection of enteric fever, attention may be drawn to the value of anti-typhoid inoculation, as illustrated in the experience of British troops in India, and facilities may be offered to those wishing to avail themselves of this provision.

It must be borne in mind that a large increase of hospital accommodation for enteric fever, and possibly also for small-pox, may be needed. As regards small-pox especially, you should make all necessary arrangements for dealing at once with any outbreak that may occur. Among other precautionary measures, it may be advisable to extend the list of notifiable diseases to chicken-pox for a period of (say) a year. For this purpose the provisions of Section 7 (6) of the Infectious Disease (Notification) Act, 1889, will be available.

The medical staff of the Local Government Board will be prepared to consult with medical officers of health on any points arising in connection with this work, and a medical inspector will consult locally as to prospective arrangements when the need for this is indicated.

THE ENEMY'S TREATMENT OF THE RED CROSS.—Loth as every thinking man must have been to believe the atrocities alleged against the German army, and willing as he must have been to believe that the first reported cases of firing on the Red Cross were accidental, it must regretfully be admitted that it is difficult any longer to maintain that attitude. The accounts of those returned from the front are numerous and independent, the evidence of private letters from combatant officers is to the same effect, and the number of members of the Royal Army Medical Corps whose names occur in the casualty lists is testimony which cannot be overturned. These lists are as yet very incomplete; the names of non-commissioned officers and privates are known in only a few cases, but among the officers it is known that, up to the time of writing, one has been killed and six wounded, while thirty-three are missing, some of these in all likelihood being also wounded. If, in the as yet incomplete lists, such are the casualties among the officers, there must be a very much larger number of non-commissioned officers and of privates whose names have yet to be revealed, and the total numbers will apparently be in excess of those which might be due to the usual accidents of warfare.

The *British Medical Journal* for 12th September speaks of the capture and continued imprisonment of two British Red Cross surgeons who were proceeding to the front at the request of the Belgian authorities. We are glad to record that Lieutenant H. C. D. Rankin, M.B., Ch.B., who is mentioned as missing in the lists of 10th September, has since reported himself. Lieutenant Rankin, who took his degree at Glasgow University in 1911, was a house physician in the Western Infirmary and a house surgeon in the Royal Infirmary of Glasgow. He served with the Red Cross in the Scottish Balkan Unit during the Balkan War of 1912-13, receiving from the Servian Government the Order of Saint Sava (4th Class), and he also received the medal of the Red Cross Society presented by Queen Alexandra. He became a commissioned officer of the Royal Army Medical Corps in 1913.

THE BRITISH RED CROSS SOCIETY: TRANSPORT WORK.—We have received from Mr. J. Inglis Ker, editor of *The Motor World*, an appeal to motorists throughout Scotland on behalf of the transport work of the Red Cross Society. Its expenses have so far been largely borne by the members of the transport committee and their helpers, in order to keep intact the general fund, but as they are daily increasing, and as the running of the private cars and other motor vehicles so freely given to the committee demands a steadily augmented revenue, the present appeal to motorists is made. Mr. R. J. Smith, secretary of the Scottish Automobile Club, is convener of the transport committee, and under his experienced guidance the work will be effectively carried through. The appeal has the heartiest approval of the Scottish Automobile Club and the Automobile Association, and medical members of these bodies and other medical motorists may be confidently looked to to support its object. Subscriptions, which are limited to £1, and will be acknowledged in the columns of *The Motor World*, should be sent to Mr. Inglis Ker, at 73 Dunlop Street, Glasgow.

THE USE OF VACCINES ON ACTIVE SERVICE.—The letter which appears in the *British Medical Journal* for 12th September over the signatures of many of our most eminent medical and scientific men makes an urgent appeal for the compulsory inoculation of our forces against enteric fever. The figures given make its efficiency apparent, and it should now be a matter of common knowledge among the medical profession that anti-typhoid inoculation does protect from enteric fever. The difficulty is to persuade the general public; but when it is remembered that no less than 57,000 cases, with 8,000 deaths, occurred in our forces during the Boer War, it ought to be possible to secure the passing of an Act enforcing inoculation, which is already compulsory in the French army, in the army of the United States, and even in the Turkish army. The development of sepsis in connection with wounds is also more to be dreaded in military than in civil practice, and Sir Almroth Wright strongly urges its preventive treatment by an appropriate "antisepsis vaccine." The vaccine is available, and "all that is required is to create a general demand for its application." The Department for Therapeutic Inoculation, St. Mary's Hospital, Paddington, has already supplied gratuitously to the British army and navy, and also to the French military hospitals, over 180,000 doses. In warfare in the past deaths from disease have always been more numerous than deaths from wounds, and it is evident that any effective measures to reduce the liability to disease are worthy of the most vigorous support.

THE TERRITORIAL FORCE AND SERVICE ABROAD. — The universal response of the country to the demand for an army large enough to be of effective weight in the present tremendous war has been eagerly shared in by the Territorial Force, many battalions of which have volunteered as units for foreign service. Their names have appeared in the daily press. Amongst them the medical profession will recognise with a personal thrill that the Lowland Mounted Brigade Field Ambulance, the 1st Lowland Field Ambulance, and the 2nd Lowland Field Ambulance have volunteered as units, and have been accepted by the War Office. The names of the officers of these units were published in our September issue, and are familiar to each of us as the names of personal friends. It is our duty and our pride to tell them how highly we estimate their courage and self-sacrifice, and under what a debt of gratitude they have placed not only us who must remain behind, but the country to whom they render such devoted service.

LONDON SCHOOL OF CLINICAL MEDICINE (Dreadnought Hospital, Greenwich, London, S.E.).—We are requested to announce that in consequence of the war, and in the absence of so many of the teachers, it has been found necessary to abandon the clinical teaching for the next session. Classes in operative surgery and pathology will, however, continue as usual, and particulars as to dates and hours can be obtained on application to the Secretary, Seamen's Hospital, Greenwich, London, S.E.

The London School of Clinical Medicine has long been very favourably known to graduates of Glasgow University, many of whom have profited in particular by the special facilities which it gives for the study of operative surgery and pathology. It will be noticed that these are the classes which are to be continued, and we do not doubt that in spite of the temporary limitation of the field, Glasgow graduates will be found to take advantage of these classes. It may be added that various clinical appointments are open to those attending the courses of study.

THE DR. ROBERT POLLOK LECTURESHIP.—Our readers will find, under the heading of " Appointments," the intimation that Walter J. Dilling, M.B., Ch.B., has been appointed to the Robert Pollok lectureship on materia medica and pharmacology. Dr. Dilling, who is an honours graduate of the University of Aberdeen, where he took his degree in 1907, has since then had a career of much distinction. He was the Carnegie Scholar in physiology from 1907 to 1909, and also assisted Professor MacWilliam in the teaching of the subject. From 1909 to 1910 he was Carnegie Fellow, and while Scholar and Fellow he studied at Rostock under Professor Kobert, to whom he ultimately became first assistant. During this period he superintended the researches in the pharmacological laboratory of Rostock, and himself engaged in research both independently and on behalf of the German Government. In 1910 he was appointed ·lecturer on pharmacology in the University of

Aberdeen. His published contributions to medicine, mainly pharmacological, have been numerous, and have appeared both in German and English periodicals. He is the author of an *Atlas of the Crystalline Forms and Absorption Bands of the Hæmochromogens*, published at Stuttgart in 1910, and the ninth edition of Bruce's *Materia Medica and Therapeutics*, which appeared in 1912, was entrusted to his editorship.

GLASGOW EYE INFIRMARY.—Our readers will learn with regret of the resignation of Dr. James Hinshelwood, who joined the staff of the Eye Infirmary in 1890 and has been one of its surgeons since 1896. Although the institution thus loses one of its most distinguished officers, 'we are glad to be able to state that Dr. Hinshelwood is continuing to devote himself to his private practice.

GREENOCK: VITAL STATISTICS.—The report of Dr. W. S. Cook, Medical Officer of Health for Greenock, on the health of the burgh during 1913, issued on 5th August, states that the birth-rate, though still relatively high compared with other towns, was lower than in the previous year—30·96 per 1,000 of the population as against 31·41. The corrected death-rate was 18·22, which is too high, and it will probably remain so until housing conditions are improved. The infantile death-rate was 116·78, and the death-rate from phthisis 1·45 per 1,000 of the population. The population is estimated at 79,278. The natural increase during the year was 983, against 967 last year.

ILLNESS OF THE ACTING MEDICAL OFFICER OF HEALTH.—We regret to announce that Dr. William Wright, whose appointment as Acting Medical Officer of Health for Glasgow was announced in our September issue, has been compelled to relinquish his new office owing to an attack of appendicitis, for which he has undergone a successful operation. His place, as will be seen from our intimation under " Appointments," has been filled by Dr. Alexander M'Lean, a native of Glasgow and a graduate of our University, who for five years has been a member of the medical staff of the Sanitary Chambers, and for three years has been an Assistant Medical Officer of Health.

PATENT MEDICINES: REPORT OF THE SELECT COMMITTEE.—
The Select Committee on Patent Medicines, whose sittings
extended during three sessions of Parliament, have issued
their report. They find that the existing law is chaotic,
that the state of things is intolerable, and that new legislation
is urgently needed in the public interest.

They recommend that the laws governing the advertisement
and sale of patent, secret, and proprietary medicines and
appliances be co-ordinated and combined under the authority
of one Department of State. That there shall be established
a register of manufacturers, proprietors, and importers of
patent, secret, and proprietary remedies, and that every such
person be required to apply for a certificate of registration,
and to furnish the principal address of the responsible manu-
facturer or representative in this country, and a list of the
medicine or medicines proposed to be made or imported. That
an exact statement of the ingredients and their proportions in
every patent remedy, of the alcoholic strength of every
medicated wine, and of the therapeutic claims of such remedies;
and a specimen of every therapeutic appliance other than
recognised surgical appliances be furnished to the Department.
That a special Court be constituted, with power to permit or
prohibit the sale and advertisement of any patent, secret, or
proprietary remedy or appliance. That the President of the
Local Government Board have power to institute the necessary
proceedings to enforce compliance with the law. That in the
case of a remedy the sale of which is prohibited the proprietor
or manufacturers be entitled to appeal to the High Court.
That the Department be empowered to require the name and
proportion of any poisonous or patent drug to be exhibited
upon the label, and that an annual fee be payable in respect
of every registration.

Among other things the Committee recommend that the
Indecent Advertisement Act be amended on the lines of Lord
Braye's Bill, that the advertisement and sale (except the sale
by doctors' order) of medicines purporting to cure the following
diseases be prohibited:—Cancer, consumption, lupus, deafness,
diabetes, paralysis, fits, epilepsy, locomotor ataxy, Bright's
disease, rupture (without operation or appliance). That it be
a breach of law to change the composition of the remedy

without informing the Department. That the period of validity of a name as a trade mark for a drug be limited, and that it be a breach of law to give a false trade description of any remedy, to invite sufferers from any ailment to correspond with the vendor of a remedy, to make use of fictitious testimonials, and to promise to return money paid if a cure is not effected.

The Committee say that no measures of smaller scope will secure the public protection.

SUPPLY OF CHEMICAL PRODUCTS.—Mr. Runciman, the President of the Board of Trade, has appointed a committee to consider and advise as to the best means of obtaining for the use of British industry sufficient supplies of chemical products, colours, and dyestuffs of kinds hitherto largely imported from countries with which we are at present at war. The Lord Chancellor (Viscount Haldane of Cloan) is the chairman of the committee, and the following is a list of the other members:—Dr. George T. Beilby, J.P., F.R.S., LL.D.; Dr. J. J. Dobbie, F.R.S., LL.D.; Mr. David Howard, J.P.; Mr. Ivan Levinstein, Professer Raphael Meldola, D.Sc., LL.D., F.R.S.; Mr. Max Muspratt, J.P.; Professor W. H. Perkin, Ph.D., D.Sc., LL.D., F.R.S.; Mr. Milton Sharp, Sir Arthur J. Tedder, Mr. Joseph Turner, Mr. T. Tyrer, together with Mr. John Anderson, of the National Health Insurance Commission, and a representative of the Board of Trade. The Secretary of the committee is Mr. F. Gosling (of the Patent Office), to whom all communications should be addressed at the Commercial Intelligence Branch of the Board of Trade, 73 Basinghall Street, E.C. The Committee held their first meeting at the Board of Trade on 28th August.

KILMUN SEASIDE HOME EXTENSION.—The extensive scheme of alterations and improvements which has been in progress at the Kilmun Home during the last few months, and which is now nearing completion, was inspected on 5th September by the directors and other friends interested in the work of the home. At the beginning of the year contracts were placed for the enlargement and remodelling of the kitchen and provision store-rooms, the providing of three additional bedrooms, a sitting-room, bath-room, and other conveniences for the domestic staff, and a complete installation of electric lighting for the house and grounds, power for the generation of the current to be obtained by turbine plant. Permission to form a storage dam, to furnish the necessary water supply, was generously granted by the superior, Mr. Harry G. Younger. The entire home buildings were also repainted and decorated, and other improvements effected which will materially add to the comfort of the patients and staff. While some of the tradesmen have not completed their contracts, the advanced stage of the work enabled the directors and their friends to estimate the increased facilities now provided for the carrying on of their convalescent home work. Regret was expressed at the absence of Miss Brown, the matron of the home, who has temporarily placed her services as a nurse at the disposal of the Government.

NEW PREPARATIONS, &c.

From Messrs. The Hofmann-La Roche Chemical Works, Ltd.

Iodostarin " Roche."—This is stated to be a compound of iodine with one of the higher acids of the fatty acid group, and is said to contain 47·5 per cent of iodine. It is claimed to be stable, odourless, and tasteless, and to pass through the stomach unchanged, being split up in the intestine and thus obviating gastric disturbances. It is claimed that experiments have established that 70 to 80 per cent of the iodine is assimilated, and that the toxicity is negligible. Each tablet contains 3 grains.

Sedobrol " Roche."—This is stated to be a combination of sodium bromide with fat and spicy extractives of vegetable proteins. Each tablet is said to contain 17 grains of sodium bromide, and one or two tablets dissolved in a cup of hot water form an appetising bouillon. The advantages of administering it are said to be—(1) Free dilution is ensured, which, together with the presence of the stimulating vegetable extractives, obviates gastric disturbances; (2) bromide may be given in the form of a dietetic, and the patient is unaware of the presence of a drug; (3) it enables the physician to give bromide while gradually withdrawing the daily intake of sodium chloride—this without rendering the diet insipid, an important factor in epilepsy. This is certainly a most palatable preparation.

REVIEWS.

Astrology in Medicine. The Fitzpatrick Lectures delivered before the Royal College of Physicians on 6th and 11th November, 1913, with Addendum on Saints and Signs. By CHARLES ARTHUR MERCIER, M.D., F.R.C.P. London: Macmillan & Co., Limited. 1914.

WITH an erudition that astounds, and with a lucidity that makes our own brain reel, Dr. Mercier unfolds in these lectures the principles and practice of medical astrology. It is a marvellous achievement. Syren-like he lures us on with the Signs of the Zodiac, the Seven Planets, and the Houses of Heaven, and we are deluded into thinking that it is going to be plain sailing after all; ere long, however, we are battling, if not for dear life, at least for very sanity, as we are swept into the maelstroms and rapids of elementary qualities, humours, aspects, jurisdictions, conjunctions, oppositions, sextiles, circles, cycles, trines, trigons, *et hoc genus omne.* But this wonderful man somehow or other pilots us through, and once again we perpend, though mere wrecks of our former selves.

To erect a scheme of the heavens at a nativity—we now know enough to avoid speaking of casting a horoscope—or to cast a decumbiture is, according to our candid author, just a little more difficult than lying, provided you be not obsessed "by a punctilio of needless scrupulosity," and take the precaution of selecting "a person whose career is closed." Thus, for example, if you make yourself familiar with all the minutiæ of Nelson's life, there is no reason in the world why you should not foretell to a nicety, not only his wounds and ailments, but also all that befell at Trafalgar; indeed, taking your courage in both hands, you may even go the length of predicting that strange and almost incredible incident of "Kiss me, Hardy!"

If any man, after perusing these *Lectures,* be still athirst for astrological lore, then we would strongly advise him to consult Dr. Mercier with the least possible delay, for such is the very

kind of case in which this cultured Fellow specialises. It must
not be thought, however, that *Astrology in Medicine* is a prosy
performance. Dr. Mercier could not be dull if he would; and
here, as elsewhere, we find him "wearing all that weight of
learning lightly like a flower," while executing many a mad
capriole after the fashion of happy boy or "troutlet in a pool."

As we read these Fitzpatrick Lectures we blush for our
colleagues who will be talking of the strenuous life, and are
forcibly reminded of what we ourselves too often forget,
namely, that medicine was once a learned profession. "It's
fair Itchybob, O man!" as Mr. Polly would have remarked.
Nevertheless, on closing this work, we feel pervaded by a sense
of gratitude almost too deep for words, gratitude that we were
not called on to practise physic in those brainy, blood-letting,
star-considering times, when the exact science of astrology was
a compulsory subject of the medical curriculum, and thankful-
ness that we are doctoring a people who demand nothing more
from us than the rough and ready methods of the nineteenth
and twentieth centuries.

It is but meet that a book by our readiest, cleverest, and
wittiest controversialist should be embellished by one example
of his incomparable skill. That the supply may never be cut
off is our fervent prayer; all the same that antagonists, or
victims, should still be found to offer themselves is for us an
inscrutable mystery, unless it be perhaps connected in some
remote sort of way with that statistical calculation as to the
number of fools born every minute. The jurisdiction of Luna
is evidently still operative. You know how Dr. Mercier plays
the game! Who amongst you has not applauded and envied,
as you watched him sparring for points rather than boxing for
knock-outs, and converting into the lightest of light farcical
comedy what his opponent had intended should be tragical-
historical!

The moment the mercurial Mercier gets off the chain of these
Fitzpatrick Lectures, he gambols and riots in an ecstasy of fun
on the subject of "Saints and Signs" in an addendum, which
was *not* delivered to the Royal College of Physicians, but read
to the fortunate, if less dignified, Casual Club. Such are the
penalties of greatness! Humour, wit, and satire follow here
so close, they gall each other's kibes. Dr. Mercier, though full

of surprises, never disappoints; he keeps us all the time on the tip-toe of expectancy, yet far surpasses our wildest hopes. The man with heart bowed down by panel woes will here find both solace and tonic, and with that rare modesty so characteristic of all true explorers, be made free of momentous and far-reaching discoveries, the fruit of untiring research. To describe what these mysteries are would be a very questionable kindness, since to be appreciated in all their savour they must be partaken of in the Mercier atmosphere. All hail! Great wit, scholar, doctor, droll! Fellow of infinite jest, of most excellent fancy! We are all the better for you. Long may you be spared to point out that this world and even the physitians and chirurgeons thereof are very much funnier than some douce sober folk would have us believe !

Therapeutics of the. Circulation. By Sir LAUDER BRUNTON, Bart., M.D., D.Sc., F.R.S. Second Edition. London: John Murray. 1914.

THE second edition of a work already so favourably known as Sir Lauder Brunton's *Therapeutics of the Circulation* might be dismissed with a brief recapitulation of the praises which its first appearance had called forth, were it not that in the intervening years there have been many changes and advances in our knowledge of the heart and vessels, advances in conformity with which the book has undergone substantial alteration. Originally published in the form of lectures, which as they were delivered in the University of London were illustrated by experiments, the arrangement of the subject-matter was a little irregular. A more systematic grouping has now been followed, and chapters have taken the place of lectures. Much description of apparatus has been omitted, while the newer methods of cardiac examination have received due attention, and so much new matter has been added that, as its author claims, the book has practically been rewritten. But it preserves the features which made the former edition so distinctive. Sir Lauder Brunton's conception of the teaching of therapeutics is that it must be based upon a thorough knowledge of physiology, pathology, and pharmacology, and much of his book is thus a preparation for the more strictly therapeutic sections which occupy its latter part. It is a preparation not wasted, for whoever reads will know not only what measures to adopt but why he adopts them, and will rise from his perusal with no merely empirical knowledge of the subject. He will be aided in his task by the easy and seductive style of which the author is so distinguished a master.

Guy's Hospital Reports. Edited by F. J. SEWARD, M.S., and HERBERT FRENCH, M.D. Vol. LXVII. London: J. & A. Churchill. 1913.

THE present volume of *Guy's Hospital Reports* will have a touching interest for all Guy's men, for its opening article, by Dr. Hale White, is a commemoration of the life of Samuel Wilks, by whose death in 1911 the medical profession suffered so grievous a loss. Sir Bryan Donkin, Dr. Jessop, and Sir George Savage add their remembrances of him to Dr. Hale White's sympathetic account.

The medical articles in the *Reports* are of varied interest, and realise the expectations which we form on opening a volume of this famous series. The first of them, on carcinoma of the gall-bladder associated with gall-stones, by Messrs. Fawcett and Rippmann, demonstrates that the usual text-book description of the symptoms is inaccurate in many points. Thus biliary colic is seldom present in such cases, jaundice only in three out of every five cases; tumour is often absent, and when it is present is not usually of characteristic shape; and, further, gall-stones do not play an important part in the production of cancer of the gall-bladder. Mr. Mollison and others report some interesting cases from the ear and throat department, and these are followed by a series of brief neurological studies under the editorship of Dr. Hertz, who makes a valuable point in the diagnosis of neuritic sciatica when he refers to the loss of ankle-jerk on the affected side. Mr. E. P. Poulton contributes a review of recent work on creatine and creatinin, with an account of personal observations which in some important points controvert previous findings. He concludes that though none of the theories of creatinine metabolism is entirely satisfactory, creatinine is a product of endogenous nitrogen metabolism, and has no relation to the nitrogen of the food. The apparent excretion of creatine in many pathological conditions is probably due to an error in analysis, and the origin of urinary creatine is at present unknown. Other articles of importance are Dr. E. L. Kennaway's, on the excretion of acetone bodies, Mr. Tanner's study of four hundred and forty cases of inguinal hernia, and Mr. A. Read Wilson's paper on parasyphilis of the nervous system, which has special reference to some of its rarer manifestations. The volume for 1913 fully maintains the reputation of its predecessors.

The Bacterial Diseases of Respiration, and Vaccines in their Treatment. By R. W. ALLEN, M.D., B.S.Lond. London: H. K. Lewis. 1913.

DR. ALLEN has brought together in the present volume a series of articles which he contributed to the recently established *Journal of Vaccine Therapy,* and by the addition of much new material, and revision of the old, has made of them a book which forms a thoroughly practical guide to the vaccine treatment of respiratory diseases. Its first four chapters are preliminary, and are occupied with the bacteriology of the respiratory tract, and with methods of staining and culture. Chapter V is devoted to general considerations in connection with the use of vaccines in respiratory diseases, to questions of dosage, and to methods of preparing and administering the vaccine. With the sixth chapter the special part of the work begins, and the rest of it is concerned with the treatment of disease of the upper respiratory tract, of bronchitis and asthma, pneumonia, whooping-cough and other febrile conditions, and of tuberculosis. Dr. Allen claims that his is the first adequate book upon its subject "in the English language, or, indeed, in any tongue;" and although there have been numerous scattered articles on the vaccine treatment of particular respiratory diseases, the claim both to priority and to adequacy is, we believe, substantiated. The book is more than adequate, it is authoritative, for Dr. Allen speaks from a long personal experience of the methods of treatment he advocates; and his tone is not that of indiscriminate advocacy, but remains throughout judicial in its statement of indications and contra-indications. Those who read the volume carefully, and apply its teaching with judgment, will find that they have gained a new resource in the management of respiratory diseases.

The Students' Pocket Prescriber and Guide to Prescription Writing. By A. AUBREY HUSBAND, M.B., C.M., B.Sc., F.R.C.S.E., M.R.C.S. Fourth Edition. Edinburgh: E. & S. Livingstone. 1914.

EVIDENTLY this little "waistcoat pocket prescriber" has been found useful. It is on quite orthodox lines, and can be criticised as to its contents in the usual way, but sins committed will probably be regarded as more in evidence than sins of omission. By that it is meant that no two prescribers of experience will agree anent the value of many of the included prescriptions; and, on the other hand, that, its size considered, the book gives a remarkably good selection of formulæ. These are arranged under headings of the diseases of the various systems. Tables of weights and measures, incompatibilities, a Latin vocabulary, &c., are added at the end.

Altogether it is a very satisfactory specimen of its kind, and well worth the small price charged for it.

Treatment of Tuberculosis. By ARTHUR ROBIN. Translated by DR. LEON BLANC, assisted by H. DE MERIC. London: J. & A. Churchill.

IN these days there is perhaps a tendency to attribute every-thing to the power of the all-conquering tubercle bacillus, and to neglect the soil as a factor in the development of tuberculous lesions. Dr. Robin, on the other hand, very properly emphasises the vast importance of the soil in the question of infection. Robin claims to have discovered certain physical phenomena which he would have us accept as criteria of the resisting powers of the patients.

We have first an increased consumption of O, but without a corresponding increased excretion of CO_2, giving a diminished respiratory quotient $\frac{CO_2}{O}$. This stage is pathognomonic of the pre-tuberculous stage as well as the actively tuberculous stage.

Cod-liver oil, arsenical preparations, &c., prevent this increased oxygenation, and so are beneficial.

The difference between his figures for the normal individual and the phthisical person are not sufficiently great to make his proof very convincing.

The other important phenomenon of the pre-tuberculous stage is an increased excretion of mineral matter. All aspects of the treatment of the disease are dealt with at considerable length in the subsequent chapters of the volume.

The Ideals and Organisation of a Medical Society. By JAMIESON B. HURRY, M.A., M.D. London: J. & A. Churchill. 1913.

TOWARDS the close of last year we received a small volume entitled *The Ideals and Organisation of a Medical Society.* The author is a member and past president of the Reading Pathological Society, and in his preface he tells us that "this booklet is born of an enthusiastic appreciation of the value of such professional organisations, and of a desire to contribute to their efficiency."

Dr. Hurry is of the opinion that a medical Society exists for the advancement of medicine, and for the cultivation of good fellowship in the medical profession; and after enlarging on these ideals he proceeds to consider the organisation of a society. This chapter takes up in order the office-bearers, members, meetings, library, museum, &c. He is a firm believer in every society printing an annual record of its proceedings, and he also favours the publishing when the society has reached a ripe age, of its history *ab initio.*

Following on this chapter he formulates a code of model rules and regulations for library and museum.

It is an unusual form of publication, but the views expressed by the author are worthy of the consideration of all who may wish to organise a medical society, and they are not without value and interest to those concerned with existing societies.

Plain Rules for the Use of Tuberculin. By R. ALLAN BENNETT, M.B.Lond. Bristol: John Wright & Sons, Limited. 1914.

THIS little book is all that it claims to be, and can be confidently recommended as a reliable guide to those who are ignorant of how and when to administer tuberculin in phthisis pulmonalis.

The Fæces of Children and Adults. By P. J. CAMMIDGE, M.D. Bristol: John Wright & Sons. 1914.

THIS work deals with the examination of the fæces, the diagnostic significance of the results obtained, and indications for treatment derived therefrom.

Dr. Cammidge's book on fæces contains over 500 pages, with 13 full-page plates, the majority of these being in colour, and 96 illustrations in the text. These figures give some idea of the minuteness with which the subject is dealt, and serve as a reminder that as time goes on every separate detail connected with the subject of clinical diagnosis appears to be capable, like a perfect gas, of indefinite expansion.

Why the title should differentiate, or appear to differentiate, between the fæces of children and adults is not clear at first, but is explained in the book itself by the fact that the present work is an amplification by Dr. Cammidge of Dr. Adolph F. Hecht's *Die Fæces des Säuglings and des Kindes*, but it appears that in future editions the simple title of " Fæces " may be found appropriate and ample. In addition to Dr. Hecht's work Dr. Cammidge has drawn largely upon that of Schmidt and Strasburger (*Fæces des Menschen*), but the book is no simple translation or combination of translations of these two German works. Dr. Cammidge has succeeded in bringing into existence a new work which can only be described as stupendous in its completeness of detail.

Nowadays it is imperative that every practitioner should .know where to find information as to the advantages to be derived from the examination of every fluid and every secretion and excretion of the body. No longer can a simple routine examination of the urine be held as all that is usually required, save in the most exceptional cases of doubtful diagnosis.

It may be that less information is to be obtained from an examination of the fæces than of the urine in the great majority of cases, but still there is the undoubted fact that in a certain proportion of cases definite information on certain points may be obtained *only* from an examination of the fæces, and once this is recognised there remains only the æsthetic objection to such a rather unsavoury line of clinical investigation.

With Dr. Cammidge's name as sponsor for the work, it follows that the latter is done exhaustively and thoroughly in every detail; and the reader is bound to wonder why such an important, in many cases vital, line of investigation has for so long received but scant treatment, limited in the majority of cases to simple visual inspection, with, in some cases, a more or less perfunctory examination of the fæces microscopically.

The introductory chapter is well worthy of the most careful study; it indicates the general conditions of the fæces in a state of health, and gives indications as to collection and preliminary treatment of the fæces. The next chapter deals with macroscopic examination. In this chapter will be found many points of the greatest interest and value, such as the method of distinguishing between mucus and connective tissue particles, and the striking statement that by no method whatever has fibrin ever been demonstrated in intestinal exudates. Mucous casts and concretions are also dealt with in this chapter. The following chapter (Chapter III) deals with the microscopic examination, mainly with regard to the various food residues usually present. In the explanation of Plate I in this chapter a reference should be given to page 61 for an explanation of the term "verschollte zellen," as up to this point no mention has been made of these cell "ghosts." On page 51 is an excellent test (Hecht's) for mucus, a micro-chemical one.

The chapter on parasites and pseudo-parasites is, of course, of necessity a very long one, but its importance is so great that the author is to be commended in his effort to make it as comprehensive as possible; in this he has succeeded. Again, the following chapter, on the bacteriological examination of the fæces, is, from the same cause, a long one, but the author has wisely restrained himself from making this altogether a too prominent feature of the book. It must be evident at once that the bacteriological results from the examination of fæces are too prone to erroneous deductions to make it profitable to go into detail, which could only lead to confusion and doubt.

In dealing with the chemical examination of the fæces, Dr. Cammidge devotes a separate chapter to the examination of fresh and of dried fæces. In these two chapters will be found a mine of information which may well lead to a much more extensive use of this method of investigation. On the whole, it is probable that more information can be obtained by chemical investigation of the fæces than by any other method, although the processes involved are usually tedious and complicated.

To the ordinary medical reader perhaps the most interesting chapters are IX and X, on the diagnostic value of examinations of the fæces and indications for treatment therefrom. Dr. Cammidge devotes scant space to the consideration of the applicability and value of vaccine treatment of diseases by autogenous vaccines derived from organisms present in the fæces, and probably he is right in refusing to be carried away by the super-enthusiast, who would treat every known condition with a more or less appropriate vaccine.

There is a very valuable appendix on foods and diets. The index is copious, and this remark applies also to the very full bibliography at the end of each chapter.

The illustrations are well selected, ample without being redundant, and where the addition of colour is more helpful this finds expression in the coloured plates, the latter being remarkably correct in their colour values.

In fine, Dr. Cammidge can be congratulated upon the production of a work which must, of necessity, prove of more and more value every day to the practitioner who seeks the aid of additional methods of assistance in clinical diagnosis, and a second edition is certain to be called for at no distant date.

Practical Prescribing, with Clinical Notes. By ARTHUR H. PRITCHARD, M.R.C.S., L.R.C.P., R.N.(Rtd.) London: Henry Frowde and Hodder & Stoughton. 1913.

THE author states that his first object is to supply a number of prescriptions and to explain them, giving, by way of explanatory notes, reasons for employing the various constituents, their particular actions, and any special points concerning them.

His method is to select a certain case and give a short history of symptoms and signs, and then follows a copy of the "prescription sheet," showing the various drugs used, and alongside of this is a column headed "treatment," under which the progress of the case, diet, and methods of treatment other than by drugs are particularised. Next, there are "notes" on the drugs used, the reasons for their use, and their methods of use. Finally, there is what is designated "comments," which states more particularly the exact influence of the treatment employed in the case of the patient dealt with. In all, thirty-five illustrative cases are given, so that the book is by no means exhaustive; but those dealt with have been happily selected to suit the author's design, as the majority are cases of acute or fairly acute conditions.

The book might be described as a group of clinical lectures on treatment, reduced to print. In it the reader is shown how to plan a campaign of treatment in certain selected cases. As is not unusual in clinical lectures of the kind, there is a tendency to be dogmatic; but this cannot be called altogether a defect, as it is more a book for a medical student or a junior practitioner, and a certain dogmatism about the methods adopted will prevent confusion in the minds of the inexperienced.

The form of the book is somewhat unusual, but it suits the subject; and we congratulate the author on something new, and suggest that he might at a future date increase the number of cases, for while these thirty-five cases are perhaps enough to exemplify methods of treatment, a larger number would be still more useful. It might perhaps be possible to reduce the amount of blank space in the book, and thereby permit more cases to be dealt with without much increasing its bulk.

Clinical Electrocardiography. By Thomas Lewis, M.D., D.Sc., F.R.C.P. London: Shaw & Sons. 1913.

This little volume forms a companion and supplement to its author's already well-known *Clinical Disorders of the Heart Beat*, and it may be safely said of it that its importance, like that of its precursor, is not to be measured by its size. Its appeal will necessarily be to a more limited public than that of the former volume, for the practice of electrocardiography must remain in the hands of the expert, and the electrocardiograph, on account of its cost, is likely to be distributed only among laboratories and large hospitals. To that selected public, however, and also to those who wish to understand the significance of electrocardiographic tracings, although they are not in a position to take them for themselves, the present work must prove of the greatest use. It gives a succinct, yet admirably clear, account of the electrocardiographic method, of the normal electrocardiogram, and of the deviations from the normal standard found in such conditions as heart-block, premature contraction, paroxysmal tachycardia, auricular fibrillation, and "auricular flutter." The last of these "in its untreated state can rarely be diagnosed by any method other than the electrocardiographic," and our acquaintance with the others becomes by this method more intimate and accurate than even by the use of the polygraph. Yet, great as is the light which the polygraph and the electrocardiograph have thrown upon cardiac problems, it is well to recognise that these methods have their limitations. They illuminate for us the normal and abnormal modes of action of the cardiac musculature, but, as Dr. Lewis himself admits, "electrocardiography has little to do with valvular lesions." To recognise their limitations is not to belittle the immense importance of the results which have accrued from these methods of investigation. To overstate the case in their favour, on the other hand, is apt to excite prejudice against them ; and Dr. Lewis is perhaps guilty of such an overstatement when he says, "Those cardiac patients are few in whom an electric examination is superfluous.'

Enthusiasm is, however, a better quality than the lack of it; and Dr. Lewis's work is open to no other than this trifling cavil. It handles a difficult subject with the utmost clarity, and its exposition is aided by an excellent and abundant series of reproductions of electrocardiograms. Dr. Lewis speaks with all the authority of a pioneer in the modern developments of cardiology—developments with which his name must be constantly associated in the minds of all those who will profit by them.

Defective Ocular Movements and their Diagnosis. By E. and M. LANDOLT, Paris. English Translation by ALFRED ROEMELE, M.B., Ch.B., and ELMORE W. BREWERTON, F.R.C.S. London : Henry Frowde and Hodder & Stoughton. 1913.

PROBABLY no man in the ophthalmic world has done more to diffuse a knowledge of the subjects with which this little book deals than Dr. Landolt. He is a clinician of very great ability, and his clinical researches have largely run in the direction of the study of squint, of paralysis of the muscles, and of other similar defects. This book, therefore, is specially interesting as a *résumé* of his individual work, and as such it is of very great value.

The authors first begin with an anatomical and physiological study, in which the range of fixation is amply discussed and important definitions given. They next discuss various forms of strabismus. They divide this affection into the following groups :—(1) Paralytic or spastic squint ; (2) concomitant ; (3) associated paralysis ; (4) paradoxical affections. The methods of diagnosis and treatment of these various conditions are amply and adequately discussed.

Altogether, this is a book which we can thoroughly recommend.

Food and Feeding in Health and Disease. By CHALMERS WATSON, M.D., F.R.C.P.E. Second Edition, Revised. London and Edinburgh : Oliver & Boyd. 1913.

THE first edition of this book was issued three years ago. To the present one is added an account of methods of flour bleaching and other methods which may impair the nutritive value of food.

The first three chapters are devoted to considerations regarding food—its functions and digestion, and the daily amount required. . The seven following chapters deal with milk and eggs, animal and vegetable foods, mineral constituents and accessories, beverages, patent and proprietary foods, preservatives, and the adulteration of, and diseases caused by, food. In two chapters diets are given for different periods of life, the effects of under-feeding and of over-feeding are described, and rules are laid down for the framing of a dietary. There is a chapter containing general rules on serving food to invalids, and details regarding rectal feeding. Two chapters on infant feeding are by Dr. Dingwall Fordyce. The fifteen following chapters are on diet in diseased conditions. There is a chapter on special diet cures, and another on hospital dietaries.

In the appendix there is a series of twenty-two papers by the author and seven collaborators—"a record of experimental observations on the influence of diet on the structure of tissues." The index is very full. There are over 200 recipes, besides a great many diet charts.

We cannot speak too highly of the book ; as a practical guide to the student of dietetics it is invaluable, and should be in the hands of all who have the care of invalids or children.

The author gracefully acknowledges his indebtedness to the assistance of Mrs. Chalmers Watson.

ABSTRACTS FROM CURRENT MEDICAL LITERATURE.

EDITED BY ROY F. YOUNG, M.B., B.C.

MEDICINE.

The Diagnosis of Subtentorial Tumours. By G. W. Howland, M.D. (*The Canadian Medical Association Journal*, July, 1914).—The study of the diagnosis of subtentorial growths resolves itself into three distinct divisions —(1) The determination of the anatomical site, whether cerebellar, extra-cerebellar, or pontine; (2) the differentiation between the various morbid conditions which occur in these regions—namely, tumour, abscess, vascular, thrombosis and hæmorrhage, labyrinthine disease, meningitis, sclerosis, and atrophy, and, finally, uræmic manifestations; (3) the nature of the new growth.

The disturbance of function may be divided in eight divisions—(1) General signs of increased intracranial pressure; (2) cerebellar and cerebellar tract signs; (3) brain stem nuclei and nerve signs; (4) motor and (5) sensory tract signs; (6) affections of the bladder and rectum; (7) reflexes and (8) signs of increased ventricular pressure.

The first cardinal sign is headache. This is usually an early sign in cerebellar and extra-cerebellar tumours, but usually late in pontine and medullary growths. It is most characteristically felt at the back of the head, although it may be frontal or both. If the basal tumour causes pressure on the fourth ventricle, with dilatation of the lateral ventricles, great internal pressure with occasionally burning sensations may be complained of.

The second cardinal symptom is optic neuritis. In cerebellar and extra-cerebellar growths this is frequently early and intense, while in pontine ones it is late in appearance. It may be entirely absent. In supratentorial growths all degrees of optic neuritis occur.

The third sign—vomiting—is usually present in cerebellar and extra-cerebellar growths, and yet it may be absent for months and then recur. In pontine it is usually less severe, while in supratentorial growths it is variable.

The sensation of general giddiness due to increased intracranial pressure is frequent. True vertigo is probably due to interference with the semi-circular canals or their connection *via* the pons to the mid-brain.

Physiologically the cerebellum is probably the great centre of tone. It receives as a sensory centre the sensation of tone from all parts of the motor mechanism; it supplies constant amount of tone to the motor mechanism at rest; and in correlation with cerebral and cortical action, it supplies the necessary tone for prolonging contraction when an action is performed.

Three classes of symptoms may arise in cerebellar diseases—(1) These due to loss of tonic afferent stimuli, and in this case the cerebral action may be excessive ; (2) those due to loss of tonic and of efferent stimuli at rest, resulting in a general atonia and asthenia of motor structures; (3) those due to loss of tonic efferent stimuli, when cortical motor action is performed, leading to tremulous movement dependent on the absence of constant tonic stimulation.

One may outline the disturbances due to interference with the cerebellum by tumours under the above mentioned headings.

1. Disturbances due to excessive cerebral action owing to the absence of cerebellar afferent stimuli.

Asynergy.—This sign is not often present, but is characterised by the difficulty in performing movements of groups of muscles usually associated together.   The cortical cells find it impossible to associate a proper degree of tone for each group of muscles, and therefore simple movements which should be combined together are each performed separately.

Adiadococinesia.—This is usually tested by rapid pronation and supination of the fore-arms.   It is defective and is a valuable sign in unilateral cerebellar disease.   It depends on the facts that the cortex is unable to change rapidly from one simple movement to the other.

Cerebellar catalepsy.—This is tested by the patient lying on the back, and elevating the legs flexed at the knees.   In this case while tremor may occur before this position, when once they are held there, in cerebellar disease there is more than usual ability to keep them firmly in such position.

Loss of power of measured movements.

2. Cerebellar asthenia and hypotonia are of great value as signs if one side is only or principally affected.

3. The third group of signs is apparently dependent on the fact that a normal action of the cerebral motor cells and a continuous tonic supply from the cerebellum are necessary in order that the movement may be continuous and not intermittent.   These cardinal signs occur not only in cerebellar disease, but in disease of the tracts from the cerebellum to the nuclei in the mid-brain, to the red nucleus and probably to the thalamus.   A true intentional tremor may occur, and, if one-sided, will be on the side of the tumour.   Nystagmus is probably due to the same cause.   It is rapid on the side opposite the tumour, and slow and jerky on the side of the tumour.

4. Afferent and efferent defects may be present in cerebellar affections. There may be a marked asynergic gait owing to the patient's inability to perform the separate movements necessary in walking.   There may be, on the other hand, marked titubation, the patient staggering from side to side with a tendency to fall.   Again, in standing the patient may fall to one side from static ataxia.   The head may show marked tremblings and may be held over to one side, usually, but not always, having the occiput on the same side, depressed towards the side of the tumour.   These typical signs may recur in extra-cerebellar tumours from the growths pressing into a lobe.   They may occur in pontine tumours.   In the latter case the gait is more likely to be spastic.   As a general rule, complete paralysis of the cranial nerves issuing from the subtentorial region is diagnostic of extra-cerebellar or pontine tumours, and partial paralysis may be due to cerebellar, extra-cerebellar, or pontine causes, or cross pressure from the opposite side, or to displacement of the cerebellum itself.

The third and fourth nerves arise above the tentorium, and yet, especially with a displaced cerebellum, may be severely affected, causing loss of power of the eyes and ptosis.   The fourth nerve may be affected by a tumour growing forwards, and cause difficulty in looking downwards. Paresis of the external rectus muscle is one-sided, and is diagnostic in extra-cerebellar growths. In pontine ones it also occurs, and rarely in intra-cerebellar tumours, and then is due to pressure.

The fifth nerve may be affected in either its sensory or motor courses.

The seventh nerve is usually affected in all forms of tumour to some degree.

The eighth nerve is frequently affected in extra-cerebellar and pontine growths. Deafness, noises in the ear, giddiness, and loss of equilibrium may occur.

The ninth nerve is rarely affected in any but pontine tumours. The same applies to the vagus, spinal accessory, and twelfth nerves.

The motor power of the body, apart from that due to cerebellar disturbances in function, does not show any change. Changes in sensation of touch, pain, and temperature on the side opposite to the tumour, when they are present, are strongly diagnostic of a lesion in the pons.

Bladder and rectum disturbances are characteristic of pontine disease.

Symptoms, local and general, due to intra-ventricular pressure may be present. The value of reflexes in the diagnosis of these three lesions is not great.—D. ROSS KILPATRICK.

DISEASES OF CHILDREN.

La dentition chez les enfants. By Dr. Jules Comby (*Archiv. de Méd. des Enfants*, May, 1914, p. 335).—In this article Comby adversely criticises the opinion that dentition in the healthy infant is responsible for any pathological manifestations. He concludes from a very extensive experience that, if a healthy infant be correctly nourished, the teeth erupt early, appearing between the seventh and ninth months, and that by the twenty-second or twenty-sixth month dentition is complete. If, however, the child is bottle-fed, retarded in its development, or rachitic, then the first teeth may not make their appearance till the tenth or even the fifteenth month, and the completion of the process may be delayed till the thirty-sixth month.

To the questions whether primary dentition exerts a pathogenic *rôle*, and whether it is able to engender diseases or to aggravate those already existent, he would reply in a definite negative. Apart from gingivitis, caries, and periostitis, dentition cannot cause fever, diarrhœa, bronchitis, convulsions, or meningitis. These various conditions are rare in properly nourished infants, but common in those badly nourished.—LEONARD FINDLAY.

Préservation de l'enfant du premier âge contre la tuberculose. By Drs. P. Nobecourt and G. Schreiber (*Archiv. de Méd. des Enfants*, April, 1914, p. 241).—In view of the undue prominence being given at the present moment in the British medical press to the question of bovine tuberculosis in man, the above article is a welcome contribution. In it we are reminded that, after all, the vast majority of cases of tuberculosis are of human origin, and that it is against this type of infection that the strongest prophylactic measures are required. Now, since it has been shown, from autopsies and the results of tuberculin reactions in children, that the incidence of the infection rapidly increases with each year of life, our attention ought to be specially directed to the very young, in fact the infants. These authors advise the institution of creches and children's homes, as first suggested and carried out by Grancher, in the country, in the mountains, or by the seaside, where all infants and healthy children of tubercular parents could be isolated and reared under advantageous conditions. In this way they claim that an enormous reduction in the prevalence of phthisis and other tubercular affections in the future population would be brought about.—LEONARD FINDLAY.

Acute Bacillus Infection of the Urinary Tract in Children.

By R. G. Gordon, M.D. (*The British Journal of Children's Diseases*, June, 1914, p. 252).—In this paper the author draws attention to the various manifestations of this very common and important infection of infants. He classifies the cases under five headings according as the patients present—

1. Symptoms of general feverish disorders, without any indication that one special system was affected.
2. Cerebral symptoms.
3. Pulmonary symptoms.
4. Abdominal symptoms.
5. Urinary symptoms.

Examples of each type are given. The article is concluded with the remark that since such divergent symptoms can occur from the same cause careful examination of the urine in all doubtful cases of illness in young children is most necessary.—LEONARD FINDLAY.

A Study of the Results of Tonsil Operations on Public School Children in New York City.

By Dr. Gerhard H. Cocks (*Archives of Pediatrics*, February, 1914, p. 144).—This communication records the results of the examination of some 100 children selected from the Department of Health, and recently operated upon in the local hospitals and dispensaries. Of 107 children referred by the school medical officer for treatment 17 evaded the operation; of the 90 operated upon a general anæsthetic was known to have been used in 33, in 14 the operation was performed without anæsthesia, whereas in 43 no definite information on this point could be obtained. Thirty-one of the 107 children were suffering in addition from some nasal affection which had not been treated.

The school teachers noted that in many cases the operation had cured the child of recurring sore throat, earache, mouth breathing, &c., and that in many instances the general physical and mental condition of the child was improved.

Of the 14 cases operated upon without anæsthesia the results were with one exception uniformly bad, whereas in the 33 operated upon with anæsthesia the operation had been well performed in 24. The author makes a strong plea for the use of anæsthetics in all tonsil and adenoid operations, and says that dispensaries and cliniques, where facilities for such are not present, should be prohibited from undertaking these operations. The absence of anæsthesia acts in a two-fold manner; the operation is performed too hurriedly to guarantee efficiency, and the resulting shock has a most deleterious effect on the child's nervous system. —LEONARD FINDLAY.

The Metabolism in Osteogenesis Imperfecta with Special Reference to Calcium.

By A. Bookman, M.D. (*American Journal of*

Diseases of Children, June, 1914, p. 416).—In this paper the results of meta-holism experiments conducted in a typical case of osteogenesis imperfecta are compared with those obtained by other workers in the same condition and also in healthy infants. The patient was aged three months, and had presented curvature of the bones with a tendency to spontaneous fractures from birth.

. The author's conclusions are—

1. In active cases the calcium retention is somewhat below or decidedly below the normal. (This diminution in calcium retention is not nearly so severe as is found in the active stage of rickets.)

2. It is probable that variations in the course of the disease cause changes in the calcium metabolism.

3. The deficient retention of calcium is apparently favourably influenced (as in rickets) by cod liver oil and phosphorus, and still more strongly by calcium lactate.—LEONARD FINDLAY.

DISEASES OF THE EAR.

The Protective Mastoid Operation: An Operation of Election. By W. Sohier Bryant, of New York (*Journal of Surgery*, &c., December, 1913).—Aural surgeons in their attitude towards mastoid operations may be roughly divided into two classes—those who operate on cases of aural suppuration only when they are forced to do so, and those who anticipate more or less serious complications by operation. The present paper is a plea for more frequent operation, both in regard to acute and chronic middle-ear suppuration. As the aim of the oculist is the preservation of sight, so the aural surgeon should more carefully consider the function of the ear in his attitude towards operation. We cannot help thinking insistence on this is justified. The operative procedure adopted should be conditioned by the clinical signs and symptoms. Without sharing in the enthusiasm of the author for various methods, it can certainly be accepted that a "punishment graduated to fit the crime," or, in other words, an operation in proportion to the extent of the disease, and having regard to the aim in view—the retention or improvement of the hearing, for example— may in many cases lead to more satisfactory results than the expectant treatment hitherto frequently adopted. Nowadays one is not limited either to the simple opening of the mastoid cells, or to the performance of the complete radical mastoid operation. The author refers to various methods, showing a natural predilection (especially naturally, shall we say? in an American) for his own. He insists on the value of skiagraphy of the mastoids, especially in acute cases, from the point of view both of prognosis and of the indications it may give as to the best surgical procedure to adopt.—W. S. SYME.

Indications and Technique of Labyrinthectomy. By Falgar, of Barcelona (*Archives Internationales de Laryngologie, d'Otologie, et de Rhinologie*, January-February, 1914).—This is a thoughtful and timely contribution to a difficult subject. In it the author endeavours to lay down the indications for operating on the labyrinth, and the manner in any individual case by which this should be accomplished. Labyrinthectomy is not many years old, and it is only in accordance with the nature of things that its advocates should have gone to the extreme. It cannot be denied that in middle-ear suppuration with labyrinth symptoms the inner ear has been opened up without sufficient justification, and though it is very true that involvement of the labyrinth by the suppurative process adds greatly to the gravity of the aural lesion, and much increases the risk of intracranial complication, it is becoming more evident that operation on the labyrinth is itself fraught with a good deal of danger. Moreover, though labyrinth symptoms may arise in the course of middle-ear suppuration, it does not by any means follow that the suppurative process has itself invaded the internal ear. It is especially necessary to guard against this conclusion in acute cases, and we agree with Falgar that an acute serous labyrinthitis may arise in the course of acute middle-ear suppuration, may entirely abolish the labyrinth functions, and yet may quite pass off and the functions return to normal. Such a result was at one time not conceded. In chronic middle-ear suppuration the sudden abolition of the labyrinth functions would be more probably due to actual purulent invasion. So that Falgar contends that a more expectant attitude as regards labyrinthectomy should be adopted in acute than in chronic cases. The condition of the labyrinth wall found on the performance of the mastoid operation may also give indications.

Falgar then describes the various methods of labyrinthectomy, and endeavours to fix the indications for each method. He reports ten cases on which he has operated, describing the procedure adopted. In one case the facial nerve was raised from the aqueduct and held aside (Uffenorde's method, he says). In a similar case where the nerve was already exposed to the disease we adopted this procedure, and it certainly gives a freer field for operation. Neumann's method is undoubtedly the best procedure when there is a probability of an intracranial complication in the posterior fossa being also present.—W. S. SYME.

DISEASES OF THE EYE.

Nystagmus.—At a combined meeting of the Neurological, Ophthalmological, and Otological Sections of the Royal Society of Medicine, held on 26th February, 1914, there was a demonstration of cases of nystagmus, followed by a discussion upon the subject. Many cases of nystagmus of various types were shown by members of the different sections, with special reference to the symptoms from the particular point of view of the observer, and this part of the *Transactions* makes interesting reading.

The discussion which followed seems to have brought out little that is new upon the subject.

The particular type of nystagmus which is of greatest interest, possibly, to ophthalmic surgeons is that met with in miners. The paper which deals most fully with this branch of the subject is that of Dr. Lister Llewellyn. The writer takes as his text "The relation of miner's nystagmus to general nystagmus," and seeks to show that there are several points in which the two resemble one another.

The principal etiological factors in the causation of miner's nystagmus seem to be fairly well agreed upon. The macula has a feebler perception of light than the perimacular retina where rods and cones are placed together. The miner, working in exceedingly feeble illumination, seeks, more or less unconsciously, to utilise a portion of the retina which can appreciate both light and detail ; the result is that some portion of the retina, near the macula but not in it, is brought to such a position that the image of the portion of the working at which he is striking falls on it. As this part of the retina is not a fixed point like the macula, the eye is feeling as it were round the macula all the time of work in the feeble illumination, and hence the eye automatically takes on a slightly swinging or rotatory motion.

This may go on for a long time without interfering with the miner's ability to use his eyes above-ground, ceasing, as it were, of its own accord when the illumination is increased and the macula can be utilised satisfactorily.

When, however, the habit becomes so fixed that the eyes continue to move even in good illumination, it is manifest that the vision above-ground becomes interfered with, and the macula becomes of less and less use. Before this stage has been reached, however, it is probable that some of the associated symptoms of miner's nystagmus—giddiness, head-movements of compensatory nature, &c.— have been developed, and the man is no longer able for work.

Generally speaking, the nystagmic habit becomes deeply rooted before the miner has to cease work, and hence the extreme difficulty experienced in getting rid of it even after a more or less prolonged period of rest. According to the duration of the habit the period required to get rid of the tendency to nystagmus is greater or less. Of course no definite rule can be laid down to define the period of cessation of work required by any individual who has suffered from miner's nystagmus, but it seems to be agreed that about a quarter of the period of duration should intervene between the last sign of nystagmus and the first attempt to work in the pit again. It is also agreed upon that a man who has once suffered from miner's nystagmus is never quite free from risk of relapse.

Llewellyn makes an interesting observation regarding the illumination of the face of the coal, quoting from Trotter's work on "Illumination." He shows that the amount of light falling on the coal in a safety lamp mine may be only about one-fiftieth of a candle-power per square foot, or even less. The proportion of this light which may be reflected into and utilised by the eye is only about 3 per cent.

The discussion is very interesting, and should be read by all ophthalmic surgeons.—LESLIE BUCHANAN.

The Diagnosis and Treatment of Sympathetic Ophthalmitis.
—In the *Transactions* of the Royal Society of Medicine (Section of Ophthalmology), 4th February, 1914, there is some interesting information regarding the early diagnosis and preventive treatment of sympathetic ophthalmitis, and, as this is one of the most important matters for consideration in ophthalmology, a brief account of the discussion will be given here.

The subject was brought up during a discussion upon the use of salvarsan in ophthalmic practice, which was opened by Mr. Lang. In the course of his remarks, Mr. Lang alluded to the fact that, some three years ago, Mr. Browning had informed him of the fact that the blood count in cases of sympathetic ophthalmitis was much the same as it was in cases of syphilis and some other conditions of protozoal origin. This caused Mr. Lang to say at once, "If so, may the same method of treatment be of use in sympathetic ophthalmitis as in syphilis?" The result was that the next case in which sympathetic ophthalmitis was present which occurred under his care was treated by injection with salvarsan. The result seemed to be moderately favourable.

Mr. Lang points out that ophthalmic surgeons are deeply indebted to Mr. Browning as the discoverer not only of a new means of establishing the fact of the presence of sympathetic disease, but, still more important, of foretelling its occurrence and possibly of preventing it.

Mr. S. H. Browning then takes up the theme, and tells how he came to the conclusion that sympathetic ophthalmitis was in some way allied to the recognised protozoal diseases. He shows, in a tabular statement, the differential blood counts, in average, of several diseases, and gives a normal blood count for comparison. This table shows that there is a marked increase of the number of non-granular leucocytes and a diminution in the number of granular leucocytes.

Mr. Browning points out the fact, which is, of course, easily understood, that in making a diagnosis of sympathetic disease, syphilis must first be excluded.

The clinical result of treatment by salvarsan in sympathetic disease was sufficiently good to justify its continuance, but what was of great importance as an indication was the fact that after such treatment the differential blood count always tended to revert to the normal. In the intervals of treatment, the count again became of the protozoal type.

The results in twenty cases treated are given both in descriptive statement and in tabular form, and are not very striking as a demonstration of the beneficial results of the treatment. The ordinary course of sympathetic affections must be taken into account, however.

There is another point which must be alluded to, namely, that in a few of the cases the diagnosis of sympathetic disease was made on a comparatively slender foundation of fact. For instance, Case IX is as follows :—Right anophthalmos, cause unknown ; sympathetic irido-cyclitis in left, &c. Case XVI is precisely similar.

Mr. Lang then described a case of sympathetic uveitis which was treated by salvarsan, and in which an unusually good result was obtained. The exciting eye was injured by gunshot.

Mr. Fisher alluded to a case of sympathetic affection in which he waited, before doing any operation, until the blood count was normal and then got a good result.

Mr. Lawford alluded to a case of what he terms post-operative plastic irido-cyclitis which gave a good result after treatment by neo-salvarsan.

Mr. Henderson spoke of the use of salvarsan in two cases in which late infection had occurred after cataract extraction, and raised the point as to the benefit of the drug as possibly having a beneficial effect on the exciting as well as the sympathising eye. In this connection it is important to note that in several of the cases described by Mr. Browning the sympathising eye was ultimately excised.

Replying to a question by Mr. Parsons, Mr. Browning said that one could get a typical blood count before the sympathetic disease developed in the second eye.

The record of the entire discussion should be read by any one specially interested, as a brief note like this cannot correctly convey the feeling of the members who entered into the discussion, but the general feeling seemed to be that this was a very important matter, and one which might be only the beginning of something much larger.

A point which at once will strike the reader is this, that it requires a specially trained hæmatologist to give a correct reading of the blood count, as the differentiation of the leucocytes is not an easy matter.—LESLIE BUCHANAN.

Books, Pamphlets, &c., Received.

Manual for Women's Voluntary Aid Detachments, by P. C. Gabbett, M.R.C.S., Lieut.-Col., I.M.S. Second edition, revised and enlarged (reprinted 1914). Bristol: John Wright & Sons, Limited. 1913. (1s. net.)

Public Health Laboratory Work, by Henry R. Kenwood, M.B., F.R.S.Edin., D.P.H., F.C.S. Sixth edition. With illustrations. London: H. K. Lewis. 1914. (10s. net.)

The Vaccination Question in the Light of Modern Experience: An Appeal for Reconsideration, by C. Killick Millard, M.D., D.Sc. London: H. K. Lewis. 1914. (6s. net.)

Nature and Nurture in Mental Development, by F. W. Mott, M.D., F.R.S., F.R.C.P. With diagrams. London: John Murray. 1914. (3s. 6d. net.)

A Text-Book of Insanity and other Mental Diseases, by Charles Arthur Mercier, M.D., F.R.C.P., F.R.C.S. Second edition, entirely rewritten. London George Allen and Unwin, Limited. 1914. (7s. 6d. net.)

The Operative Treatment of Fractures, by Sir W. Arbuthnot Lane, Bart., M.S., F.R.C.S. Second edition. London: The Medical Publishing Co., Limited. 1914. (10s.)

Forty-fourth Annual Report of the Operations of the Sanitary Department of the City of Glasgow for the year ending 31st December, 1913, by Peter Fyfe, Chief Sanitary Inspector. Glasgow: Robert Anderson.

Elements of Surgical Diagnosis, by Sir Alfred Pearce Gould, K.C.V.O., M.S. Lond., F.R.C.S.Eng. Fourth edition, revised and enlarged by the Author, with the assistance of Eric Pearce Gould, M.A., M.Ch.Oxon., F.R.C.S.Eng. With 10 radiographic plates and other illustrations. London: Cassell & Co., Limited. (10s. 6d. net.)

Tuberculosis of the Bones and Joints in Children, by John Fraser, M.D., F.R.C.S.E., Ch.M. With 51 full-page plates (2 in colour) and 164 figures in the text. London: Adam & Charles Black. (15s. net.)

A Manual of Minor Surgery and Bandaging (Heath and Pollard), for the Use of House Surgeons, Dressers, and Junior Practitioners. Fifteenth edition. By H. Morriston Davies, M.D., M.C.Cantab., F.R.C.S. London: J. & A. Churchill. (7s. 6d. net.)

Practical Medical Electricity: A Handbook for House Surgeons and Practitioners, by Alfred C. Norman, M.D.Edin., Sunderland. Profusely illustrated. London: The Scientific Press, Limited. (5s. net.)

Standard Prescriptions for Insurance Practice, compiled by C. H. Gunson, M.B., Ch.B. London: The Scientific Press, Limited. (1s. net.)

A War Cookery Book for the Sick and Wounded, compiled from the Cookery Books by Mrs. Edwards, Miss May Little, &c., &c., by Jessie M. Laurie. London: T. Werner Laurie, Limited. (6d. net.)

GLASGOW.—METEOROLOGICAL AND VITAL STATISTICS FOR THE FIVE WEEKS ENDED 19TH SEPTEMBER, 1914.

	WEEK ENDING				
	Aug. 22.	Aug. 29.	Sept. 5.	Sept. 12.	Sept. 19.
Mean temperature, . .	59·2°	59·8°	60·3°	57·2°	52·8°
Mean range of temperature between highest and lowest,	19·5°	17·8°	16·3°	21·6°	13·3°
Number of days on which rain fell, ...	1	6	1	3	5
Amount of rainfall, . ins.	0·13	1·03	0·02	0·37	0·79
Deaths (corrected), . .	300	303	363	354	336
Death-rates, ...	15·0	15·1	18·1	17·6	16·7
Zymotic death-rates, . .	1·0	1·4	0·9	1·2	0·8
Pulmonary death-rates, .	2·9	2·8	2·5	2·7	2·5
DEATHS—					
Under 1 year, . . .	74	93	104	125	107
60 years and upwards, .	72	56	87	70	65
DEATHS FROM—					
Small-pox, ...	...	...	...	...	...
Measles, ...	1	1	2	...	2
Scarlet fever, . . .	3	6	2	7	4
Diphtheria, . . .	5	3	1	3	...
Whooping-cough, . .	9	12	13	13	6
Enteric fever, . . .	5	6	...	2	2
Cerebro-spinal fever, . .	1	..	1	1	...
Diarrhœa (under 2 years of age),	26	46	61	67	54
Bronchitis, pneumonia, and pleurisy, . . .	34	34	38	34	32
CASES REPORTED—					
Small-pox, ...	...	...	...	...	...
Cerebro-spinal meningitis, .	...	1	1	3	3
Diphtheria and membranous croup, ...	15	20	13	23	28
Erysipelas, . . .	24	31	21	29	21
Scarlet fever, . . .	113	107	104	117	136
Typhus fever, . . .	...	...	...	...	...
Enteric fever, . . .	23	16	10	12	11
Phthisis, ...	37	39	31	47	87
Puerperal fever, . .	2	5	1	1	2
Measles,* . . .	8	10	33	20	6

* Measles not notifiable.

SANITARY CHAMBERS,
GLASGOW, 23rd *September*, 1914.

THE

GLASGOW MEDICAL JOURNAL.

No. V. NOVEMBER, 1914.

ORIGINAL ARTICLES.

SIX CASES OF DISEASE OF THE LOWER ABDOMINAL ORGANS, SOME OF WHICH SIMULATED TUMOURS OF THE UTERUS AND ADNEXA.*

By J. M. MUNRO KERR, M.D.,

Muirhead Professor of Obstetrics and Gynæcology, University of Glasgow.

FOUR years ago I brought under the notice of this Society a number of cases of disease of the cæcum and sigmoid which simulated affections of the uterus and adnexa. To-night I propose to refer to some interesting examples of affections more particularly of the lower part of the abdomen and pelvis which I have encountered in my hospital and private practice. They are of sufficient rarity to justify my bringing them under your notice and putting them on record.

CASE I.—*Right-sided hypernephroma—Nephrectomy—Full-time pregnancy a year later.*

The specimen which is here shown was demonstrated by Dr. Shaw Dunn to the Society on 13th December, 1912,

* Read at a meeting of the Medico-Chirurgical Society of Glasgow held on 6th March, 1914.

along with a number of others of a similar nature. It was removed from a woman, aged 32 years, who was placed under my care in the Western Infirmary on 5th September, 1910. She had been seen by Dr. Holmes when on holiday, and he was specially interested in the tumour because it so closely resembled an ovarian cyst. On admission to my wards the patient informed me she had been married for ten years and had four children. The tumour in the abdomen had been noticed first three years before, but caused no pain or discomfort, although recently it had slightly increased in size. It could be felt in the right side close by the pelvic brim, and was about the size of a "grape fruit." It was only moderately movable. A day or two after admission the patient was anæsthetised, and a very careful bimanual examination made. At this examination I was quite satisfied the tumour had no connection with the uterus, for the latter could be entirely isolated from the tumour. I could also feel with difficulty a small body close by the uterus, which, on the whole, I was inclined to think was the right ovary. I could not, however, altogether exclude the possibility that the tumour was of ovarian origin, although I was inclined to think that it was connected with the right kidney. There was nothing abnormal discovered in the urine.

A few days after the examination under anæsthesia I opened the abdomen in the middle line and removed the tumour, which proved to be of renal origin. This was done without difficulty. Some gauze was introduced into the cavity from which the tumour was enucleated, and the end of the gauze was brought out through a counter opening in the loin. Her temperature remained absolutely normal for the first twenty-two days, but on the twenty-third day it went up, and was more or less disturbed for the succeeding ten days. She ultimately made an excellent recovery.

Her urinary outflow for the first fortnight after the operation averaged 30 oz.; during the last few days before she left she was sometimes passing as much as 60 oz. per diem.

She had a confinement a year later. Her pregnancy was undisturbed, and when I last heard of her, her health was excellent.

In this case it was only possible to exclude the ovarian

origin of the tumour by determining an ovary apart from the tumour. This, as I have indicated, could not be done with absolute certainty, although I thought the small body I felt to the right of the uterus was the right ovary.

The tumour is a typical example of an encapsuled "hypernephroma."

CASE II.—*Retro-cœcal myoma—Enucleation.*

The second case was also a tumour in the region of the cæcum. The patient was brought to me on account of a hard swelling in the right iliac region. She was a woman of 54 years of age, and had reached the menopause a year or two before.

On abdominal examination the tumour was very hard and fixed, and felt exactly like a fixed fibroid tumour of the uterus. On bimanual examination, however, it was found quite unconnected with the uterus. It projected slightly down into the pelvis. I could not define the right ovary, and was inclined to think that the growth might be a malignant tumour of the right ovary, although the fact that it had been present for some time and had not been increasing much in size raised doubts in my mind regarding its malignancy. Upon opening the abdomen I found the uterus and ovaries of both sides perfectly normal. The tumour was situated behind the cæcum, which was stretched over its upper and inner margin. It was readily enucleated from the cellular tissue, and proved to be a fibro-myoma, which, I think, had probably been at one time connected with the uterus but had become detached. The patient made an excellent recovery.

CASE III.—*Polypus of the ileo-cœcal valve—Removal of cœcum—Lateral anastomosis between ileum and cœcum.*

This particular case was one of special interest because she had been under the care of several physicians and surgeons in the Royal and Samaritan Hospitals. I kept her under observation in my wards for ten or twelve days before operating, as I could not decide what the nature of the condition was.

She was placed under my care by Dr. Wilson, of Shettleston. She complained of attacks of pain in the lower part of the abdomen.   There was nothing special in her menstrual or obstetric history.   Some months before admission she had a vague paralytic stroke and slight facial paralysis.

On questioning her very carefully she stated that with the pain a lump rose in her abdomen, and that these attacks were cured by castor oil.   Generally her bowels moved regularly every second day if she took a mild laxative.   The motions were rather dark in colour, and were often very offensive in odour.   She stated, however, that there was no pain when the bowels moved.

When the spasms come on there is great pain, then something like an explosion occurs inside her, and the pain ceases and the swelling goes down.

I happened to be at her bedside one day when she informed me she had an attack of pain, and on turning down the bedclothes and examining the abdomen I discovered a small swelling rise up in the lower quadrant of the abdomen rather more to the right of the middle line, and just above the symphysis.   As the spasm passed off the abdomen became quite soft and flat.

It was perfectly obvious after seeing the abdomen during an attack that there was some intestinal obstruction, and when I palpated over the region of the cæcum I thought I could feel a distinct fulness and resistance in that region.   I determined, therefore, to open the abdomen.   When this was done I found the whole region of the bowel in the neighbourhood of the ileo-cæcal valve thickened, especially the ileum. I removed the cæcum, and then established a lateral anastomosis between the ileum and ascending colon.

The specimen which you see was examined and mounted by Professor Teacher.   It shows a polypus situated at the valve, and, in addition, a small ulcer in that area.   I have not the slightest doubt that this polypus occasionally obstructed the fæcal matter passing from the ileum into the cæcum, and was the cause of the attacks of pain the woman had suffered from for so many years.

She has reported herself several times since the operation, and says she is free from all abdominal discomfort.

CASE IV.—*Calcareous gland, right-sided, simulating stone in right ureter.*

It is hardly necessary to take up time with this particular case, as the stereograph speaks for itself.

The patient came under my care complaining of pain in passing urine of fourteen weeks' duration. The pain was never very severe, but just as micturition was finishing it came on and continued for about an hour. About four weeks before admission she was seized with acute pain in the right side accompanied by sickness and vomiting. On questioning her she stated that she had had several slight attacks of a similar nature. Bimanual abdomino-vaginal examination revealed nothing, but a stereograph made by Dr. Riddell showed a shadow just above the brim of the pelvis on the right side. Nothing abnormal was found in the urine.

I felt almost certain I had to do with a case of stone in the ureter. When I opened the abdomen, therefore, and examined the ureter I was very much suprised that there was no stone present, and that I had really to deal with several calcareous glands of the mesentery. These I dissected out along with the appendix, which was adherent to the cæcum. The patient has had no return of her symptoms.

CASE V.—*Greatly distended double ureter on the left side simulating a cyst in the broad ligament—Nephrectomy.*

In some respects this is the most interesting case which I have to bring before you to-night.

This patient came into my wards in the Royal Infirmary on 19th March, 1913. She was 34 years of age and married, but she had never been pregnant.

The history of her illness was as follows :—A fortnight after marriage (about six years ago) she commenced to have pain in the left side. This pain was associated with great sickness and was generally worse at the time of her periods. She had been twice in the Samaritan Hospital, and on one occasion a slight operation was performed. Her bowels were constipated, and once or twice she had a little blood and a slimy discharge in her motions. The pain in her left side often extended round to her back and into her left hip. On examining her under an anæsthetic I discovered that the uterus was slightly retroflexed, and that on the left side there was some indefinite thickening. As her discomforts were so great I determined to open the abdomen.

When the abdomen was opened I found that the left ovary was cystic; I therefore removed it. The right ovary and appendix were normal. Not being satisfied, however, that this small cyst could account for all the patient's discomforts, I examined with my fingers the right broad ligament and pelvis generally, and I thought I could detect a slight fulness towards the base of the broad ligament. I therefore determined to examine the condition more carefully, and so I split open the broad ligament. Having done this I found a sausage-shaped swelling running towards the bladder in the exact position of the ureter. It was about the thickness of my thumb. I was inclined to think I had to deal with some condition obstructing the ureter.

Proceeding with my dissection I came across a normal ureter.

The position of the distended sausage-shaped ureter was as follows:—It ran along close by the normal ureter on its inner aspect. At the kidney end it opened into the pelvis of the kidney above the normal ureter. At the lower end it terminated on the bladder wall, but there was no opening into the bladder as far as I could discover, and I tested this very carefully by passing a sound into the bladder and a probe into the ureter. It contained very clear fluid. The normal ureter, as I have said, ran close by the outer aspect of the distended one. Its upper end was connected with the lower part of the pelvis of the kidney, while its lower end, as it approached the bladder, curved over the anterior surface of the blind distended one.

The kidney was large and lobulated. I also examined the other kidney, which seemed to be of normal size and shape.

By this time I had spent a considerable time in dissecting off the sausage-shaped ureter, so I simply removed it, and tied it off above and below. I am extremely sorry that I adopted this procedure. I should have removed the kidney; for four or five days after the operation, although the patient's temperature was perfectly normal, I began to be suspicious there was a leak going on from the pelvis of the kidney, and that I had torn the insertion of the distended ureter. I therefore on the seventh day removed the left kidney by a lumbar incision. I found the perirenal tissues sodden.

The nephrectomy presented no great difficulty, and the patient seemed for a little to improve, but she gradually sank and died a fortnight after the second operation.

As already mentioned, I regretted afterwards that I had not performed nephrectomy at the first operation, but my idea was that I might possibly be able to leave behind a functionating kidney.

CASE VI.—*Chronic inflammation in sigmoid and pelvic colon simulating malignant tumour—Resection of pelvic colon—An end to end anastomosis.*

This case raises several interesting questions in connection with the surgery of the pelvic colon in women.

The patient was seen by me with Dr. Napier, of Crosshill, who informed me that she was a healthy woman who had six or seven of a family, but recently had been complaining of pain in the lower part of the abdomen, more especially when the bowels moved. During the last few weeks the pain had been increasing in severity, and the doctor was satisfied that she was losing weight, and certainly she herself informed us that she thought she had become much weaker, and altogether felt very miserable.

On bimanual vaginal examination I could readily detect an irregular hard swelling behind and to the left of the uterus. It was absolutely fixed and extended a little way above the brim of the pelvis. On rectal examination nothing more could be felt. There was no bleeding from the bowel, but occasionally there was some slimy mucus in the motions. I made a diagnosis of tumour of the ovary, probably malignant in nature, and I was doubtful if I could do a great deal for her by operating. However, we determined to operate, so she was removed to a nursing home.

On opening the abdomen, I discovered the uterus pushed forward by a swelling to which it was loosely adherent. It was obvious that the tumour was not of ovarian origin, for both ovaries, although adherent to it, could be readily separated.   I now thought I had to deal with a malignant tumour of the lower part of the sigmoid and pelvic colon.

I found I could get beyond the tumour below; indeed, I could leave behind about 2 inches of what seemed to be sound bowel.   I therefore divided the pelvic colon below the tumour. I then dissected off the tumour and cut across the sigmoid beyond the growth.   I was now in rather an awkward position, for I had a greatly distended sigmoid to attach to a small portion of pelvic colon of normal calibre situated deep down in the pelvis.   I knew it would be futile to attempt an exact end to end anastomosis, but it occurred to me, and no doubt it has occurred to others in a similar difficulty, that if an exact end to end anastomosis of two-thirds of the circumference of the bowel ends could be secured, the other one-third, which was imperfectly brought together, would heal by granulation tissue.   I therefore attached the two ligatures to the lower part of the pelvic colon and pulled it up as far as possible.   I then stitched the upper cut end of the sigmoid to the rudiment of the pelvic colon as carefully as possible round the anterior two-thirds.   I then overstretched the sphincter ani.   Having done this I opened through the vaginal fornix widely and packed in gauze round the imperfect anastomosis.

The patient was then put back to bed, and I gave instructions that she was to be kept slightly under the influence of morphia, and on no account were the bowels to be moved for ten days.   I removed the gauze gradually from the sixth to the eighth day.

On the tenth day I gave her a large dose of castor oil, and told the nurse that she was not to be astonished if a great deal of fæcal matter came by the vagina.   As I expected, the most of the fæcal material came by the vagina.   In about a fortnight, however, all the fæces had ceased to come by the vagina, and in the end the wound in the vaginal cavity healed up, and the patient's bowels moved normally per rectum. She made an uninterrupted recovery.   I have not seen her for some months, but when I last saw her she was in very good health indeed.

TWO CASES ILLUSTRATIVE OF SPLENIC ANÆMIA AND SPLENECTOMY.

By WILLIAM R. JACK, M.D.,

Physician to the Glasgow Royal Infirmary ; Lecturer in Clinical Medicine, Glasgow University;

AND

D. T. C. FREW, M.B., CH.B.,

Extra Dispensary Physician and Clinical Assistant to the Glasgow Royal Infirmary.

THE following cases, one of splenic anæmia, the other of portal thrombosis simulating it in its clinical features, illustrate some points in the diagnosis of the disease, while the former is also of interest from the successful result of splenectomy.

Mrs. D., aged 37, was admitted to the Glasgow Royal Infirmary on 7th January, 1914, having previously been under the care of Dr. J. C. Middleton in the Outdoor Department. She complained of debility, loss of appetite, attacks of bronchitis, breathlessness on slight exertion, and of a "lump" or swelling in her left side, while for a few days before admission she had had pain in the lumbar region and difficulty in micturition. She had been healthy until, at the age of 25, she suffered from rheumatic fever; and since then she had "never felt the same," having suffered from debility and from frequent attacks of bronchitis. During the last three years she has had several attacks of diarrhœa, and the swelling in her side was first noticed about three years ago. Within this time she has become pale, and in the past year she has twice had attacks of lumbar pain with difficult micturition. Her food has always been sufficient, and her lodging adequate.

She has been ten times pregnant. Four of the pregnancies resulted in still-births, and of the six children born living only three survive. Her family history revealed nothing of importance.

On admission she was found to be thin and pale, with a distinct yellow tinge in the skin. The sclerotics, however, were bluish and free from icterus. There was no pain, and she lay comfortably in any position. There were no deformities; œdema was absent, and there was no cutaneous eruption, nor, although the history of her pregnancies was suspicious, was there any other evidence of previous syphilis in the history or in the presence of cicatrices. The Wassermann reation was also negative. Her cardio-vascular system showed little change beyond what was to be expected from her anæmia. There was a moderate degree of bronchitis, with a mucous expectoration in which no tubercle bacilli were found. There was no evidence of enlargement of the thyroid or thymus, and nothing to suggest disease of the pituitary or adrenal glands. The external lymphatic glands were not enlarged. The urine contained a faint trace of albumen, but was not otherwise abnormal. Menstruation was normal, but scanty. The nervous system presented no abnormality.

The teeth were decayed; there was some degree of pyorrhœa alveolaris; and the tongue was dry, fissured, and furred. The stomach was apparently of normal size; and while there was some flatulent distension of the intestine there was no evidence of obstruction or of thickening of the colon. Ascites was absent. She had well-marked hæmorrhoids, both internal and external, but they had never bled, nor had there been other hæmorrhages from the alimentary tract or elsewhere.

The left epigastric and left upper lumbar region were occupied by a firm, smooth, flat swelling, projecting somewhat into the umbilical region, and having a sharply-defined anterior border, with a notch; thus conforming to the characters of an enlarged spleen. There was no pain here, and but little tenderness. The measurements were—length, 9½ inches; breadth, 2½ inches. The liver was enlarged, and palpable an inch below the costal margin in the right nipple line. It was smooth, firm, and free from nodules.

On examination the blood showed—

Red cells, ...	2,600,000 per c.mm.
Hæmoglobin, ...	35 per cent.
White cells, ...	1,100 per c.mm.
Colour index, ...	0·675.

Films showed a remarkable scarcity of white cells, but, so far as could be judged, no alterations in the normal proportions of their different varieties. No myelocytes were found. There were very few blood platelets. The red cells showed some anisocytosis and poikilocytosis, but megalocytes and megaloblasts were entirely absent. Only one or two nucleated cells were found in several films, and these were normoblasts. There was little polychromatophilia, and no stippled cells were found. The staining was less intense than usual, and ring staining was frequent.

Treatment by arsenic was instituted, and nuclein was also given with the object of increasing the number of leucocytes. As a result the red cells increased to some degree in number, averaging, from 13th February onwards, 3,500,000, but the white cells remained at about the same figure, varying between 1,500 and 1,000 per c.mm. The percentage of hæmoglobin was virtually unaffected, and the colour index was consequently somewhat reduced.

The blood-picture was therefore that of an anæmia of moderate degree and of the chlorotic type, with a remarkable diminution of leucocytes, a leucopenia of extreme degree. It conformed in every respect to the picture of splenic anæmia, and this diagnosis was supported by the presence of a considerable chronic enlargement of the spleen without enlargement of the lymphatic glands and without any obvious cause, and by the practically afebrile course of the disease. There were one or two transitory elevations of temperature in the first fortnight after admission, once to 100·6°, once to 100·2°, but all other temperatures were below 100°, and for the last four weeks the temperature was normal.

The failure of medicinal treatment led to operative measures, and on 27th February the spleen was removed by Professor Robert Kennedy. It was found to be greatly enlarged, weighing 1 lb. 10 oz., but the operation itself was chiefly notable for the extreme friability of the vessels, which led to very considerable loss of blood. The anæmia was thus temporarily aggravated, and within a few days of the operation she unfortunately developed a patch of pneumonia at the left base. She made, however, a fair recovery, and early in April was sent to the Convalescent Home. Since then her general condition has steadily improved. She has been able to resume housework, has become less breathless on exertion and of better colour, and, though her bronchitis has to some extent persisted, and she has had an occasional attack of colicky pain, the amelioration of her condition has been very striking. A slight degree of œdema of the ankles was present for some time after she began to go about, but when she was last seen, on 24th July, it had disappeared, and the enlargement of the liver which was present before the operation had also ceased to exist.

On 24th July, 1914, the blood showed—

Red cells, ...	3,500,000
White cells, ...	10,000
Hæmoglobin, ...	60 per cent.
Colour index, ...	0·85

There was a remarkable increase in the mononuclear white cells and the transitional type, while here and there were found cells indistinguishable from myelocytes.

The red cells showed better staining than before, though there were still some ring forms. Poikilocytes and microcytes were still found, and several crenated cells and cells with central staining were seen. Polychromatic staining was also visible here and there, while one or two stippled cells were present, and two normoblasts. Thus it would seem that while the blood showed regeneration, there was still some difficulty in disposing of effete and degenerating corpuscles, and perhaps also some defect in the control of leucocyte formation.

The spleen excised was firm, showed many dilated vessels, and seemed congested. There was some evidence of perisplenitis of slight degree, and friable adhesions had formed. Sections showed that the main increase was in the reticulum of the pulp itself and its contents. The supporting tissues were increased only in a minor degree; and the condition seemed a hyperplasia of the pulp with some degree of congestion. The Malpighian corpuscles appeared to be slightly (if at all) enlarged. The vessels were thin-walled and dilated. Fresh films of the pulp showed mainly mononucleated cells, in great numbers and of all sizes, together with red corpuscles, some few of which were nucleated.

The diagnosis of splenic anæmia made in this case would appear to be justified by the symptom-complex, by the pathological findings in the spleen, and by the favourable result of splenectomy. Rolleston[1] defines chronic splenic anæmia as a condition presenting the following characters :—"(1) Chronic splenomegaly which cannot be correlated with any recognised cause ; (2) absence of enlargement of the lymphatic glands ; (3) chlorotic anæmia, namely, with a low colour index ; (4) absence of leucocytosis, and usually the presence of leucopenia ; (5) liability to copious gastro-intestinal hæmorrhages from time to time ; (6) the prolonged course without any tendency to spontaneous cure, though splenectomy (if successful) is usually curative." To all of these conditions the present case- conforms, with the single exception of number (5), with regard to which it may probably be assumed that gastro-intestinal hæmorrhages would have appeared at a later stage, had the case been allowed to run an uninterrupted course. The duration of a case of splenic anæmia is long ; as Rolleston states, it was over ten years in half of Osler's series of fifteen cases ; and a patient who has suffered for not more than three years may be looked upon as still in the early stages of the disease. Other conditions which might simulate splenic anæmia—leukæmia in an aleukæmic stage, syphilis of the liver and spleen, &c.—may in this case be excluded by the results of examination of the blood, by the absence of enlargement of lymphatic glands, and by the negative Wassermann reaction. The diarrhœa, which was noted as having been present on several occasions during the past three years, is a symptom which according to Banti "occurs in the transitional stage between splenic anæmia and Banti's disease," and this statement would accord with the fact that there was a slight enlargement of the liver, which is not commonly present in uncomplicated splenic anæmia. The condition of the spleen would also bear out this assumption ; although there was slight thickening of the trabeculæ, the main increase was in the reticulum of the pulp and its contents—the condition, in fact, of *fibro-adénie*, which is a precursor of the development of portal cirrhosis.

To justify splenectomy, the diagnosis of splenic anæmia must be certain, and medicinal treatment must have failed. The operation is a severe one, and has a considerable mortality, which, however, may possibly be lessened by its performance at an early stage of the disease. Its results in other forms of splenic disorder are at' least questionably beneficial, and in certain instances it may be directly harmful. But the diagnosis is often a matter of some difficulty, and the following case may be adduced as an instance :—

J. A., æt. 17, admitted to the Glasgow Royal Infirmary on 12th April, 1914, suffering from hæmatemesis. He had been in good health till the end of February, when one morning on his way to work, after some preliminary nausea, he vomited a quantity of dark red blood. The attack passed off in five minutes, when he went on to his work and worked all day. He remained well till three weeks before admission, when a similar attack, lasting about three minutes, caused him to go to bed, where he stayed until admitted to hospital. There was no recurrence till 11th April, when he noticed blood in his stools, and on the 12th, previous to admission, he had a third hæmatemesis, of brief duration but preceded by faintness. He had never had epistaxis or bleeding from the gums, nor had he suffered from breathlessness. During the last eighteen months he had occasionally vomited, usually after meals, and particularly after taking eggs, but until the end of February he had never vomited blood. The vomiting was not preceded by pain, nor has he had any other symptoms of gastric disorder. In childhood he had had scarlet fever and measles, but otherwise he had always been healthy. The family history had no bearing on the case.

On admission his temperature was 100.8°, his pulse 112, and his respirations 28. He was thin, with a yellowish pallor of the skin, but no jaundice, and his mucous membranes were distinctly anæmic. The skin was dry. The vessels were normal, the pulse full, regular, and of medium tension, and the systolic blood-pressure was 130. The cardiac dulness was normal, but there was a blowing systolic murmur over the mitral and pulmonic areas, partly replacing the first sound. The lungs were normal to percussion and auscultation.

The tongue was covered by a white dry fur, and the breath was bad. The teeth were in fair condition, and there was no pyorrhœa. There was a tendency to constipation. There was no gastric tenderness or other abnormality, the hepatic dulness was normal, and its lower border could not be palpated below the costal margin. The spleen was much enlarged; its lower border with the notch could be felt 4 inches below the costal margin, and the percussion note over it was uniformly dull. There was no tenderness over the spleen or in any other part of the abdomen. The abdominal veins were slightly distended, especially in the lower part, and there was a slight degree of ascites. The stools presented the characters of melæna. The superficial lymphatic glands were not enlarged. The nervous system presented no abnormality except that the tendon-jerks were defective; and the urine was normal. Examination of the blood gave the following results :—

	On admission.	18th April.	25th April.	28th April.
Red cells,	1,800,000	1,800,000	600,000	1,500,000
White cells,	6,500	5,000	2,000	4,000
Hæmoglobin,	16 °/₀	15 °/₀	10 °/₀	14 °/₀
Colour index,	0·45	0·42	0·83	0·46

On 12th April and 28th April differential counts were made, with the following results:—12th April—Polymorphonuclear cells, 40 per cent; lymphocytes, 33 per cent; transitionals, 27 per cent. 28th April—Polymorphonuclear cells, 49 per cent; lymphocytes, 31 per cent; transitionals, 18 per cent; eosinophile myelocytes, 2 per cent.

By 16th April melæna had ceased, but the temperature continued to swing between 99° and 101°. On the morning of the 24th melæna reappeared, and in the evening there was a large hæmatemesis, 28 oz. of blood being vomited. The third blood count was taken on the following day, which accounts for the low figures presented. Melæna continued till the 28th, but there was nevertheless an improvement in the blood condition. On the 30th, however, a small hæmatemesis (5 oz.) occurred, which was sufficient to complete his exhaustion, and he died on the morning of 2nd May.

The treatment consisted in feeding by rectal injections of glucose in normal saline; hypodermic injections of morphia for the hæmorrhage, and strychnine for the collapse; the local application of ice to the epigastrium, while ice was also given by the mouth; and latterly calcium lactate was given orally in doses of 15 grains, and normal saline was also given subcutaneously.

Post-mortem, the body was anæmic and emaciated. There was hypostatic œdema of the lungs, but no local lesion. The heart showed an extreme degree of fatty degeneration, but no valvular lesion, and the vessels were healthy. The abdomen contained a little clear serous fluid, and the peritoneum looked dull, as if slightly thickened. The liver was anæmic and slightly fatty, but otherwise normal. The gall-bladder was large and thick, its walls being œdematous. The bile passages were open. The portal tract was much thickened, and externally showed small congested blood-vessels. The upper part of the duodenum adhered to it for fully an inch from the pylorus, and the adhesion contained many vessels. Vessels were also abnormally numerous in the suspensory ligament at the back of the liver.

The spleen, which weighed 16 oz, was greatly enlarged, but soft, fibrous, and rather anæmic. At its upper end the capsule was attached to the diaphragm by a broad and very vascular adhesion. The splenic veins were tortuous, and plugged with loose red thrombi. On dividing the portal fissure there was found a thrombus, principally white, almost completely filling the main trunk of the portal vein. It extended out to the spleen and down into the mesentery, but upwards it did not pass beyond the portal fissure. Apparently it completely obstructed the vein, although it was contracted and loose in places.

The kidneys were anæmic. There was no ulceration of the stomach, but there was marked compensatory dilatation of the œsophageal veins. The pylorus was normal. The duodenum and the rest of the intestine were not ulcerated, but about an inch beyond the pyloric ring, in a situation corresponding exactly to the adhesion to the portal tract, there was an oval slightly depressed area which might possibly be the cicatrix of an ulcer. It lay very close to the thrombosed portal vein.

There was a marked erythroblastic reaction of the bone-marrow. The lymphatic glands were perhaps slightly larger than normal. The brain was rather anæmic.

Here, then, we have a case which fulfilled nearly all the conditions postulated by Rolleston in his definition of chronic splenic anæmia. There was a chronic splenomegaly which could not be correlated with any recognised cause. There was absence of enlargement of the lymphatic glands. There was a chlorotic anæmia, with a low colour index. Although leucopenia was not present, except on the one occasion, just after a severe hæmorrhage, when all the elements of the blood were much reduced, there was an absence of leucocytosis. Copious gastro-intestinal hæmorrhages were present; and if we assume that the occasional vomitings which preceded them were early symptoms of the disease, it had lasted at least eighteen months. Yet there were features in the case which appeared to make the diagnosis uncertain. One·of us (Frew), from the clinical features, was inclined to consider the symptoms as due to thrombosis of the splenic vein, possibly complicating splenic anæmia; the other, from the results of the differential blood-counts and from the constant presence of sub-febrile temperatures, which are unusual in splenic anæmia, leaned rather to the view that we had to deal with an acute leukæmia in an aleukæmic stage. As will be seen from the account of the *post-mortem* examination, the former opinion proved more nearly in accordance with the anatomical lesions; but the true diagnosis, namely, an old-standing and extensive portal thrombosis, which from the character of the thrombus must have been in existence at least for several months, and which may possibly have originated in the irritation of a long obsolete duodenal ulcer, was not suspected during life.

It is unnecessary to do more than indicate that if, on a merely probable diagnosis of splenic anæmia, the operation of splenectomy had been performed in such a case as is described above the results could not have been other than disastrous.

REFERENCE.

[1] Rolleston, "Chronic Splenic Anæmia and Banti's Disease," *The Practitioner*, April, 1914. The paper reviews the whole subject, and gives a full bibliography.

PRACTICAL POINTS IN ABDOMINAL SURGERY, BEING
THE "JAMES WATSON LECTURES" DELIVERED BEFORE
THE ROYAL FACULTY OF PHYSICIANS AND SURGEONS,
11TH AND 14TH MARCH, 1913.

By T. KENNEDY DALZIEL, M.B., F.R.F.P.S.,
Surgeon to the Western Infirmary, Glasgow.

(*Concluded from* p. 262.)

Adhesions to the liver.—Should perforative peritonitis arise
in such a case, it may be a most difficult matter to detect the
source of escape, and even if discovered it is no easy matter
to close such a perforation. In some cases it is only possible
to pack the region and trust to the formation of adhesions,
while a gastro-enterostomy should be done.

Apart from pain associated with perforation, we have
undoubtedly a group of ulcers in the stomach so painful as
to call for relief by operation, provided medicinal and dietetic
treatment have failed. The degree of pain is by no means
commensurate with the size of the ulcer. A minute ulcer in
the pylorus may give rise to more pain than a large and
perhaps a more chronic one.

Hæmorrhage in ulceration.—Lastly, it is necessary to operate
for hæmorrhage in ulceration. One finds varying statements in
text-books as to the mortality from hæmorrhage, and I at once
grant that it is comparatively small. That fatal hæmorrhage,
however, does occur there is no doubt. Death occasionally
takes place from persistent bleeding from a coronary artery,
or it may be that recurrent hæmorrhage saps the patient's
vitality and leads to death from intercurrent causes, or
devitalises the tissues locally and hastens perforation. There
can be no doubt that in recurrent hæmorrhage following the
indication of progressive ulceration one should operate. The
line of treatment to be followed, however, in acute progressive
hæmorrhage is a more difficult matter. Doubtless the clinical

features may in some cases indicate the urgent necessity of action. In three cases I have been able to expose the bleeding artery and ligate it; it is best done by transfixing the edge of the ulcer by a stitch, thereafter making a by-pass. One of three terminated fatally by an extraordinary thrombosis of pulmonary and systemic veins about three weeks later; the others made good recoveries.

In conclusion, I do not think ulceration of the stomach is ever to be treated lightly, and I believe that as our technique advances, and the safety of surgical proceedings is more completely demonstrated, ulceration of the stomach, just as much as trouble in the appendix, will be looked upon as a signal for interference. The unfortunate thing is that it is often a matter of extreme difficulty to diagnose ulceration of the stomach before serious complications have ensued.

That malignant disease tends to affect a chronic ulcer there can be no doubt. One can give many cases already where the immediate relief afforded by gastro-enterostomy for chronic ulceration of the pylorus, and a cessation of all symptoms for several years, was followed by recurrence of a cancer. This raises the question whether it is not good surgery to excise the chronic ulcers of the pylorus, in the hope that the resulting scar may be less liable to cancerous change. Needless to say, in such a matter a definite conclusion can only be reached after long experience.

Hyper-acidity of the stomach.—The genesis of this condition is wrapped in obscurity. That a temporary hyper-acidity will follow indiscretions of diet there can be no doubt; but that some patients have constant and persistent hyper-acidity with congestion of the mucous membrane is also true, a condition with which every physician is familiar. It seems likely, and in my experience has invariably occurred, that the mucous membrane becomes extremely red and chronically thickened; and while alleviation may be obtained by the use of alkalies and modification of diet, the condition may be an extremely inveterate one, rendering the life of the patient utterly miserable.

It seems probable that, whatever the origin of the complaint may be, undue retention of the food in the stomach intensifies the condition.   I had one patient recently of this kind in my wards, sent me by Drs. Cowan and Armstrong, of Kirkintilloch ; she had suffered for years from symptoms of acidity in a very exaggerated degree.   The congestion of her stomach was reflected in her face, which gave one the impression of a lady who habitually used, or rather abused, alcohol, every part of her countenance being a most vivid red.

Tumours of the stomach.—These, for the most part malignant, are usually epithelial; only two cases of sarcoma have come under my observation.   As previously indicated, such tumours frequently have a preceding history of ulceration, and their situation corresponds in frequency to that of simple ulceration, the lesser curvature near the pylorus being the favoured seat. There can be no doubt of the propriety of operation in such cases, and the rules which guide one apply here as elsewhere, the earlier the operation the more favourable the issue, and so the best results are obtained in cancer of the pylorus where obstructive symptoms early call for interference.

The symptoms of cancer of the stomach elsewhere, like those of simple ulceration, may be extremely vague ; indeed, a loss of appetite and gradual inability to take much at a time may be the only symptoms apart from the gradual loss of strength and weight, and the development of anæmia, which is so characteristic of malignant disease.   One is amazed sometimes to find with so little complaint the entire stomach converted into a cancerous mass.   In such cases palpation is of little use unless the tumour be in the pyloric third of the stomach.   Fortunately the great majority of cancers occurring in this zone may be readily felt, especially if the patient be examined under an anæsthetic. When operation is practised it must be carried out fearlessly, and on exactly the same principles as guide us in the treatment of cancer elsewhere.

Palliative operations can be done where the pylorus is obstructed, and where secondary growths or peritoneal infection debar radical treatment.   One obtains, however, better results from radical treatment.   It is quite extraordinary how much a patient will stand if one has removed the cancerous tumour, and how disappointing the result may be, whatever operation may be done, when the tumour is left.   Many mistakes in diagnosis occur in tumours of the stomach, not only on external examination, but even when exposed by a laparotomy.

Such a case I heard of recently. A woman was sent to me by Dr. Barr, of Carluke, with a large palpable tumour which we exposed and, finding it adherent to the liver, deemed inoperable. She was therefore sent home with a bad prognosis. Some months afterwards she returned to the hospital with the tumour hardly perceptible, and now at the end of two years she is quite well. This was a case of mistaken diagnosis; we thought it to be cancerous, but it was not. Whether the operation had an influence in causing it to disappear I leave to your imagination.

It has been gravely asserted by some that laparotomy may cure cancer; I think not, though even advanced cases of cancer seem to be relieved for a time by laparotomy. I take this to be an evidence of faith healing. Perhaps it may be that other causes are brought to bear. In the simple cases a more strict attention to diet, &c., and in the truly malignant, occult influences may lead to the improvement.

Chronic interstitial enteritis.—I have pleasure in drawing your attention to this condition, which, I think, has not yet been fully described.

Twelve years ago I saw a professional colleague suffering from obstruction of the bowels of a fortnight's duration, previous to which he had had for several weeks numerous attacks of colic, slight attacks of diarrhœa with no tenderness over the abdomen, very slight rise in temperature, and no appreciable alteration in the pulse-rate. When seen by me the abdomen was not distended, nor were the muscles rigid, but to the hand they gave a sense of putty-like resistance. As vomiting was persistent I concluded that there might be an obstruction high up, and so opened the abdomen and found the whole of the intestines, large and small alike, contracted and rigidly fixed, so that when a loop was lifted from the abdomen it sprang back into its sulcus. That the wall of the whole intestine was chronically inflamed there could be no doubt. In parts the peritoneum seemed œdematous, as were also the omentum and mesentery, and the glands in the latter could be felt enlarged. Nothing could be done to restore the function of the canal, and the patient died a few days afterwards.

We were not then familiar with the condition, and it was supposed to be tuberculous, though this was negatived by microscopic examination, the only information we obtained from the pathologist being that the condition was a chronic inflammatory one.

A few years later, with Dr. Gibb, of Paisley, I saw an exactly similar condition in a young man of 32 years. His symptoms were somewhat more acute than in the previous case, but practically the same. He also died. No examination was allowed.

In these two fatal cases the whole of the small and large intestines were involved.

The following five cases, being localised and therefore excisable, permitted operation, and excision of the affected portion was in all cases followed by complete restoration to health :—

The first of these cases I saw with Professor Gemmell in 1905. Mrs. T. was admitted to the Western Infirmary with symptoms of partial obstruction, and one could palpate a coil of intestine, rigid and thickened. Treatment was of no avail, attacks of pain becoming more frequent. Progressive emaciation and general malaise led to operative interference, when a portion of jejunum, over 2 feet in length, was found to be affected, and was excised. The patient made a complete recovery. Subsequently, I removed from two other cases the caput cæcum and the adjoining portion of the ileum ; in another case the sigmoid ; and in another the transverse colon. Lastly, from a child of 10 years, the specimen which I now show, and which even now indicates the great thickening of the bowel wall. This was from the middle of the ileum.

The following is the pathological report, from the laboratory in the Western Infirmary, of the condition in the specimens obtained from the ileum, jejunum, and colon —:

Histologically, there is much in common in the three cases —indeed, they form a graded series in which all the stages from acute to chronic may be traced. The most acute lesions are found in Master W. G., and the most chronic in Mrs. N.

The following description is based upon a study of numerous sections from each case :—

The earliest change in the bowel appears to be that of acute congestion. The vessels throughout are dilated, and there is much œdema of the submucosa. As evidences of the acute inflammation the vessels are seen to be rich in polymorpho-nuclears, and there is considerable infiltration of all the coats with similar cells. Here and there, too, in mucosa and submucosa irregular hæmorrhages have occurred. These changes also implicate the mesentery in a lesser degree. It is noteworthy that the lymphoid aggregations are singularly free from pathological change. .

With increasing infiltration the next phase arises, namely, cellular and fibrinous exudation within the gut lumen, and bile-stained to the naked eye. Still later, the mucous membrane is denuded of epithelium, and, the muscularis mucosæ being obscured by infiltration and necrosis, the appearance is that of a few islets of glandular tissue lying in a semi-purulent collection which abuts upon the much altered submucosa. There is, however, no great sloughing of the bowel wall, and the muscle is not laid bare—indeed, it is in a way protected, as shown by a new formation of capillaries in the more superficial layers of the submucosa.

In the specimens from Mrs. T., the regenerative process is in the ascendency, although the condition is still fairly acute. The serous and muscular coats are slightly œdematous, markedly congested, even slightly hæmorrhagic, and consider-ably infiltrated with both polymorphs and mononuclear cells. The submucosa is also œdematous and infiltrated, mononuclear cells, however, predominating. The muscularis mucosæ is definable as the outer limit of a broad zone of young granula-tion tissue which is evidently replacing the now thin layer of purulent exudate within the gut lumen.

A still further advance in the healing process is seen in the sections from Mrs. N. There is, within the lumen, scarcely any purulent exudate, it (and the mucosa) having been replaced by granulation tissue in which the vessels are numerous and well formed, and fibroblastic transformation is well marked. There is less œdema of the tissues than in the two previous cases, and though leucocytic infiltration of all the coats is still great, it is definitely a mononuclear one. Further, there is a notable number of eosinophiles throughout; and a few giant cells are also present in the granulation tissue.

From the acute case (Master W. G.) coliform bacilli were isolated in pure culture from the depths of the affected bowel wall under circumstances which suggest an etiological relationship. They were also demonstrable in suitably stained sections.

A careful search has failed to reveal micro-organisms of any kind in the depths of the other two cases, the ordinary bacterial flora of the gut alone being visible in the most superficial part of the exudates.

The clinical symptoms in all the cases were similar, the characteristic and most striking feature being most violent colic, causing vomiting and occasionally an escape of some blood, also constant mucus from the bowel. The bowel becoming exhausted, or the contents being forced through the rigid portion, the patient then would be at rest, quite comfortable, and cheerful for a time. In the case of the child even ten or twelve hours might elapse between the attacks of pain, which were truly distressing in their intensity. In the young one would naturally suspect intussusception, except that the obstruction was not complete, while the intensity of the pain put a chronic intussusception out of the question. Above the affected portion of the bowel peristalsis could be observed. During a painful attack the inability to retain food and the constant suffering led to steady emaciation. The temperature only occasionally rises during the intervals of pain, and the pulse is quiet. In all the cases one could determine an area of resistance in the colon and sigmoid, naturally giving rise to the supposition that we might have to deal with a diffused and malignant growth. As far as I am aware the prognosis is bad except in cases where the disease is localised, and even there it seems hopeless unless operation be had recourse to. As regards etiology we have obtained no direct clue by histological or pathological examination. The cases give the impression that they are probably tuberculous, and yet from the uniform character of the affection it is evident it is not so, because the affected bowel gives the consistence and smoothness of an eel in a state of *rigor mortis*, and the glands, though enlarged, are evidently not caseous.

In vol. xx of the *Journal of Comparative Pathology and Therapeutics*, M'Fadyen draws attention to Johne's disease, a chronic bacterial enteritis of cattle which was called pseudo-tuberculous, in which the histological course and naked eye appearances are as similar as may be to those we have found in man. The condition was first described by Henny and Frothingham in 1895, since which time numerous observers in various parts of the Continent have noted its course, and M'Fadyen examined six cases found in England in 1911. M'Fadyen, however, describes an acid-fast bacillus similar to but demonstrably not the tubercle bacillus, differing in size and not giving rise to tuberculosis in guinea-pigs. This bacillus is found not only in the tissues, but also on the surface of the mucous membrane which in animals seems to be more affected (presumably because they die earlier) than in man, so that the disease is not so advanced. In my cases the absence of the acid-fast bacillus would suggest a clear distinction, but the histological characters are so similar as to justify a proposition that the diseases may be the same. As far as I know the disease has not been previously described, but it seems probable that many cases must have been seen and been diagnosed as tuberculous, and possibly nothing done for their relief.

With regard to treatment, these cases which have come under observation have pursued their course uninfluenced by dietetic or medicinal treatment, and apparently operation alone can afford relief, and then only if the disease be limited. Five out of the seven made a perfect recovery after the operation. The subject has been for some years one of great interest to me. My friends, the pathologists, prefer to call it "hyperplastic enteritis," and I can only regret that the etiology of the condition remains in obscurity, but I trust that ere long further consideration will clear up the difficulty.

The last specimen I show of this disease I obtained recently from a patient of Dr. Revie, of Kilmarnock, a lady on whom I had performed colostomy on the right side a year previously with the object of arresting the intestinal current to enable us freely to flush the diseased colon. The symptoms were those already described, with an exaggerated degree of pain, and persistent and most painful diarrhœa, with blood and mucus. Distinct improvement followed the colostomy and lavage, though during the year she had on two occasions exacerbations. When seen at the end of the year she had been extremely ill again for one month, and was so evidently losing ground that I advised complete removal of the colon, which, shrunk to its present dimensions, I now show you. The histological character is similar to those found in the previous specimens. The patient has made an uninterrupted recovery so far, and I hope at no distant date to transplant her caput cæcum, which alone was unaffected and was left, on to the rectum.

Adhesions.—Recently considerable attention has been drawn by numerous writers to congenital adhesions and their effects. These are mostly found at the four corners of the abdomen— that at the hepatic flexure being associated with the name of Jackson, at the splenic flexure with Payr, and near the caput, involving the lower end of the ileum, with Lane, while those involving the sigmoid flexure have been recognised for many years. I am also well familiar with adhesions of a somewhat similar character involving the first part of the duodenum and the gall-bladder.

The subject of these adhesions has recently been most excellently considered in a monograph by Gray of Aberdeen, with whose view I am inclined to agree that they are the result of "the excess of physiological fusion," and rarely, if ever, acquired as the result of plastic peritonitis. They differ in character, and are represented by a clearly defined web with a well-arranged circulation, and easily separable from the sub-jacent blood-vessels.

Such bands bind down the intestine, or sling it up at the splenic and hepatic flexures, in some cases profoundly interfering with peristalsis, and the consequent overloading of the bowel causes enteroptosis. In early life these adhesions may give rise to little or no disturbance, but as age advances constipation with, it may be, intercurrent attacks of diarrhœa, lead on the one hand to intestinal indigestion and toxæmia, and on the other to very profound neurosis. Symptoms of toxæmia can be readily recognised by the feeble circulation, somewhat dusky skin, tendency to perspiration, progressive emaciation, dull and restless habits, and, frequently, troublesome headaches and painful joints.

The patient complains of a distended feeling in the abdomen, with colicky pains and borborygmi. Not infrequently there is a sense of obstruction, and often actual visibly distended coils of intestine may be seen. The constipation is troublesome, requiring often large doses of purgatives, and is a condition which may be helped materially by massage. The congestion of the bowel may occasionally lead to a certain amount of bleeding. In the more acute cases the pain is frequently referred to the seat of the adhesions. Not infrequently such cases are mistaken for malignant disease. Indeed, in one week about three years ago I operated on two farmers—one sent me by Dr. Saunders, of Lochmaben, the other by Dr. Reid, of Forth—who presented symptoms so characteristic of malignant disease of the sigmoid, namely, discharge of blood and mucus, swelling and tenderness over the sigmoid, and emaciation, that one had no hesitation in advising operation, when we found in both cases no malignant disease but a tight congenital adhesion band, so anchoring and interfering with the intestine as to give rise to the symptoms complained of. In both cases the correction of the adhesion restored the individuals to the perfect health they now enjoy.

The first case of sigmoid adhesion upon which I operated occurred fourteen years ago, and was that of a merchant from Greenock whose symptoms were those of abdominal neurasthenia, with constant complaint of local pain and persistent constipation. Since then I have frequently operated for adhesions in this region and at the splenic flexure—less frequently at the hepatic flexure. Curiously, I have but rarely seen the adhesions at the end of the ileum, though it may be that the interesting and instructive work of Mr. Lane in drawing particular attention to their presence may lead us to find them more frequently in future.

Acquired adhesions resulting from plastic peritonitis present infinite varieties, not only in their anatomical arrangements, but also in the effect produced in some tuberculous cases. Very extensive adhesions seem to produce a minimum effect, especially in the young, while one slight band may cause immense trouble.

Nine years ago I operated on a patient of Dr. Whiteford, in Greenock. The patient suffered from continual abdominal discomfort, and occasional symptoms of obstruction, these symptoms being relieved, as a rule, by the use of morphia.   We found the whole of the alimentary canal welded into what seemed a solid mass, but from which we were enabled to enucleate the whole length of the small intestine, as if the bowel had worked itself loose whereby it lay like a worm in its burrow.

This mass of fibrous tissue—which embodied the whole of the small intestine, and had resulted from peritonitis due to perforation of a gastric ulcer—was evidently shrinking on the bowel, and mechanically constricting but not interfering with its muscular activity.   The operation gave great relief to the patient, though we had much trouble afterwards with the acquired morphia habit.

There is no doubt that an appreciation of the disordered function and neurosis which may attend the presence of acquired and congenital adhesions will lead to surgical relief, just as in gastric cases surgery has restored to well-being many miserable sufferers.

The following cases illustrate what one may term the "curiosities of adhesions":—

One patient, from Dr. Dobie, of Crieff, came to me with a history suggesting gastric disorder, and generally presenting the features of "habitus enteropticus."

J. S., age about 40 years, a well-developed but poorly-nourished man, complaining of attacks of pain and occasional vomiting, loss of appetite, general weakness, and constipation, his symptoms being increased after exertion.   Occasionally coils of small intestine could be seen.   Observation clearly indicated that the stomach was not at fault, and on operation we found that practically the whole of the small intestine herniated into the lesser sac of the peritoneum, the posterior wall of which, fixed at one part by an adhesion band, had gradually formed a sac which projected into the lesser peritoneal cavity.   The lumen of the neck being about 2 inches in diameter, the intestine could easily be withdrawn; thereafter the orifice was closed by a number of catgut sutures, the result being complete restoration to normal health.

Another interesting and unusual result of adhesions came under observation a few years ago with Dr. Reid, of Forth. The case was that of a lady who had had peritonitis, presumably from old gastric ulceration, leading to adhesions which extended from the posterior abdominal wall to the mesentery of the small intestine. She was thrown from a dog-cart, and a few weeks later developed symptoms of obstruction, found to be due to a hernia of the small intestine through a hole in the mesentery, caused by a tearing at the seat of the adhesion. She made a perfect recovery; but two years later was again thrown from a dog-cart, and within forty-eight hours acute abdominal symptoms supervened, necessitating a laparotomy, when we found the freely movable bowel had torn the mesentery close to the seat of the suture, and again a hernia had formed. In this case, unfortunately, collapse was profound, and although the parts were rapidly restored to position, no reaction took place, and the patient died within a few hours.

Adhesions are also found connecting the gall-bladder with the duodenum, and occasionally with the colon. Such adhesions may lead to kinking of the gall-bladder, and give rise to local pain and attacks of bilious vomiting, simulating early gall-stone suppuration. Separation of such adhesions, and fixation of the gall-bladder by suture, has in three cases completely relieved long-standing troublesome dyspepsia, which was presumed to be due to gall-stones.

Obituary.

HENRY SHERWOOD RANKEN, M.B., Ch.B.

We regret to announce the death, from wounds received in the fighting of 22nd September, of Captain H. S. Ranken, Royal Army Medical Corps. Captain Ranken, who was the son of the Rev. Mr. Ranken, Parish minister of Irvine, was educated at Irvine Academy, of which in 1889 he was the head boy, and thereafter he proceeded to the study of medicine in the University of Glasgow and in Anderson's College. He took the degrees of M.B., Ch.B., in 1905, at the age of 21, after which he spent a year in the Western Infirmary as house physician and house surgeon. He was also for a time Assistant Medical Officer to the Brook Fever Hospital, Metropolitan Asylums Board. In the examination for entrance to the Royal Army Medical Corps, open to the whole Empire, in which he competed about six years ago, he took first place. He was a member of the Sudan Sleeping Sickness Commission, and was sent by the Egyptian Government to the Lado Enclave, Uganda, to study the disease. The results of his investigations are embodied in the reports which, along with Mr. H. G. Plimmer and Captain W. B. Fry, he presented to the Royal Society, and which appeared in its *Proceedings*, 1910-11, under the title of " Reports on the experimental treatment of trypanosomiasis." About a year ago he had the honour of delivering a lecture on the subject to the Royal Society, and thereafter returned to continue his work in Uganda. He was home on furlough at the outbreak of war, and at once offered his services for work at the front. He survived his wounds only a few days, and died on 25th September in a base hospital between Soissons and Rheims, having shown gallantry so distinguished that he was recommended for the Victoria Cross by the officer commanding the 1st Battalion King's Royal Rifles, to which he was attached. Dr. Ranken was universally popular, and many friends will mourn the premature close of a distinguished career.

DAVID M'CRORIE, L.R.C.P. & S.E., L.R.F.P.S.G., Glasgow.

WE regret to announce the death of Mr. David M'Crorie, which took place on 25th September at his residence in Pollokshields. Mr. M'Crorie, who was born in Kilwinning, entered upon the study of medicine at a later age than usual, his former profession having been that of a teacher. After completing his curriculum in the training college he was appointed second master in Henderson Street Public School, and afterwards became headmaster of Laurieston School, near Falkirk. His bent towards medicine, however, induced him to abandon this profession, and he entered upon his new studies in St. Mungo's College. He took the Triple Qualification in 1891, and, obtaining the Foulis Scholarship in 1895, he devoted himself more particularly to the subject of bacteriology, for which purpose he made the journey to Berlin. He was for a time in practice with his brother, Dr. Archibald M'Crorie, but he abandoned practice to give himself to laboratory work. In 1896 he was appointed assistant pathologist to the Glasgow Royal Infirmary, and in 1901 he became bacteriologist to that institution and lecturer on bacteriology at St. Mungo's College, in which positions he did much valuable work. In spite of his devotion to medical subjects, he maintained his interest in education, and was a Fellow of the Educational Institute of Scotland. His published papers, contributed to the *Glasgow Medical Journal* and to the *British Medical Journal*, were concerned with pathological and bacteriological subjects. His death, which occurred at the age of 58, had been preceded by a considerable period of ill-health, for which he had been granted nine months' leave of absence from his duties.

WILLIAM WALKER, M.D.Glasg., Buenos Ayres.

WE regret to announce the death of Dr. William Walker, a graduate of the University of Glasgow, who had for long been settled in South America. Dr. Walker was a native of Kilbirnie, where his father was a medical practitioner for many years. He studied at the University of Glasgow, and took the degree of M.D. in 1863. In 1864 he was house physician and house

surgeon in the Glasgow Royal Infirmary with Dr. Fraser and
Mr. Lister respectively. Shortly afterwards he took a voyage
as ship's surgeon to South America, but just before reaching
Uruguay the boat became a total wreck on the coast during a
violent gale. The sole survivor, "with nothing in the world
but the clothes I had on me," he was rescued by the members of
a small English colony in the vicinity, and became medical
adviser to the few scattered families engaged in cattle-ranching,
for which he ultimately abandoned the medical profession,
amassing a large fortune in his new pursuit. Still mindful of
his native town, he gave to Kilbirnie only last year the sum of
£2,000 for a free site for a public hall. His death, as intimated
by cable, took place at Buenos Ayres on 1st October.

WILLIAM HALDANE, M.D.Glas., F.R.F.P.S., F.R.C.P.E., BRIDGE OF ALLAN.

WE regret to announce the death of Dr. William Haldane, of
Bridge of Allan, which took place at his house after a few days'
illness. Dr. Haldane, who was born in 1847, was a native of
Bridge of Allan, and received his school education in Stirling.
His professional studies were carried out in the Universities of
Edinburgh and Glasgow, and at the latter University he took
the degrees of M.B., C.M., with honours, in 1872, and that of
M.D. in 1876. In 1876 he also became a Fellow of the Faculty
of Physicians and Surgeons of Glasgow, and in 1895 the Royal
College of Physicians of Edinburgh, of which he had become a
member in 1894, honoured him by electing him a Fellow
without examination. After his graduation in 1872 he
became resident surgeon in the Glasgow Royal Infirmary
under the late Sir George Macleod. He was also resident
physician there with the late Sir Thomas M'Call Anderson,
to whom, as Professor of Clinical Medicine, he for a time was
assistant in the University of Glasgow. He also acted as house
surgeon to the Glasgow Lock Hospital.

Dr. Haldane began practice in Braemar. He was soon known
as the first man of the district, and he had the honour of attending the late King Edward there before he ascended the throne.

He removed at a later date to Bridge of Allan, and there acquired a practice which was not limited to the town, but extended throughout the county of Stirling, his services being on all hands required in consultation. He was consulting physician and surgeon to Stirling Royal Infirmary, and was widely known as an authority on climatology and balneology, his numerous contributions to which subjects led to his being appointed Vice-President of the British Balneological and Climatological Society.

Dr. Haldane was as conspicuous in the public affairs of Bridge of Allan and the county of Stirling as he was in medicine. He was a Justice of the Peace for the county; he was chairman of the Bridge of Allan School Board and of its gas and water companies; and he was a member of its Parish Council. At one time, too, he was Surgeon-Major in the local Volunteers. Nor did he neglect the social side of life; and his admirable social qualities brought him the chairmanship of the Edinburgh and Glasgow Club, a position which he was eminently qualified to adorn. He was known, indeed, in so many capacities, and in all of them so much esteemed, that it may truly be said of him that when he died on 18th October he left friends to mourn him throughout the whole of Stirlingshire, and far beyond its borders.

CURRENT TOPICS.

UNIVERSITY OF GLASGOW: GRADUATION IN MEDICINE.—A graduation ceremony was held at Glasgow University on 8th October, when degrees were conferred on over fifty graduates in Medicine and Science. Professor Noël Paton, Dean of the Faculty of Medicine, presented the medical graduates for the capping ceremony, and Professor Graham Kerr presented the science graduates. The ceremony was performed by the Vice-Chancellor, Sir Donald MacAlister, K.C.B., who intimated that Mr. James William Moffatt had gained the Brunton Memorial Prize of £10 awarded to the most distinguished graduate in Medicine of the year. On the close of the ceremony, the Vice-Chancellor asked the audience to stand and sing a verse of the National Anthem on that special occasion. This was done with great heartiness. The following is the list of the medical degrees conferred:—

BACHELORS OF MEDICINE AND BACHELORS OF SURGERY
(M.B., Ch.B.)

I. WITH HONOURS.

James William Moffatt.

II. WITH COMMENDATION.

John Bowes M'Dougall.	Alexander Hislop Hall.
Dagmar Florence Curjel.	Donald M'Intyre.

III. ORDINARY DEGREES.

Grace Gillies Turnbull Anderson.	Walter Thompson Currie.
Andrew Duffield Blakely.	Fritz Vivian Daeblitz.
Abraham Blashky.	John Nairn Dobbie.
Maurice Smith Bryce.	Alexander Moffat Dunlop.
John Cameron.	Dugald Ferguson.
James Campbell.	Thomas Ferguson.
Robert Clark, M.A.	James Bryan Fotheringham.
Andrew Climie.	Walter Weir Galbraith.
Agnes Elizabeth Mary Cooke.	John Aitken Gilfillan.
James Paterson Crawford.	Ethel Winifred Gompertz.
Thomas Muir Crawford.	Peter Gordon.
William Cullen.	Joseph Graham.

David Cochrane Hanson.
Joseph Welsh Park Harkness, M.A.
Hugh Douglas M'Crossan.
Kenneth Norman MacLean, M.A.
William Martin.
Gladys Montgomery.
Laurence Sebastian Morgan.
Hugh Quigley.
Frederick Powlett Rankin, B.Sc.
Adam Rankine.
Robert Ray.

Thomas Forbes Brown Reid.
James Gordon M'Gregor Robertson.
John Kenneth Smith.
Edward Napier Thomson.
James Walker.
William Herbert Nairne White.
Marguerite Wilson.
John Wylie.
Gavin Young.
John Miller Young.
Isabella Henrietta Younger.

APPOINTMENTS.—The following appointments have recently been made:—

John Alexander, M.D.Aber., to be Consulting Physician to Belvidere Fever Hospital.

A. W. Harrington, M.D.Glasg. (M.B., 1900), F.R.F.P.S., to be Consulting Physician to Ruchill Fever Hospital.

David Macdonald, M.D.Glasg. (M.B., 1906), to be Consulting Physician to Ruchill Fever Hospital.

Adam Patrick, M.A., M.B., Ch.B.Glasg. (1908), to be Consulting Physician to Belvidere Fever Hospital.

James Russell, M.B., Ch.B.Glasg. (1902), F.R.C.S.E., to be Assistant Surgeon to Victoria Infirmary, Glasgow.

Indian Medical Service (gazetted 22d September): Captain J. Forrest, M.B., Ch.B.Glasg. (1901), to be Major.

Royal Army Medical Corps (23rd September): To be Lieutenant on probation—W. F. Wood, M.B., Ch.B.Glasg. (1912). Granted the temporary rank of Lieutenant—J. M. Renton, M.B., Ch.B.Glasg. (1905), F.R.C.S.E.; J. M'I. Morgan, M.B., Ch.B.Glasg. (1909); R. R. K. Paton, M.B., Ch.B.Glasg. (1910).

25th September: Granted the temporary rank of Lieutenant —D. Y. Buchanan, M.B., Ch.B.Glasg. (1909); M. M. Rodger, M.D.Glasg. (M.B., 1907); J. F. Smith, M.B., Ch.B.Glasg. (1911); A. Currie, M.B., Ch.B.Glasg. (1901); A. Lindsay, M.B., Ch.B.Glasg. (1913).

Royal Regiment of Artillery, R.A.M.C.: To be Lieutenants on probation—K. D. Murchison, M.B., Ch.B.Glasg. (1912); J. C. Pyper, M.B., Ch.B.Glasg. (1912).

Royal Army Medical Corps (29th September): Granted the

temporary rank of Lieutenant—W. Rankin, M.B., Ch.B.Glasg. (1904); H. F. Warwick, M.B., Ch.B.Glasg. (1904).

Royal Army Medical Corps, Territorial Force (attached to other than medical units): Lieutenant Eric D. Gairdner, M.B., Ch.B. (1902), to be Captain.

Royal Army Medical Corps (2d October): The undermentioned officers of the Home Hospital Reserve to be temporary Captains (at Maryhill)—A. T. Campbell, M.B., C.M.Glasg. (1886); J. G. M'Coll, L.R.C.P. & S.E., L.R.F.P.S.G. (1894); W. Westwood Fyfe, M.D.Glas. (M.B., 1893). To be Lieutenant on probation— Norman Cameron, M.B., Ch.B.Glasg. (1912).

5th October: To be Lieutenants on probation—R. P. A. Kirkland, M.B., Ch.B.Glasg. (1912); J. E. Black, M.B., Ch.B.Glasg. (1911).

6th October: To be temporary Lieutenants—K. C. Middlemiss, M.B., Ch.B.Glasg. (1908); J. L. R. Philip, M.B., Ch.B.Glasg. (1913).

8th October: To be temporary Lieutenant—W. Macewen, M.B., Ch.B.Glasg. (1910).

13th October: To be temporary Lieutenant—M. A. Macdonald, M.B., Ch.B.Glasg. (1910).

15th October: To be temporary Lieutenants—J. S. K. Boyd, M.B., Ch.B.Glasg. (1913); D. M. Borland, M.B., Ch.B.Glasg. (1909); R. M. Hill, M.B., Ch.B.Glasg. (1906); H. L. Neil, M.B., Ch.B.Glasg. (1911); J. J. Sinclair, M.B., Ch.B.Glasg. (1909); W. R. Snodgrass, M.B., Ch.B.Glasg. (1913).

THE "BRITISH PHARMACOPŒIA."—Advance copies of the *British Pharmacopœia,1914,*the publication of which was delayed. by the outbreak of war, are now accessible to the public for inspection, and may be consulted at the offices of the General Medical Council in London, Edinburgh, and Dublin, from 10 A.M. to 4 P.M. daily. The official publication of the work, of which a review will be found upon another page, will be made by notices in the *Gazettes* on Thursday, 31st December, 1914, on which day copies will be on sale at the price of 10s. 6d. net.

MEDICAL SOCIETIES OF GLASGOW.—The following gentlemen have been elected office-bearers of the various medical societies of Glasgow for the session 1914-1915 :—

MEDICO-CHIRURGICAL SOCIETY.

President,	. . . . . .	Mr. A. Ernest Maylard.
Vice-Presidents,	. . . . .	{ Dr. W. F. Gibb. Dr. Douglas W. Russell.

Council.

Section of Medicine.	Section of Pathology.
Dr. Frank J. Charteris.	Dr. J. Shaw Dunn.
Dr. J. S. M'Kendrick.	Dr. J. Arch. Campbell.
Dr. G. Morris Crawford.	Dr. A. M. Kennedy.
Dr. Leonard Findlay.	Dr. John Anderson.
Section of Surgery.	**Section of Obstetrics.**
Dr. Thos. Kay.	Dr. G. Balfour Marshall.
Dr. Duncan Macartney.	Dr. J. Nigel Stark.
Dr. J. Ewing Hunter.	Dr. Peter M'Bryde.
Dr. Wm. Rankin.	Dr. R. D. Hodge.

Treasurer,	. . . . .	Dr. James H. Martin.
Editorial Secretary,	. . . .	Dr. Robert Speirs Fullarton.
General Secretary,	. . . .	Dr. Archibald Young.

OBSTETRICAL AND GYNÆCOLOGICAL SOCIETY.

Owing to the dislocation of work caused by the war, to the additional work which it has thrown on many shoulders, and to the absence on active service of many members of the profession, the office-bearers of the Obstetrical and Gynæcological Society for the session 1914-15 have not yet been elected. No meetings of the Society for the transaction of public business will be held before the New Year—if, indeed, such meetings are to be held at all this session. But a meeting for the election of office-bearers is to be held at an early date, and a list of those elected will appear in a future issue of the *Journal.*

SOUTHERN MEDICAL SOCIETY.

Hon. President,	. . . . .	Dr. Eben. Duncan.
President,	. . . . .	Dr. David Lamb.
Vice-Presidents,	. . . . .	{ Dr. Arch. M'Crorie. Dr Jas. R. Drever.
Secretary,	. . . . .	Dr. Jas. Russell.
Editorial Secretary,	. . . .	Dr. Robert Adam.
Treasurer,	. . . . .	Dr. W. H. Manson.
Seal Keeper,	. . . . .	Dr. R. N. Dunlop.

Extra Members of Council.

Dr. Aitken.
Dr. Stewart.
Dr. Graham.

Dr. M'Donald.
Dr. Paton.

Court Medical.

Dr. Yuill Anderson.
Dr. A. Miller.

Dr. Peden.
Dr. Robertson.

EASTERN MEDICAL SOCIETY.

President, ...	Dr. Joseph Green.
Past President, ...	Dr. David Glen.
Vice-President, ...	Dr. Alex. Johnstone.
Secretary, ...	Dr. Hugh A. M'Lean.
Reporting Secretary, ...	Dr. A. P. Granger.
Treasurer, ...	Dr. J. Wallace Anderson.
Seal Keeper, ...	Dr. J. W. Turner.
Auditors, ...	{ Dr. H. M. Wilson. / Dr. W. H. M'Walter. }

Council.

Dr. J. Miller Semple.
Dr. J. W. Mathie.
Dr. Thos. Russell.

Dr. W. H. Brown.
Dr. Neil Keith.
Dr. John P. Granger.

NORTHERN MEDICAL SOCIETY.

President, ...	Dr. Alex. Dickson.
Past President, ...	Dr. James B. Miller.
Vice-Presidents, ...	{ Dr. Lewis MacLachlan. / Dr. J. Horne. }
Treasurer, ...	Dr. James H. Martin.
Secretary, ...	Dr. Charles Bennett.
Reporting Secretary, ...	Dr. R. D. Hodge.
Seal Keeper, ...	Dr. Arthur M. Crawford.
Auditors, ...	{ Dr. John Baird. / Dr. Malcolm Campbell. }

Council.

Dr. A. J. Ballantyne.
Dr. Stanley Richmond.
Dr. R. G. Inglis.
Dr. R. Langmuir.
Dr. J. A. C. Macewen.
Dr. John Ritchie.

Dr. A. T. Campbell.
Dr. J. Gray.
Dr. Jas. Todd.
Dr. J. G. Connal.
Dr. Robert Grieve.
Dr. T. D. Waddell.

PARTICK AND DISTRICT MEDICAL SOCIETY.

President, ...	
Vice-Presidents, ...	{ DR. FARQUHAR GRACIE. / DR. W. S. PATERSON.
Treasurer, ...	DR. T. DOUGLAS BROWN.
Secretary, ...	DR. EDWARD J. PRIMROSE.
Recording Secretary, ...	DR. JAMES GIRDWOOD.

Council.

DR. J. HAMILTON CAMPBELL.	DR. JOHN MORTON.
DR. J. GIBSON GRAHAM.	DR. E. J. HENRY.
DR. JAMES WYLIE.	DR. W. H. KIRK.
DR. A. E. WARD.	DR. JAMES SCOTT.

MEDICO-CHIRURGICAL SOCIETY OF GLASGOW.—The following circular has been issued by the Council to members of the Medico-Chirurgical Society :—

" At a meeting of the Council of the Society, held on Friday, 25th September, it was resolved unanimously that the general disturbance of professional activities arising out of the European War crisis made it inexpedient to attempt, for the present, to carry on the ordinary work of the session.

" Apart from the fact that many of the members, and some of the office-bearers, of the Society are already on active service, while others may be called upon at an early date, it is certain that, for some considerable time, the war, and events directly or indirectly connected therewith, must form an all-engrossing preoccupation.

" Recognising this, the Council have decided to delay the opening of the session, at least until January.

"The members of Council earnestly hope that this suspension of the Society's activity may not be prolonged further than the date presently contemplated.

" Due notice will be given when meetings will be resumed."

ROYAL HOSPITAL FOR SICK CHILDREN, GLASGOW. — The following statement, received too late for insertion in our October issue, gives an account of the educational facilities afforded to students by the Royal Hospital for Sick Children :—

Hospital (Yorkhill), 206 cots. Visiting physicians and surgeons attend 9.15 A.M. daily.

Dispensary or Out-patient Department. Over 12,000 cases treated annually. Physicians and surgeons attend 11.30 A.M.

Country Branch Hospital (Drumchapel, Dumbartonshire), 26 cots.

For the clinical instruction of students the year will be divided into three terms. A special course of lectures and clinical instruction on the medical and surgical diseases of children (meeting the requirements of the Medical Ordinance) will be given in each of said terms. The class will meet daily at 11 A.M., and will consist of 15 medical and 15 surgical meetings.

Students attending the hospital in their third year of clinical study will be given every opportunity of taking part in the regular clinical work in the wards under the supervision of the visiting physicians and surgeons.

Hospital fee (admitting to hospital and dispensary for purpose of clinical instruction, and attending said special course, &c.), for one term, £1, 1s.; or for whole year, £2, 2s.; fee for clinical instruction and said special course for one term, £1, 15s. Fees are payable to, and further information may be obtained from, the Medical Superintendent, The Hospital, Yorkhill.

ARRANGEMENTS FOR DOING THE WORK OF DOCTORS SERVING WITH THE FORCES.—The Local Medical and Panel Committees for the Burgh of Glasgow have adopted the scheme outlined below for dealing with the work of doctors who are on active service. It is to be understood that the Committees have no wish to interfere with whatever private arrangements may have been made, but are anxious, in every possible way, to assist, and to conserve the interests of, colleagues who have gone, or who may contemplate going on service.

1. A list of doctors volunteering to act for absent doctors is to be drawn up.

2. Insured persons to be transferred temporarily to the "volunteers" in blocks, to be held in trust for the absent doctor, and restored to him on his return.

3. Payment to be made at the rate of 9d. *per caput* per quarter.

4. All records to be kept in the ordinary way.

5. Every reasonable effort to be made by doctors to

discourage permanent transference of patients from lists of absent doctors.

6. Arrangements for temporary transference and for adjustment of Insurance accounts to be made by the Clerk to the Insurance Committee, who has agreed to do so.

7. For private work, doctors are advised to make their own arrangements, wherever possible.

8. If arranged through the Committees, payment to be half the fees received, including midwifery.

9. Accounts to be rendered on the absent doctor's forms, either by the substitute or by the doctor's representative, as may be arranged.

10. Visits and consultations to be distributed among the "volunteers" by the doctor's representative strictly in rotation, as far as possible, bearing in mind geographical convenience; or a list of the volunteers may be given to the patient, who may then exercise a choice.

11. Some steps should be taken by the absent doctor's representatives to inform patients by circular, or notice displayed in the consulting rooms, or otherwise, that the work is being done, so as to prevent patients drifting.

Those who are willing to volunteer under the above scheme should notify the Secretary, Dr. James R. Drever, as soon as possible, and indicate which class of work they are willing to do, viz.—(*a*) Insurance work; (*b*) all private work; (*c*) private work, exclusive of midwifery.

It will be a convenience if they will indicate also whether they wish the work for which they volunteer to be confined to a particular district.

NATIONAL INSURANCE: EXPENDITURE ON MEDICINES IN SCOTLAND. — A memorandum regarding expenditure on medicines and appliances has been issued by the Scottish National Insurance Commissioners. The Commission, with a view of ascertaining the causes which underlay the varying experiences of insurance areas, obtained the services of Mr. J. F. Tocher, D.Sc., F.I.C., Aberdeen University, to inquire and report as to the prescribing and dispensing of medicines under the insurance scheme. A careful scrutiny was made by Mr. Tocher of 156,424 prescriptions selected from burgh and county areas, out of 3,018,598, the total prescriptions for 1913, with respect to the character and quality of the drugs ordered for the insured. It was found that insurance practitioners throughout Scotland had, as a rule, selected the most modern drugs and those of best repute, denying to their insured patients no medicines usually available in private practice. There were, however, wide differences between the drug accounts of different committees, which seasonal variations could not account for. Nor could these differences be wholly ascribed to local circumstances affecting the incidence of sickness in one area as compared with another. Prescription frequency was one of the respects in which methods of prescribing revealed variety. High prescription frequency, where it was known to exist, might usefully form the subject of a conference between the insurance and panel committees. A similar difference was found to obtain as regards the price of prescriptions. In several areas an investigation was made with a view of discovering whether high charges against the drug fund, in so far as due to prescribing customs, were the result of methods followed in the area by the practitioners as a whole, or were due to the procedure of a section of the profession, or of individual practitioners. In the view of the Commissioner's reporter, it was a minority of the profession in any area who ran up a drug bill beyond the expected limits, but startling examples of extravagant prescribing were nevertheless adduced.

As the legitimate claims upon the drug fund of a committee might from time to time be high owing to the price of certain indispensable remedies, it appeared to the Commission to be matter for regret that any portion of the fund should be consumed in defraying the cost of prescriptions which were excessive in quantity or which included preparations whose action, if any, was mainly nutritive. Waste, under such conditions, would appear to be almost inevitable and the risk of misappropriation great.

Certain drugs and medicinal substances were relatively cheap, while others were comparatively costly. Expense by itself should never be a bar to the supply of a drug under national insurance, but, in order that the insured person might receive proper and sufficient medicines, restrictions must be imposed on improper or excessive prescribing. Suggestions were made in the memorandum as to how insurance and panel committees might act in the matter. After pointing out that repeat prescriptions often tend to carelessness or excess, the memorandum stated that if any committee after consideration were to resolve that repeat orders, bearing such words only as "repeat," "repeat mixture," or their equivalents, and showing no prescription written out in due form, should not be paid for if dispensed by chemists, the Commission would raise no objection. Unscheduled appliances had been ordered, but if supplied these should not be paid for by an insurance committee. Consideration of the prescriptions investigated indicated a certain amount of overlapping between medical and sanatorium benefits. The result was that the drug fund would be called upon to bear a burden from which it should be immune, and the general tendency to shortage would be accentuated.

One consequence of the state of war now existing in Europe had been to produce in this country a shortage in the supply of certain drugs and prescribed appliances. In the case of some preparations it was probable that no further consignments could be obtained from Continental firms until the termination of hostilities; in the case of others it might be possible to procure quantities from sources not hitherto drawn upon. The duration of shortage would vary with different substances, to an extent which it was not possible at this juncture to foresee. The question at issue with regard to the use of such articles was not wholly or mainly one of price. Nor was it one which solely affected the insurance medical service. Apart from these considerations, it was essential at present that all existing stocks of remedies for disease should, as far as possible, be husbanded by reserving drugs in which there was a shortage for cases to whose treatment they were indispensable, and endeavouring to provide for the needs of others by other remedies of similar action.

HEALTH OF THE ARMY.—The War Office has issued the following through the Press Bureau :—

The Director-General of the Army Medical Service reports a highly satisfactory state of health of the Armies camped, billeted, or quartered in the various commands at home. Nowhere is there any undue prevalence of preventable disease, and the massing of large numbers of men in the military and other stations under difficult conditions has not been accompanied by any untoward results.

Concerning the health of the Expeditionary Force, the Director-General reports an equally satisfactory state of affairs. He is satisfied that the utmost vigilance is being exerted to maintain the present position. To ensure still greater security Lord Kitchener has decided to establish at the War Office a Sanitary Committee, consisting of military and civilian members, to advise him on all matters affecting the health and well-being of troops at home and abroad.

He is also sending the Director-General, Sir Arthur Sloggett, overseas to make a thorough inspection of the medical arrangements and co-ordinate the work of the Army Medical Services with the St. John Ambulance and Red Cross societies, of which he will be Chief Commissioner. Sir Arthur Sloggett will be accompanied by Colonel Burtchaell, Royal Army Medical Corps, as staff officer. During his absence at the seat of war Sir Alfred Keogh will act as Director-General at the War Office.

THE SICK AND WOUNDED: HOME HOSPITAL ARRANGEMENTS.— The following statement, showing how the sick and wounded of the Expeditionary Force are being received and distributed after their arrival in this country, was issued by the Press Bureau at the end of September:—

All the hospital ships proceed to Southampton, where there is a special staff for the reception and distribution of the sick and wounded officers and men who are being sent home on them. The arrangements are under the control of a Surgeon-General, who holds the appointment of a deputy-director of medical services. He has at his command 12 ambulance trains specially constructed for the conveyance of 4 officers and 96 men lying down, or for a considerably greater number of patients sitting up. Twice weekly telegrams are received by him from all the larger military and Territorial Force general hospitals stating the number of beds vacant in each. With this information before him he arranges convoys of sick and wounded on arrival, and dispatches them to their destination in one or more of the ambulance trains.

Already the sick and wounded from overseas have been comfortably placed under treatment in most of the large military or Territorial Force hospital centres. At the railway stations of these localities arrangements are made by the military authorities for conveying sick and wounded in motor or other ambulance vehicles from the railway stations to the hospitals. Voluntary Aid Detachments have already done useful work in connection with this stage of the movements of the sick and wounded, and it is expected that the scope for utilising voluntary aid in this direction will be extended as its value becomes better known.

As the military hospitals get filled up arrangements have been made for transferring sick and wounded from them to various hospitals arranged by voluntary effort. Many schemes have been submitted to the War Office, through the British Red Cross Association, in accordance with Field Service Regulations. At present the opportunity of using private hospitals to any great extent has not arisen, as there are still several thousand beds vacant in the military and Territorial Force hospitals. There is no doubt, however, that in time private hospitals will be of much use as an overflow and also when it is necessary to set free a sufficient number of beds for future requirements in the larger military hospitals.

When sick and wounded are sufficiently convalescent to be granted sick furlough advantage is being taken of the many offers of accommodation for them in convalescent homes in different parts of the country; and, in order to prevent overlapping and to facilitate the means of placing men on sick furlough, so far as possible, in their own counties, a Central Registry of Convalescent Homes has been formed by a joint committee of the British Red Cross Society and the Soldiers' and Sailors' Help Society. This central registry acts as a clearing-house. Only convalescents who would be given sick furlough to their own homes, if they so desired, are being sent to convalescent homes. Convalescents who require continued hospital treatment will be sent either to the special home in connection with the hospital from which they are transferred (under the supervision of the medical officer of the hospital) or to one or other of the private hospitals already referred to.

In order to enable a convalescent to be placed on sick furlough in a convalescent home all that he has to do is to inform the medical officer who is in charge of him where and what county or neighbourhood he would like to proceed to. These particulars are entered on a form and sent to the central registry. The address of the nearest railway station to the convalescent home in the neighbourhood is entered on the form, and it is immediately returned to the medical officer of the hospital. Whenever the convalescent is ready to leave on sick furlough the medical officer sends word to the convalescent home, stating the hour of the man's arrival at the railway station, where arrangements are made to meet and take him over. This arrangement has been working very well, and already over 100 convalescents have been received in various convalescent homes.

It may also be of interest to know that in all the hospitals arrangements are made for replenishing any deficiencies in the men's kits and for giving them any additional clothing which it may be desirable for them to take with them when they go on sick furlough. The hospitals are, for this purpose, receiving many generous gifts of pyjama suits and other articles of clothing.

At the end of their sick furlough the men are required to rejoin the depôts of their regiments in order to be refitted, until arrangements are made for their rejoining their units, either in this country or abroad. They are provided with railway warrants to enable them to go to convalescent homes and to rejoin at their depôts. Arrangements have also been made that they shall receive their pay both while they are in hospital and while they are convalescent.

SCOTTISH RED CROSS HOSPITAL.—The staff of the Scottish Section of the British Red Cross Hospital was entertained to tea in the City Chambers on 30th September before its departure for France. Its medical officers are Messrs J. W. Struthers, M.B., Ch.B.Ed., F.R.C.S.E.; J. A. G. Burton, M.B., Ch.B.Glasg., D.P.H.Cantab.; and A. U. Webster, M.B., Ch.B.Aber. Five of its nine orderlies are medical students, and there are nine nurses under the charge of Miss Katherine Young as matron. The Lord Provost, who presided over the meeting, was accompanied to the platform by the Duchess of Montrose, Lady Stirling Maxwell, Sir George T. Beatson, and Mr. R. D. M'Ewan. Interesting speeches were delivered, and the staff left in the evening for France.

It was originally intended that the site of the hospital should be Rouen, and at the time of departure it was understood that Rouen was its destination; but, owing to the improved military situation, the site was fixed in Paris, where the hospital is established on the second floor of the Hotel Astoria, in which its staff is fully occupied. Rouen, however, remains the base for supplies, which are shipped from Glasgow by Messrs J. & P. Hutchinson's steamers. Of the 50 beds practically all are endowed, and have been named in accordance with the wishes of those who have endowed them.

Of the motor ambulance waggons required for the Mobile Field Hospital in France the first batch of seven, five of which were Argyll cars and two Wolseleys, were despatched by boat on 15th October. The cost of six of them had early been guaranteed by generous donors, and on 13th October at a largely attended meeting of the Scottish Automobile Club in their rooms in Blythswood Square, Glasgow, an appeal for £20,000 to provide a fleet of motor ambulances was made to Scottish motorists and others interested. Sir J. H. A. Macdonald, who presided, strongly commended the appeal. Sir George T. Beatson, chairman of the Scottish Branch of the British Red Cross Society, who followed him, gave a detailed explanation of the methods of transport and of removing the wounded from the fighting line to the general hospitals. The increase of impedimenta in modern warfare had made the transport question one of the chief problems of a campaign. For the general supply of food, ammunition, medical stores, &c., to an army there were three zones of operations. The first started from the reserve depôt and base supply and went up to the railhead; from there another zone went forward to what was called the refilling point; and then there was the zone of the fighting line. In each zone a different vehicle of transport had to be employed. In the present war stores were taken up by rail to the railhead; motor vehicles conveyed them thence to the refilling point, and the remaining journey was made by horse transport belonging to the different units in the fighting line. The next point which required to be explained was the medical assistance to the wounded. Immediately behind the fighting line were the regimental bearers (two men per company) and the medical officers with a supply of small panniers on the back of a mule

or pony.   Their duty was to give immediate assistance in cases
of hæmorrhage, &c., and to direct the wounded to the collecting
zone, where they got into touch with the field ambulances,
which were divided into a bearer division and a tent division.
When the field ambulances had done their work they had to get
rid of the wounded in order to move on with the fighting units,
and accordingly they formed a clearing hospital to which the
wounded might be brought down by the field ambulances
themselves, or in carts or in vehicles belonging to the supply
column.   From the clearing hospital the wounded were taken to
the railhead station and then conveyed to the general hospital.
The whole of these operations took place within three zones—
the collecting zone, the evacuating zone, and the distributing
zone, which had its base hospital in the case of the present war
at Southampton, the men being brought across the Channel in a
hospital ship.

The principle underlying the general transport arrangement
of an army was that each department must adapt itself to the
general system, and undoubtedly the medical arrangements for
bringing down the wounded could be assisted by utilising the
supply waggons which returned empty after they had discharged
their contents.   These arrangements, however, had broken down,
not from any fault of the authorities but simply as the result of
the war.   The railways had been more or less destroyed, and the
main roads by which the wounded would have been brought
down had been done away with.   He had been told that between
Laon and Paris about 170 bridges had been destroyed.   In
consequence of that the only way to bring the wounded from
the clearing hospital to Paris as quickly as possible was by
motor ambulance.   A great many had been brought down in the
supply waggons—men lying on stretchers on the top of straw in
trucks which were probably open and not very comfortable.
Many of them had spent two or three days in these trucks,
having to be removed from one train to another at places where
bridges had been destroyed.   That entailed very great suffering.
If therefore they could provide a supply of motor ambulances that
could go from Paris to wherever the clearing hospital was situated,
they would be doing a very great service in giving the wounded
a better chance.   There was another very important point.   Men
were dying from lockjaw owing to the tetanus microbe, which

flourished in rich soil, getting into their wounds and being allowed to remain there too long without treatment. If the wounds were quickly cleaned and if an injection of anti-tetanic serum could be given they might prevent a good many deaths. The Scottish Branch of the Red Cross Society had sent to France a unit consisting of three doctors, ten nurses, six medical students, and three general orderlies. They had been located in Paris, but owing to a difficulty with regard to a hotel they would probably make their headquarters at Chantilly, which, however, would be advantageous, as the distance to Braine, where the clearing hospital was to be placed, was much less than the distance from Braine to Paris. They had sent out at present only 50 beds; but he hoped that contributions would enable them to increase the hospital to 100 beds. If they had a good fleet of motor ambulances it would make a very great difference to the wounded and be a material help to the general system of evacuation. The principle underlying all medical assistance in time of war was to evacuate as quickly as possible down to the rear. Sir Alfred Keogh, head of the Medical Service, had informed him last week in London that what was wanted now was money in the shape of motor ambulances. With that authority to support them they would not go wrong, and if the motorists in Scotland could raise the money for these ambulances they would be giving the best gift they could make to the country.

Lord Newlands moved a resolution commending the scheme of the Red Cross Society, and in his own name and that of Lady Newlands presented the Automobile Club with a motor ambulance to be sent to the front. Sir John Ure Primrose seconded the resolution, and Mr. R. J. Smith, convener of the Transport Committee, stated that within a week they had received promises of twelve motor ambulances, which were now being got ready. The meeting separated after the formation of an influential committee to promote the object of the fund, and after the intimation, made by Mr. Inglis Ker, that subscriptions amounting to over £1,500 had already been received.

Mr. J. A. G. Burton, the representative of Glasgow on the staff of the Scottish Hospital, is a graduate of Glasgow University, where he took the degrees of M.B., Ch.B., in 1909. He has relinquished the post of Assistant Pathologist to Glasgow Royal Infirmary in order to go to the front.

Scottish Red Cross Society.—The Scottish Branch of the British Red Cross Society has issued an interesting account of the work it has been enabled to undertake since it appealed to the public for support. It recalls that on 19th August there appeared in the columns of the *Glasgow Herald* a letter from the Duchess of Montrose regarding the Scottish Branch of the British Red Cross Society and a communication headed "Advice to Helpers," in which information was given as to the organisation of the Scottish Branch. Since that date the demands which have been made on the Society in consequence of the development of the European War have been steady and various. The Scottish Section of the British Red Cross Hospital in France, and the motor ambulance units for service between the fighting line and the base hospitals, could not have been equipped, and cannot be maintained, without the aid of the committees and workers of the Scottish Branch, entrusted with the supervision of work parties, the co-ordination of stores and the arrangement and despatch of materials. These departments of the Scottish Branch have been steadily at work for two months, and during that period have despatched over 35,000 gifts in kind, clothing, and medical comforts to the Navy, to our Army in France, to Belgium, and to Serbia. The centre from which the work of these departments is controlled is situated at St. Andrew's Hall, Glasgow. The Headquarters Organising Clothing Committee, of which the Duchess of Montrose is president, and Mrs. Charles Cree convener, acts as a clearing house for the gifts in kind, deals with inquiries from workers, and keeps in touch with the district stores. Scotland is divided into four districts, with centres in Glasgow, Edinburgh, Aberdeen, and Dundee, and from these centres lists of the stocks available for despatch are supplied to the Headquarters Organising Clothing Committee from time to time. In this way a local demand on one centre can be supplied either from the central stores or from another centre if necessary, and the Organising Committee in turn can draw on the district stores when material is required for despatch to the Continent or to the Fleet.

The offices of the Society at St. Andrew's Hall are also used by the Western District Committee, which deals with gifts in kind from Glasgow and the Western Counties. Gifts from the city of Glasgow are dealt with by Lady Stirling Maxwell, while

Mrs. Charles Cree deals with those from the Western Counties. The Countess of Eglinton's Gifts in Kind Committee is situated at 216 Bothwell Street, Glasgow. At St. Andrew's Halls, Glasgow, is also situated the office of Colonel R. D. M'Ewan, the commissioner for the western district, who in addition to his work as commissioner has undertaken the purchase and despatch of stores and work in connection with the voluntary aid detachments. In the management of the stores Mrs. Kennedy, convener, is assisted by skilled labour. Whenever they are received articles of clothing are sorted out, washed where necessary, measured, and packed in labelled packages, which are available for despatch at a moment's notice. Articles range from triangular bandages to British Red Cross kit bags.

In addition to the committees to which reference has already been made, the St. Andrew's Hall is also the headquarters of the Red Cross Visiting Committee, of which Mrs. Charles Walker is the convener. The six members of this committee attend at Stobhill Hospital and place the resources of the Red Cross Society at the disposal of the patients. Similar committees are at work or in course of formation in Edinburgh, Aberdeen, and Dundee.

A visit to the offices and stores at St. Andrew's Hall, Glasgow, or to the stores at Edinburgh, Aberdeen, and Dundee will satisfy even the most critical observer that the administration of the Scottish Red Cross funds is being carried out in a businesslike manner, and that in this work the nation is indebted to the ladies, who have generously placed their personal services at the disposal of the Society from 10 to 6 daily and from 10 to 1 on Saturdays.

GLASGOW DISTRICT MENTAL HOSPITAL, GARTLOCH.—Dr. W. A. Parker, in his seventeenth annual report of the Glasgow District Mental Hospital at Gartloch, states that on 15th May last there were on the register 774 persons—407 men and 367 women—this being an increase of 21 on the whole population compared with the same date in 1913. Cases admitted during the year numbered 263, and 242 were discharged or died. There were 1016 cases under care during the year, and the average daily number of patients resident during the year was 774·2. The character of the admissions from the point of view of probable recovery was again very poor this year. Only 28·8 per cent of the admissions were first attacks of under one year's duration, and no less than 67·67 per cent were hopelessly incurable cases of chronic delusional insanity, senile and organic dements, general paralytics, epileptic insanity, and cases of congenital defect. The percentage of patients admitted above 50 years of age was higher than ever before, being 36·1 of the admissions. The recovery-rate, calculated on 263 admissions, was 35·3 per cent, the male recovery-rate being 32 per cent and the females having a recovery-rate of 38·6 per cent. The Scottish average recovery-rate for the last four years, excluding private cases, was 37·8 per cent. The deaths amounted to 76, being 9·8 per cent calculated on the average number in residence. Fourteen deaths were due to general paralysis of the insane, 12 to senile decay, 11 to cerebral hæmorrhages and softenings, 13 to diseases of the heart, 10 to lung disease other than tubercle, and 3 to tubercle.

The abuse of alcohol still headed the list of causes of insanity in the admissions. In 49 cases alcohol was put down as the determining cause of insanity, and in combination with syphilis or lactation in other 10 cases, or 59 in all, making 22·4 per cent of the admissions. To senility and adolescence were ascribed 28 and 24 cases respectively. Syphilis alone or in combination with alcohol was responsible for at least 23 cases, while cerebral hæmorrhage or softenings and bodily illness, non-syphilitic, were responsible for other 43 cases. Of the cases admitted 168 were tested for syphilis by the Wassermann reaction, and of these 38 gave a positive and 130 a negative result. As usual, the influence of alcohol as an indirect cause of insanity was very striking. Of the admissions the cases in which a history of the abuse or non-abuse of alcohol by their parents was obtained gave a percentage of parental abuse of alcohol of 51·6 per cent; but when these cases were separated into two groups, namely, those who were above and those who were not above the age of 26 on their first attack of mental illness, a history of parental abuse of alcohol was found in 80·6 per cent of those whose first breakdown took place before they had completed 26 years of age, while of those whose first breakdown took place above the age of 26, there was a history of parental abuse in only 36·6 per cent.

HEALTH OF RENFREWSHIRE.—At a meeting of Renfrew
County Council, held in Paisley on 8th October, Sir Charles B.
Renshaw, Bart., presiding, Dr. A. Campbell Munro submitted
an interesting report with regard to the treatment of tuberculosis in the county. He stated that the new phthisis
pavilion at the Johnstone Hospital was now practically in a
condition fit for the reception of patients, and it would add
16 beds to the accommodation at their disposal. The Darnley
Hospital Committee had, in compliance with the request of the
Council to have a pavilion at Darnley, not presently required,
placed one at their disposal for the accommodation of pulmonary
tuberculosis cases. The pavilion was licensed for the accommodation of 25 patients, and the charge would be 30s. per
week for each patient. With these 41 beds the accommodation
at their disposal was doubled. The County Council was thus in
a position to undertake the hospital and sanatorium treatment
of all cases of pulmonary tuberculosis in the county area, burghal
and landward. Very few places in the United Kingdom were
as favourably placed. Mr. Joseph Johnstone moved that the
Council undertake the hospital and sanatorium treatment of all
cases of pulmonary tuberculosis in the county area, burghal and
landward. He stated that the position of the county with
regard to the treatment of tuberculosis was highly gratifying.
Hitherto they had not been able to undertake the work so fully
as they would have liked, but they were now happily in a
position to do so. He also pointed out that owing to the
Insurance Committee being short of money the Council had
to deal with insured as well as uninsured persons. At the end
of the year, when the Insurance Committee prepared their
budget, the County Council would have an opportunity of
considering their further action in the matter. Mr. Johnstone
at a later stage explained the accommodation provided by their
sanatorium. Dealing with the cost of the buildings, he said
it would throw only 5-14ths of a farthing on the ratepayers so
far as the capital expenditure was concerned. The motion was
adopted.

NEW PREPARATIONS, &c.

From Messrs. Burroughs Wellcome & Co.

'*Tabloid*' *Pleated Triangular Bandages* (sterilised).—Two bandages folded and compressed into very small space, packed in an impervious container. Each bandage has clearly printed on it illustrations showing how it may be used. This is an ideal emergency dressing for use both by the profession and by laymen.

'*Tabloid*' '*Xaxa*' *Compound.*—These compressed discs are said to contain 'Xaxa,' grains $3\frac{1}{2}$; phenacetin, grains $2\frac{1}{2}$; caffein, gr. $\frac{1}{2}$. This should prove a very useful combination.

'*Tabloid*' *Colchicine and Nux Vomica Compound.*—These compressed discs are said to contain colchicine, gr. $\frac{1}{70}$; ext. nuc. vom., gr. $\frac{1}{4}$; ext. hyoscyami, gr. $\frac{1}{2}$; ext. gentian, q.s. This is also a good compound.

'*Soloid*' *Toluidine Blue.*—These pellets each contain 0·1 gram. of the stain, which, of course, is useful not only for staining bac. diphtheriæ, but also for general histological purposes. They will be convenient for those who occasionally desire to make up a fresh stain.

'*Soloid*' *Sabouraud's Medium.*—These pellets are advanced for the extemporaneous production of peptone-maltose-agar medium for the growth of various organisms associated with dermatological practice. It is claimed that these products keep indefinitely, and that the medium can be made from them in about ten minutes, though, of course, to ensure absolute sterility, it must be sterilised in the ordinary way on three successive days. For dermatologists and others who have not the resources of a laboratory at their disposal, this preparation and the other similar ones marketed by the firm should be invaluable.

REVIEWS.

***

The British Pharmacopœia, 1914.

THE fifth issue of *The British Pharmacopœia* will be published on 31st December, 1914, but advance copies have been sent out for review. The first impression made by studying it is the number of changes, necessary and unnecessary, which have been made. Since the last issue in 1898 there has been an enormous output of new drugs, chiefly synthetic, and it is an interesting comment on the value of the product that the compilers of the new *B.P.* have only found it necessary to include less than a dozen drugs to represent the much advertised commercial products. In the new edition, accordingly, we find official drugs representing such commercial preparations as aspirin, veronal, eucaine, diuretin, urotropin, purgen, lysol, heroin, trional, and eucaine. We are glad to see that there is no official recognition of organic iodides, bromine or iron preparations. The new official preparations are in most cases so thoroughly disguised by the fanciful names given to them that it will be some considerable time before they are recognised. It is a distinct lack that there is no indication of the commercial trade-name. In the *B.P.* codex this plan was adopted, and greatly facilitated the introduction of the *B.P.C.* nomenclature. Now the practitioner must learn that barbitone is chemically the same as the trade-preparation veronal, that benzamine lactate is his old friend β-eucaine, diamorphine hydrochloride, heroin, and so on. There is absolutely no indication what these preparations represent, except that the useless information is given of the exact chemical name of the drug. A number of new vegetable preparations have been incorporated, and, speaking generally, these are drugs used in the East as substitutes for drugs already official. In this way a few new astringents and anthelmintics have been officially recognised. On the other hand, only one new drug of animal origin has been included, viz., adrenalin. Neither vaccines or serums receive any official recognition.

The British Pharmacopœia fulfils a twofold function. It is alike a guide for the chemist and a standard for the physician. Roughly speaking, the numerous changes which have been made in way of altering the official descriptions and improving the tests for the various drugs are chiefly of interest for the druggists, and no doubt in due course we shall have their opinion about the changes. Similarly, the many minor changes in the composition of pill excipients interest chiefly the druggists. It is a different matter when we come to the question of the composition and doses of the official drugs and preparations. These points concern the physician. In the new edition, there are many, we believe too many, changes in composition and strength of old preparations. It is, of course, evident that this question of change in composition affects chiefly the present generation of practitioners. It is immaterial to the coming generation what is the composition of the *B.P.* preparations. To the present generation it will be a distinct hardship that so many important preparations in constant use have been altered in composition. To name but a few—paregoric, laudanum, tincture of digitalis, tincture of nux vomica, tincture of strophanthus, compound jalap powder, nitroglycerin tablet, solution of perchloride of mercury, antimony wine, in the new *B.P.* represent different preparations from those of the old *B.P.* We question whether the inconvenience of the change is really counterbalanced by the approximate correspondence of the new preparations to those recommended in the International Agreement of 1906.

The greatest change affecting the physician is the adoption of the metric system for dosage. In the old *Pharmacopiœa* the metric system was given as an alternative in the compounding of the official preparations, but the official dosage was in the imperial system. Now the metric system is alone official in the formula of the official preparation, and an alternative metric scale of dosage is given along with the older imperial doses. The compilers seem to think that the fact that students already use the metric system in laboratory work will render it an easy matter for them to adopt it to their materia medica. It is true that in the physiological work the metric system is in use, but in our experience though students glibly talk about c.c., litre, gramme, etc., they have but little conception what values these terms represent. In any case, the student does not use the terms mils, decimils, centimils, now introduced into the *B.P.*

Of greater difficulty is the fact that it is not easy to find metric whole numbers which correspond accurately to the imperial quantities usually employed in dosage. The compilers have recognised this, and in the preface state that the correspondence between the two scales of doses is one of approximate equivalence only. That the degree of equivalence may be only very approximate is shown by a few tests. The official dose of tincture of digitalis is given as 3-10 decimils or 5-15 minims. Now, one decimil is $= 1{\cdot}69$ minims, so that 10 decimils is $= 16{\cdot}9$ minims. The difference between $16{\cdot}9$ and 15 is nearly 12 per cent. The ratio of 4 mils to 1 fluid drachm is taken throughout. Now $16{\cdot}9 \times 4 = 67{\cdot}6$ minims, whereas one fluid drachm contains 60 minims—or again, roughly, an error of 12 per cent. Similarly, the fluid ounce is equal to $28{\cdot}4123$ mils, but for purposes of dosage the fluid ounce is taken to be equivalent to 30 mils, involving an error of about 8 per cent. As 1 milligram corresponds almost accurately with $\frac{1}{64}$ grain, the errors in the minute doses of solids are not so marked. To make the correspondence more accurate the doses of arsenic, strychnine hydrochloride, and other drugs, formerly with a dose of $\frac{1}{60}$-$\frac{1}{15}$ gram., have now been changed to $\frac{1}{64}$-$\frac{1}{16}$ gr. The gramme corresponds more nearly to 15 grains than the mil to 15 minims, since one gramme $= 15{\cdot}432$ grs. Thus the assumption that 4 grammes $=$ 60 grains is not so far out, since 4 grammes $= 61{\cdot}728$ grains.

Another difficulty which will certainly arise from the double system of dosage is the question of bottle supply. The present range of 2, 4, 6, and 8 oz. bottles does not readily yield itself to the metric scale.

The substitution of empirical for constitutional chemical formulæ is not a forward step.

On the whole, the new issue seems to have been carefully revised, but there are still a few errors which have been overlooked. Thus the metric doses of tincture of strophanthus and of theobrominæ et sodii salicylas are incorrectly given. On p. xxiii. cresolis is wrong. On p. 50 Bitter Orange should be Bitter-Orange. The index is defective in a few places. Troch. krameriæ is omitted, and also the trochiscus of ipecacuanha and the trochiscus of morphine and ipecac, on pp. 573 and 574.

On p. 596 confection of sulphur is erroneously stated to be a preparation of sublimed sulphur, instead of precipitated sulphur. On pp. 532 and 533 surely distilled water is meant in defining the volumes of the measures of capacity. Would it not be well to include on p. 534 an approximate equivalent for the ounce of 437·5 grs. ?

A new feature is the publication of official abbreviations of the Latin names. In it the contraction tr. is used for tincture. The official contraction—Ext. Gossyp. Rad. Cort. Liq.—is far too long ; Ext. Gossyp. Liq. is surely sufficient.

Anæmia and Resuscitation: An Experimental and Clinical Research. By GEORGE W. CRILE. New York and London : D. Appleton & Co. 1914.

THIS is a profoundly interesting book, and represents an amount of hard work, well ordered, and to be commended as an example to those about to engage in scientific research.

To those who are familiar with Dr. Crile's contributions to the literature and practice of surgery our praise will not be unexpected ; to others we recommend the present work.

Briefly put, the author's experiments go to prove the extreme susceptibility of the brain to anæmia. He lays stress on the difficulty in overcoming anæmia of the brain, and in conformity with the importance of this fact he devotes the first two chapters of the book to a consideration of anæmia of the central nervous system. Dogs were killed by chloroform and resuscitated after the lapse of a period varying from three to fourteen minutes. The author found the average limit of total cerebral anæmia admitting of recovery to be between six and seven minutes; any recovery after more than seven and a half minutes was exceptional. "The histologic evidence that, even in so-called 'recovered' animals, some or even many nerve cells are permanently lost, and that all are temporarily damaged explains the great temporary and lesser permanent loss of power following any grave anæmia of the brain " (p. 72).

The subject of anæmia of voluntary muscles occupies several chapters. From experiments in this field the author draws important conclusions. As regards muscular contractures, pressure, though usually present, is not an essential factor. Anæmia alone, nerve injury alone, or both in combination may cause contractures.

Clinical applications of experimental results are given, and there is a careful consideration of anæmia in spinal cord lesions, anæmia resulting from flap tension and from suture tension, &c.

To the surgeon, however, perhaps the most interesting subject considered is anæmia of the small intestine, with resulting production of powerful toxins and their action on the organism.

We need not dwell on the clinical application of the author's results. Suffice it to say that it has seldom been our good fortune to read so interesting a book, and we are sure that none of our readers who may peruse it will be disappointed. It is more than a mere addition to our knowledge; it is a· mental stimulant of a high order.

Anaphylaxis. By CHARLES RICHET. Translated by J. MURRAY BLIGH, M.D. Liverpool: The University Press. London: Constable & Co., Limited. 1913.

AN account is given first of all of the discovery of the phenomenon of anaphylaxis in 1902, and a summary of the main points established regarding it up to 1910. Anaphylaxis produced by alimentary absorption, and by hereditary transmission, has to be distinguished from what are merely cases of marked individual susceptibility. The incubation period varies with the dose, the type of animal, and, more especially, with the antigen used; and the results of various experiments by different observers show that the shortest period is ten days. The anaphylactic state lasts a long time, possibly, in the guinea-pig at least, during the remainder of life. The symptoms vary somewhat in different animals. They are described as they occur in dogs, rabbits, guinea-pigs, &c., and in man, the last occurring chiefly in children who have received antidiphtheritic serum on several occasions. Prophylactic intravenous second injections of horse serum in man are dangerous. Although anaphylaxis is not induced by crystalloids, there are apparently a few exceptions in the case of certain drugs in predisposed people. Colloids almost invariably induce it. Injections of heterogenous serum —that is, the serum from an animal of a different species— cause it, also albuminous substances, possibly without exception. The anaphylactising powers in general of many substances have been tested by experiment, and the effects on them of heat and of chemical processes have proved the co-existence of a *preparatory* and of an *exciting* substance, the specificity of which, from a practical standpoint, is absolute. Hence a possible application in forensic medicine. Of anaphylactising substances in particular, sera, milk, eggs, toxins, bacterial albumens, extracts of cancerous tumours, and fluid from hydatid cysts are considered. Passive anaphylaxis has been induced in the dog, rabbit, and guinea-pig by injecting serum from an anaphylactised animal. This serum contains toxigen. Subsequently a dose of antigen that would be non-toxic to a fresh animal is injected. The condition may be homogeneous or heterogeneous, and is specific.

The phenomenon of anaphylaxis *in vitro* is produced, but not invariably, by mixing the blood of an anaphylactised animal with the antigen. The fluid becomes highly toxic, owing, probably, to the formation of a substance which has been named apotoxin.

The question of the relation of anaphylaxis to precipitin formation and complement deviation, being still the subject of research, is briefly referred to.

Anti-anaphylaxis is the prevention of the appearance of anaphylaxis by intercurrent injections of antigen.

The possible use of anaphylaxis as a test for the recognition of organic fluids has already been indicated. In the diagnosis of disease it has not yet become of practical value. The sensitiveness of some individuals to certain foods and drugs may be anaphylactic reactions; likewise the occurrence of death after the escape of hydatid fluid into the peritoneum; so also eclampsia, hay fever, asthma, &c. Infection of an animal with the tubercle bacillus gives rise to preparatory substances, and tuberculin to such an animal becomes an exciting substance, giving rise to anaphylaxis. Local anaphylaxis has been seen in man, and has been produced in the rabbit. Chronic anaphylaxis, that is, death after recovery from anaphylactic shock, has been seen in some animals, and is probably due to lesions produced by the apotoxin. The artificial digestion of albumens has been investigated as regards their anaphylactising powers, but their effects are not fully understood.

Alimentary anaphylaxis sometimes occurs after certain foods in predisposed individuals, and is probably due to the presence in the blood of a toxin which reacts with the food.

General anaphylaxis—increased sensitiveness to all poisons as a result of the injection of a single antigen—has been produced in dogs.

The author's conclusions, based on the facts indicated and those ascertained by other workers besides himself, form an interesting epitome of the subject so far as it is known. For the complete bibliography for 1902 to 1911 the reader is referred to the French edition. A complete bibliography for 1910 and 1911, and of the leading papers published in 1912, is appended to the volume under review.

The translator is to be congratulated; there is almost perfect clearness, and the simplicity with which a complex subject has been presented is praiseworthy. On pp. 80 and 81 it is not quite clearly stated that albumenoids are anaphylactising substances, although it is readily inferred.

Printing and binding are most attractive.

Organic Chemistry for Students of Medicine. By JAMES WALKER, F.R.S., LL.D. London: Gurney & Jackson. 1913.

EXCELLENT in many respects as this work undoubtedly is, it suffers, from the student's point of view, by the absence of a suitable introduction. It must be remembered that the student is not always in a position to begin this complicated branch of his study by an abrupt plunge (page 2) into a consideration of the purification of organic substances.

With the subject matter no fault can be found, and if the student already knows more than a little about organic chemistry he will be able to utilise the information to the full, although it is more than probable that few medical students will be able to digest and assimilate more than a moderate amount of the material in the book.

The descriptions of many of the processes are unusually good, and an example of this is found in the description of Kjeldahl's process for the estimation of nitrogen.

As a book of reference for students and others the present work will be found invaluable.

Electrocardiographic Apparatus. Cambridge : The Cambridge Scientific Instrument Company. 1913.

WE have received from the Cambridge Scientific Instrument Company a copy of their catalogue of electrocardiographic apparatus. It constitutes a *catalogue raisonné*, and gives, besides a list of prices and illustrations of the various forms of instrument and their accessories, a brief exposition of the general principles of electrocardiography, a detailed description of the string galvanometer and of the plate· and paper cameras, time markers, and other important parts of the instrument, and a series of electrocardiograms from the different leads, illustrative both of the normal cycle and of a number of pathological conditions. An interesting modification is the phonocardiogram, by means of which a graphic record of the cardiac sounds, with their variations in pitch or tone, can be obtained, and the exact time relations of any murmur can also be accurately determined. The cost of a complete outfit varies from £200 to £290.

Physics: An Elementary Text-Book for University Classes. By C. G. KNOTT, D.Sc., F.R.S.E. London·: W. & R. Chambers, Limited. 1913.

THIS is the third edition of Dr. Knott's excellent text-book on *Physics*, and we think that it is one of the best of its kind. The book is divided into two portions—the first entitled " Matter and energy ; " the second, " Matter, ether, and energy." In the second portion we find an excellently written chapter on the electron theory and radio-activity. The book is throughout clearly and well written and easily read, and is also suitably illustrated.. We venture to think that it is one of the best books in our language for medical students while attending their courses of physics.

General Medicine. ·Edited by FRANK BILLINGS, M.S., M.D., and J. H. SALISBURY, A.M., M.D. The Practical Medicine Series. Vols. I and VI. Chicago: The Year Book Publishers. 1913.

WE find more space devoted to medical subjects in this than in the previous series, and these two volumes provide a very comprehensive review of the year's progress in the various branches. Diseases of the gastro-intestinal tract and the infections occupy much the greater part of Vol. VI, while the other sections of internal medicine are found in Vol. I.

The standard is quite up to that of last year, and the work must have entailed considerable painstaking effort on the part of the editors.

To general practitioner and specialist alike the volumes can be cordially recommended.

Practical Pathology, including Morbid Anatomy and Post-Mortem Technique. By JAMES MILLER, M.D., D.Sc., F.R.C.P.E. London: Adam and Charles Black. 1914.

THE book is one of the Edinburgh Medical Series, and, as stated by the author, is meant to give the student of medicine and practitioner in a handy form the information required for practical work in relation to pathology. It does not aim to be a book for the specialist, nor does it serve the purpose of replacing the text-book on pathology. As a student's handbook to assist him with the appearances presented by the organs as met with in the *post-mortem* room and museum, it serves well its purpose, and can be recommended as an addition to his text-books. It is well arranged and carefully written, and the author has been fortunate in allotting to each section a proportion of the book consistent with the merits of the subject discussed, and for the size of the book it contains a large amount of information of a practical nature in a small compass. The work deals with the performance of the *post-mortem* examination, with a later chapter relating to medico-legal examinations, the diseased conditions most frequently met with in the various organs, a short account of tumours, and an appendix on methods.

The appendix deserves special merit for the judicious selection of such methods as will best serve the purpose of the student without over-burdening him with alternatives. The illustrations, which are placed at the end of the volume, are entirely taken from macroscopic preparations, and are well selected and executed.

Nervous and Mental Diseases. Edited by HUGH J. PATRICK, M.D., and PETER BASSOE, M.D. Practical Medicine Series. Vol. X. Chicago: The Year Book Publishers. 1913.

THE closing volume of the Practical Medicine Series for the year 1913, like its predecessors, is highly to be commended as providing a clear and sufficient account of the advances made during 1912 in the subjects with which it deals. The series is primarily intended for general practitioners, but its arrangement in volumes devoted to special subjects makes it also convenient for the specialist, who will find in it a convenient *résumé* of work with which he is already familiar. Both in the department of neurology and in that of psychiatry the book will be a useful companion.

Diabetes: Its Pathological Physiology. By JOHN J. R. MACLEOD, M.B., Ch.B., D.P.H. London: Edward Arnold. 1913.

THIS volume, which forms one of the series of International Medical Monographs under the general editorship of Drs. Leonard Hill and William Bulloch, is essentially a review of the experimental work that has recently been done on glycogenesis and the pathology of diabetes. It is based for the most part, as its author states, upon his own researches and those of his collaborators, but it also takes into account the work of others who have given themselves to research upon these lines, and subjects their views and results to critical discussion. Beginning with an account of the sugar of the urine, for which the author considers that Nylander's and Benedict's tests are the most satisfactory, he next discusses the sugar of the blood and its relation to the urinary sugar, and then passes to a consideration of its nerve control, finding that in the presence of adrenalin stimulation of the splanchnic nerve produces hyperglycæmia, *i.e.*, that there are efferent nerve fibres controlling the glycogenolytic activities of the liver. The relationship of the ductless glands to sugar metabolism forms the subject of the next chapter, and Dr. Macleod concludes that although the pancreas, the adrenals, the parathyroids, and perhaps the posterior lobe of the pituitary body have an important controlling influence, exerted probably by hormones, it is difficult to say precisely how each gland acts. The pancreas and parathyroids facilitate and the adrenals depress the utilisation of sugar, but it is not known whether the hormones act upon glycogenesis or glycolysis. There is nothing to show that the internal secretion of the pancreas is derived solely from the islands of Langerhans.

The glycogenic function of the liver is next discussed at some length, but the conclusions reached upon this important subject seem to be as yet largely provisional, although it is shown that "the variations which occur in the process of mobilisation of sugar in the liver are not due to changes in the amount of the enzyme (glycogenase)." The environment in which the glycogenase acts must therefore change; and this leads to a discussion of hyperglycæmia, which is shown not to be a necessary accompaniment of hyperglycogenolysis. Its probable causes, and therefore the probable causes of glycosuria, are grouped in tabular form, and the author passes to consider the assimilation limit of sugars, the lowering of which indicates a fault in carbohydrate metabolism, and the determination of which is therefore of importance for the early diagnosis of diabetes. A brief consideration of the subject of glyconeogenesis

ends the volume, the importance of which for workers in carbohydrate metabolism is materially enhanced by the valuable
bibliography which is given at the close of each chapter.
Dr. Macleod's contribution to the pathological physiology of
diabetes is valuable both for its clear statement of attained
results and for its criticism of over-hasty assumptions; and
if at times the results appear but meagre to the clinician,
anxious above all things for an indication for treatment, it is
to be remembered that the removal of misconceptions is an
important step on the road to truth. The book, it may be said
in closing, is of convenient size, the type is clear, and there are
few misprints; but on p. 138, lines 15 and 16 are transposed
to the destruction of the sense.

Diseases of the Heart and Aorta. By A. D. HIRSCHFELDER,
   M.D. Second Edition. London: J. B. Lippincott Company.
   1913.

THAT the second edition of so large a work as is Dr.
Hirschfelder's upon diseases of the heart and aorta should
have been issued so soon as three years after the publication
of the first is a testimony to its merits more convincing than
any that a reviewer can give. Its explanation is to be found
not only in the unusually clear character of the author's style,
and the completeness of his presentation of the facts of cardiac
pathology and symptomatology, but also in the attention which
he devotes to the subject of treatment, and in his careful
correlation of clinical indications with physiological action.
But in the last three years many advances have been made
in the knowledge of cardiac disease, and the second edition
consequently differs from the first in several particulars. The
new subject of electro-cardiography has received detailed
consideration, the section upon arterio-sclerosis has been
rewritten in the light of recent investigations upon syphilitic
arterial disease, new drugs and new methods of treatment
have been fully discussed, and in every particular the book
has been brought into accordance with the latest results of
research. While the book is thus considerably enlarged, and

while several of its chapters have been entirely rewritten, it still presents the same qualities which gained for it immediate recognition on its first appearance. In its present form it is a very complete presentment of the subject of cardiac disease, embodying not only the author's experience, but the fruits of his wide reading, and enriched at the end of each chapter by a bibliography which must prove of great value to those who desire further information upon particular branches of the subject.

St. Bartholomew's Hospital Reports. Edited by F. W. ANDREWS, W. M'A. ECCLES, G. E. GASK, W. D. HARMER, H. THURSFIELD, and H. WILLIAMSON. Vol. XLIX. London: Smith, Elder & Co. 1914.

SOME very interesting papers are included in the present issue of the *St. Bartholomew's Hospital Reports,* which opens with obituary notices of two members of the staff of the hospital, Alfred Willett and R. B. Etherington-Smith. The first of the medical papers, by Dr. A. F. S. Sladden, details the results of a trial of some tests of pancreatic disease. The author used the tests in thirty-six cases of various forms of disease in which the diagnosis was verified either at the operation or *post-mortem,* and he finds that no reliance is to be placed on Cammidge's test, which in the presence of pancreatic disease is as often negative as positive, and in its absence is positive at least once in four times. Schmidt's and Kasiwado's "nuclei" tests are not much more satisfactory, and the most reliable indications are afforded by Loewi's adrenalin mydriasis test, the analysis of fat in fæces, the tolerance for glucose, and the finding of muscle fibres in the fæces (creatorrhœa). Mr. T. H. G. Shore writes on the prognostic value of the blood-count in myelocytic leukæmia, and finds that the ratio $\dfrac{\text{granular leucocytes}}{\text{hyaline (non-granular) leucocytes}}$ affords a useful indication of the outlook. When this ratio is above 10, the prognosis is relatively favourable, when below the reverse is the case, and before death the ratio may fall to 5 or less. Dr. Hugh Thursfield writes upon acholuric jaundice, and records the first British case of splenectomy for this condition, which in this instance was congenital. He reviews the literature, and concludes that the operation is successful in selected congenital cases, and that its mortality is low, while in acquired cases the results are not so certain. He also finds that undue fragility of the red corpuscles is pathognomonic of the congenital condition. Mr. D'Arcy Power details the results of the treatment of ulcerative colitis by appendicostomy in a series of cases. He considers that the operation is indicated in the early stages, while the condition is yet local, and as soon as local remedies have failed, and he advises the use of vaccines in conjunction with the operative treatment. Mr. A. L. Moreton records a case of post-orbital arterio-venous aneurysm successfully treated by ligature of the internal carotid, and Dr. Garnet Twigg writes upon pes cavus as an initial sign of nervous disease. He finds that the primary cause in most cases is an affection of the nervous or muscular system, and that the condition calls for careful examination of these systems. Dr. Haldin Davis contributes a paper on the use of neo-salvarsan in out-patients of the skin department; and the rest of the volume is occupied with museum catalogues and hospital statistics. It will be seen that it contains material of much clinical interest.

Reports from the Laboratory of the Royal College of Physicians, Edinburgh. Edited by G. L. GULLAND, M.D., and JAMES RITCHIE, M.D. Vol. XII. Edinburgh : Oliver & Boyd. 1913.

THE volume of these *Reports* now under review contains the contributions of workers up to the end of 1912, and consists of reprints of papers published during 1911 and 1912 in various medical and scientific journals. Many papers in anatomy, pharmacology, pathology, and bacteriology are thus united and preserved in a permanent form, which the worker on these subjects would otherwise be able to find only after a laborious search. Among them are to be found several of outstanding interest, and we may mention those of Mr. D. P. D. Wilkie, on the functions and surgical uses of the omentum ; of Drs. Ritchie and Ninian Bruce, on the suprarenal glands in diphtheritic toxæmia; and of Dr. Addis, on the pathogenesis of hereditary hæmophilia, a paper to which the subject owes its definitive elucidation. The volume, which is well got up, will be of much value for reference to workers in its special subjects.

Syphilis and the Nervous System. By Dr. MAX DONNE. Translated from the Second German Edition by CHAS. R. BALL, B.A., M.D. London: J. B. Lippincott Company, 1913.

SYPHILIS may attack either the cranium and vertebræ or the nervous system; the latter in three ways, as newgrowth, chronic inflammation, or disease of blood-vessels, these three usually occurring in combination. Primary degeneration as the result of syphilis also occurs. Each of these conditions receives some consideration, and there is also a short account of syphilitic aortitis and of differential diagnosis in specific processes. In a chapter on "Etiology of nervous lues" there are some statistics regarding the stage at which disease of the nervous system may appear, and the influence treatment, injuries, alcohol, &c., have on its appearance. Then follows an account of the symptoms and differential diagnosis of specific end-arteritis. Syphilitic cerebral meningitis and its differential diagnosis, and syphilitic basilar meningitis are each the subject of a chapter, the differential diagnosis of the latter occupying a separate one, in which also the prognosis of brain syphilis in general is described, and summarised in tabular form. In discussing the symptomatology of basilar syphilis, the relationships of the oculo-motor and trochlear nuclei are depicted. There is a chapter on neuroses and psychoses in syphilitics and in cerebral syphilis, which includes an account of the ways in which these may be caused. The relationship between general paralysis—often referred to simply as "paresis"—and syphilis is dealt with at some length. "Syphilis of the spinal cord and membranes" is the subject of three chapters; "Tabes and syphilis," "Cerebro-spinal syphilis," "Syphilitic disease of the peripheral nerves," and "Congenital syphilis as it affects the nervous system," each of one. The behaviour of the Wassermann reaction as applied to the blood and spinal fluids, phagocytosis, and the globulin test are described. The concluding two chapters are on "Prophylaxis" and "Salvarsan therapy."

There is a very comprehensive bibliography containing, we estimate, over 400 references. There are nearly 100 illustrations. We have found the arrangement of subject-matter a little confusing, but a closer acquaintance might remove this difficulty. And it took us some time to become accustomed to the peculiarity of construction which it is difficult to avoid in translating from the German.

A Synopsis of Surgery. By ERNEST W. HEY GROVES, M.D., F.R.C.S. Fourth Edition. Bristol: John Wright & Sons, Limited. London: Simpkin, Marshall, Hamilton, Kent & Co., Limited. 1914.

THE call for each subsequent edition of a book furnishes the author with a fresh opportunity of eliminating defects and of incorporating such improvements as his experience in the interval may have suggested. Still, the alterations which can consistently be made on any edition are limited largely by the original plan and scope of the work. Each edition, therefore, it may be supposed, approaches more nearly the stereotyped form.

Less than six years ago Mr. Hey Groves produced his *Synopsis of Surgery*, and already we have to welcome the fourth edition. It would be superfluous now to enter into a detailed examination of the intrinsic qualities of the work, but we may point out briefly the new features.

Complete revision has been carried out, the chapters on pathology and on bacteriology have been rewritten, recent theories of shock and new methods of anæsthesia have been added, while the scope of those sections dealing with the surgery of the spinal cord has been enlarged.

We can wish the author no better fortune for his new edition than that it may be as well received as its predecessors, and we are confident of the fulfilment of that wish.

ABSTRACTS FROM CURRENT MEDICAL LITERATURE.

EDITED BY ROY F. YOUNG, M.B., B.C.

MEDICINE.

Practical Application of the Luetin Test. By Hideyo Noguchi, M.D. (*New York Medical Journal*, 22nd August, 1914).—A little over two years ago it was shown that certain cases of syphilis give a distinct local reaction to an intradermal injection of treponema pallidum (luetin). Among non-syphilitic individuals there was no such reaction. The early experience with luetin showed that the reaction is more uniformly present in chronic cases than in primary or secondary forms of acquired syphilis. In congenital syphilis the reaction is more frequently found to be positive among late cases than among new-born infants. The observation of about fifty investigators in the last two years give the following statistical estimation of the practical value of the luetin reaction :— In primary syphilis, present in 30 per cent of cases, and usually very mild ; in secondary, in 47 per cent, and usually mild ; in tertiary, in about 80 per cent, severe, and usually pustular ; in general paralysis and tabes, in 60 per cent ; in congenital syphilis, in about 70 per cent. The Wassermann reaction is much more constant among primary and secondary cases, but the reverse holds for chronic cases, especially when under treatment.—ADAM PATRICK.

The Diet in Typhoid Fever. By Lewellys F. Barker, M.D. (*The Jour. of the Amer. Med. Assoc.*, 12th September, 1914).—Barker writes in favour of a liberal diet for enteric fever patients. It was formerly almost a universal practice to limit the diet to fluids, and to a low caloric intake. Emaciation was believed to be inevitable, and losses of weight as great as 30 per cent and 41 per cent have been recorded in extreme instances. As early as 1882 von Hoesslin had shown that foods were absorbed almost as well in typhoid fever as in health, and later observers came to the same conclusion. Shaffer and Coleman (1909) concluded that by the use of diets of high caloric value, especially rich in carbo-hydrates, it is possible to prevent not only the "febrile loss" of body protein-nitrogen in patients suffering from typhoid fever, but also that due to the so-called toxic destruction of body protein. They are inclined to believe that there is a greater need for carbohydrate in fever than in health, and that if the carbohydrate of the food intake be insufficient, the body protein will be drawn on to supply energy in an available form ; if, on the contrary, enough carbo-hydrate be given, the body protein will be protected. Kocher (1914) points out that while nitrogen loss may be compensated for by a high caloric intake, there are periods in the disease when nitrogen equilibrium cannot be maintained.

Protein may be taken in sufficient amount as eggs and milk. Schottmuller and other German writers gives as much as 100 gm. of scraped meat per day. If soup is given, it is well to add eggs and cereal. Eggs may be taken raw, or beaten up with milk, or soft boiled. From four to eight eggs may often be given in the twenty-four hours. The carbohydrate may be given partly as milk, partly as bread or toast (with butter), and partly as lactose added to the milk. Coarse cereals with cellulose are to be avoided. Boiled rice or mashed potatoes may be given as variety. Lactose is a very important article in the diet. Fat may be given, but not all patients bear fat well, especially early in the disease. It may be tried in the form of cream, butter, or yolk of egg. Fruit juices, to which lactose has been added, may be given so long as there is no diarrhœa.

It is necessary to begin this liberal diet cautiously. Coleman recommends a pure milk diet for two days in all cases. If the patient is very ill he may be kept on fluid diet—1 litre of milk, 50 cc. cream, 50 gm. lactose, up to 1·5 litres milk, 0·5 litres cream, and 1 lb. lactose, divided into eight feedings. In mild cases the patients may take from the beginning buttered toast, mashed potatoes, and cereals.

The high caloric diet will be objected to by many. The prejudice against it is contributed to by false ideas regarding the character of the intestinal contents in enteric, and their relation to the ulcers. Hæmorrhage, perforation, and relapse have been ascribed to dietetic errors, because they sometimes follow them.

—ADAM PATRICK.

Spasmodic Closing of Cerebral Arteries and its Relation to Apoplexy. By Alfred Gordon, M.D. (*Albany Medical Annals*, August, 1914). —One of the fundamental principles in the physiology of the vasomotor apparatus is the existence of a central mechanism in the medulla. A continuous flow of impulses from this area maintains the tone of the blood-vessels. Destruction of this bulbar centre is followed by abolition of the vasomotor reflex, and the blood-vessels remain dilated. For a long time there was a belief that cerebral blood-vessels have no independent innervation, and that they passively follow variations in blood pressure. This contention has been proved inaccurate, and it has been shown that in a pronounced fall of blood pressure the cerebral vessels dilate. The existence of a nerve supply to the vessels was shown also by the contraction of the cerebral vessels which follows injection of adrenalin into the carotids, and by anatomical demonstration of the nerve elements in the walls of the vessels.

This bulbar centre is not the only one which influences the vasomotor apparatus. Observations are on record which tend to prove that vasomotor disturbances may be also of cortical origin. In one case the presence of a cyst in the motor area caused vasomotor disturbance in the contralateral hand, and this passed off with the removal of the tumour. Disturbances have also followed the removal of a portion of the cortex.

There is a well-known group of clinical cases apparently due to temporary closure of cerebral arteries—intermittent or transient attacks of hemiplegia or monoplegia. The paralysis may be of any degree, and may or may not be accompanied by aphasia. The author records 14 such cases, in 8 of which he made a *post-mortem* examination. The main characteristic manifestation was a sudden onset of hemiparesis. The attacks varied greatly in frequency (three months to two years) and in duration (a few minutes to a few days). In the 8 who died the attacks became more severe, and death occurred with signs of severe apoplexy. In all these cases, *post-mortem*, softening was found in the internal capsule and portions of the basal ganglia. In 7 of the 8 cases the Wassermann reaction was positive. Administration of nitro-glycerine and anti-syphilitic remedies apparently prolonged life.

A close analysis of the cases shows that there may occur such a disturbance of the vessel wall as to interfere with the circulation in, and therefore with the function of, the nerve tissue supplied by the vessel. In a case of Lindsay Steven's (1907), in which spasmodic contraction of the main vessel occurred, no arterial disease was found *post-mortem*, but only an area of white necrosis in the vicinity of the blood-vessels. The gradual evolution of the symptoms from mild to severe, together with the *post-mortem* findings, permits the conclusion that the intermittent spasmodic contraction of the cerebral vessels gradually leads to a destruction of the tissue supplied by them through a process of softening.

—ADAM PATRICK.

SURGERY.

The Operation of Election for the Radical Cure of Inguinal Hernia. By E. A. R. Newman (*Indian Medical Gazette*, August, 1914).— After a discussion on the nomenclature used to denote the various types of inguinal hernia, the author describes the operation which he has devised and is accustomed to perform ; the incision is made ¾ to 1 inch above, and parallel to the inner two-thirds of Poupart's ligament. It is from 3½ to 4 inches in length. The canal is laid open throughout its length. When the sac is found it is cleared in the usual way, and, in the tunical variety, the funicular portion is cut off from the scrotal part. The disposal of the sac depends on whether the hernia is funicular or completely tunical ; in the former it is twisted into a cord and hoisted up through the canal after it has been transfixed by a long ligature, the latter being brought forward through the external oblique aponeurosis ; in the second case a purse-string suture is passed round the neck and tied off.

The transversalis and internal oblique, at the site of the inguinal canal, are pulled down in front of the cord, and sutured to the back of Poupart's ligament with two or three mattress sutures of silkworm gut. The outermost stitch should close the internal abdominal ring, and the innermost lessens the superficial ring round the cord. The concluding steps of the operation are conducted as usual.

—CHARLES BENNETT.

Treatment of Hernia of Muscle by Aponeurotic Grafts. By Dr. Mauclaire (*Archives Generales de Chirurgie*, 25th July, 1914).—Although observations on muscular hernia are not frequent, yet the author has noted several cases. Three of the cases which he describes refused operation. A fourth was a hemiplegic who sustained fracture of both bones of the left leg about the usual situation. The injury healed well, but the patient returned six months after his dismissal from hospital, showing now a hernia of the tibialis anticus. Doubtless the hemiplegic condition had favoured the aponeurotic distension. The author, having at this time had some experience of aponeurotic grafts in abdominal work, decided to carry out the treatment in this case by that method.

The hernial orifice was about 4 centimetres long by 3 broad. There was a cellular membrane in front of the muscle, and this was excised. A portion of the fascia lata of the same side was taken—in dimension rather larger than the measurements given above—and sutured to the edges of the aponeurotic hernial orifice.

The parts healed satisfactorily, and the limb was immobilised for three weeks, at the end of which time there was no sign of the hernia.—CHARLES BENNETT.

Abdominal Incisions. By M. J. Horan (*New York Medical Journal,* 5th September, 1914).—In this article the author describes the results of experi-ments carried out on the cadaver with the object of testing the effects of intra-abdominal pressure on abdominal incisions at different parts below the umbilicus. He begins by discussing the choice of abdominal incision with relation to nerve distribution and blood supply, and concludes that the incision which does the least damage in these respects is one through the right rectus muscle at its outer or middle third and parallel with the umbilicus.

The technique of his experiments on intra-abdominal tension is quite simple ; through an incision in the neck a tube is tied in the œsophagus, the rectum is ligated, air is pumped in with an automobile inflator, and pressure registered with a gauge.

There was no damage to the incisions of the right rectus with a pressure of 120 lb. Those in the middle line above the umbilicus withstood very high intra-abdominal pressure, while incisions in the region of M'Burney's point yielded in some cases to tension of less than 20 lb.—CHARLES BENNETT.

OBSTETRICS AND GYNÆCOLOGY.

Normal Pregnancy and Eclampsia Studied with Reference to Anaphylaxis. Eisenreich, of Munich (*Volkmann's Sammlung,* Nos. 694, 695), describes the work done to elucidate the problems connected with this subject. A long introduction gives the various hypotheses advanced to explain the occurrence of eclampsia from Hippocrates and Galen—with their more or less quantity of blood in the circulation, individual disposition, various poisons such as carbonate of ammonia or urea, variations of blood pressure, compression of the ureters, bacterial poisoning, passage of chorionic villi into the maternal circulation —down to more recent opinions, such as the ferment intoxication of Hofbauer and the fibrin ferment of Dienst. Eisenreich then discusses the principles of anaphylaxis and the history of the development of its theory. He seems to accept without question the results published by Abderhalden in regard to the digestive power on placental peptones of a ferment in the blood of pregnant women.

The author's own researches were in the direction of studying the phenomena of passive transference of hypersensitiveness to enquire whether relations of an anaphylactic nature between mother and child could be established. The work hitherto had reference to placental extracts ; his enquiries were made by means of fœtal serum, as it is difficult to work with so unstable an organ as the placenta, and it is difficult besides to distinguish the fœtal and maternal elements in it. Full details of his technique are given ; the animals used were guinea-pigs, and tables are added to illustrate the results of each experiment. In the first series the serum of a normal woman in labour or the puerperium was first injected, followed twenty-four to forty-eight hours later by an injection of serum of a normal fœtus, drawn from the placental blood. Eisenreich is of opinion that the symptoms, which followed in a few cases only, were not anaphylactic, but rather pseudo-anaphylactic. In the second series the blood of women was employed who were or had been suffering from severe but not fatal eclampsia and the blood of their own children in each case. In this series the animals nearly all suffered from marked anaphylactic shock with considerable fall of temperature. Researches were also made into the diminution of complement during normal and pathological pregnancy. In the normal women there was little or no diminution, but rather an increase from the second or third day of the puerperium. In eclamptic women the results were such that he concludes that there is no typical diminution of complement such as to permit eclampsia to be considered as a manifestation of an anaphylactic malady. In both normal and eclamptic women there was no evidence whatever of any fixation of the complement. Among his general conclusions he states that it was not shown by the passive anaphylaxis experiments on animals that there were anaphylactic relations between mother and child, nor by investigations into the diminution of the complement. With the serum of eclamptic women and of their children, however, the results show that certain biological processes have occurred which do not occur normally. The results of investigations into the deviation of the complement are so constant that there can be no question of any antibody reaction between mother and child.—E. H. L. OLIPHANT.

Theory and Practice in the Operative Treatment of Genital Prolapse. Jellet (*Dublin Journal of Med. Science*, September, 1914) delivered an address at the annual meeting of the Canadian Medical Association, in which he discussed the relation of theory to practice. He discussed the anatomy and physiology of the uterine supports, and warned his hearers against accepting descriptions of ligaments by anatomists unless they are verifiable clinically. Much of the support from ligaments can be felt *per rectum*, while the uterus is drawn down *per vaginam ;* further, the ligaments continued down the vagina can similarly be distinguished *per rectum*, while successive portions of the vaginal vault are drawn down.

The vagina is supported by the *levator ani* muscle, by the vaginal suspensory ligament, by its attachments to the cervix and by the parts of the endo-pelvic fascia which have an insertion into both cervix and upper part of the vagina. The vaginal suspensory ligament, as is demonstrable by the method above mentioned, or during Wertheim's operation, runs more posteriorly than is described by the anatomists, as for example, in Cunningham's *Anatomy*.

The uterus is supported, directly, by its vaginal attachments, by the utero-sacral ligaments, and by the different layers of the endo-pelvic fascia which pass into it laterally and anteriorly. It is supported indirectly by the pelvic floor owing to its axis lying at almost right angles to that of the vagina.

Injuries during labour affect these various supports. Thus, lacerations of the perineum tear away the levator ani from the central point of the perineum, and so permit the lateral bands to diverge outwards, while actual tearing of the muscle itself destroys the continuity of its inner edges, so that there is nothing to prevent the anterior or the posterior vaginal wall from bulging directly through the vaginal orifice. Once this process is started it tends to proceed to the middle part of the vagina, which pulls on its suspensory ligament, and this ligament is unable to withstand the abnormal strain. Jellet, however, thinks that this sequence is not often seen clinically, but that the vaginal vault rather follows the protrusion of the lower vagina, drawing the middle portion after it. The earlier descent of the upper part of the vagina is due to alterations in the uterine supports leading to uterine prolapse, which, so to speak, overtakes the vaginal prolapse, and eventually precedes it. The first direct step, so far as the uterus is concerned, is backward displacement, leading to coincidence of the axes of uterus and vagina, whereby the support of the pelvic floor is lost and the weight of the uterus is thrown on the utero-sacral ligaments and the different parts of the endo-pelvic fascia. The normal function of the utero-sacral ligaments is probably to keep the cervix in its proper relation to the posterior pelvic wall, and when they receive the full weight of the uterus they stretch and fail. Probably the usual sequence of events is, first, the prolapse of the lower portion of the anterior vaginal wall, with or without the lower posterior wall ; then, of the uterus and upper vagina ; and, lastly, of the middle of the lateral and posterior wall. This order is altered in certain cases not associated with labour, and the uterus descends first, causing a consequent inversion of the vagina. Hypertrophy of the supravaginal portion of the cervix probably occurs in cases where the vault of the vagina has prolapsed first, drawing down the uterus after it ; indeed, one may occasionally see this condition—inversion of the vagina and elongated cervix, without prolapse of the uterus.

Applying the theory to a rational method of supporting the uterus, an operation should aim at restoring the direct supports of uterus and vagina, at placing the uterus in a favourable position to resist its descent, and at the removal of complications. Thus, the shortening of the utero-sacral ligaments is indicated in all cases where they are stretched, especially where the uterus is small. In cases where the uterus is large, Jellet considers Wertheim's interposition operation to be one of the best methods of increasing the resistance of the uterus to its own descent. In this operation the uterus is placed between the anterior vaginal wall and the bladder. If the uterus is of sufficient size it is directly supported by the *levator ani* muscle, and is too large to allow the cervix to rotate round it and come down to the vulva, while the body remains in its position. But if the uterus is very small, the cervix, if free, can drop down through the vagina ; if, however, the cervix be fixed by shortening the utero-sacral ligaments, it cannot rotate and drop, while at the same time the strain on the shortened ligaments is slight.

The shortening of the bands of endopelvic fascia known as Mackendrodt's ligaments has been advised, and Jellet thinks that when they are shortened they are capable of adding to the general support of the cervix, but to be effective it must be considerable and must be done with the greatest care, or kinking of the ureters may result. He is of opinion that sufficient shortening is obtained by the insertion of the ligaments into the upper part of the vagina and uterine cavity after supra-vaginal amputation of the cervix. Apart from Stanmore Bishop's operation of fixing the vault of the vagina to the peritoneum on the front of the sacrum, there seems to be no effective way of dealing with the vaginal suspensory ligaments. The restoration of the *levator ani* muscle is an essential part of all perineorrhaphy operations, and is impracticable only where the muscle has disappeared from atrophy or retraction.

The placing of the uterus in the best position to offer the maximum resistance to its descent—that is, in ante-version—can be obtained by shortening the round ligaments or by ventri-suspension. Neither of these operations interferes with pregnancy, according to Jellet. To increase the resistance beyond the normal will inevitably interfere with pregnancy, so such an operation as Wertheim's interposition is permissible only after the natural or artificial menopause. Jellet considers this operation the most valuable procedure which has been introduced of late years for the cure of prolapse, for it also removes the prolapse of the bladder that aggravates and perpetuates the vaginal prolapse. As mentioned before, the uterus must be of sufficient size, and the utero-sacral ligaments must be shortened; otherwise the prolapse is liable to recur.

The removal of complications, such as tumours or increase in volume of the uterus, must be attended to. Erosions and lacerations of the cervix are best treated by amputation. If the uterus is hypertrophied, excision of a wedge-shaped piece is advisable, and, indeed, often necessary, in Wertheim's operation.
—E. H. L. O.

DISEASES OF THE SKIN.

Case of Schamberg's Disease: A Progressive Pigmentary Disease of the Skin.—At a meeting of the Dermatological Section of the Royal Society of Medicine, held on 16th July, 1914, Dr. E. G. Graham Little showed a case of Schamberg's disease. The patient was a man aged 56 years, in good health. He had no venereal disease; no varicose veins. The condition began twenty-five years ago with a patch on the left leg. On the right leg a patch now larger than that on the left showed itself about eight years ago. Within the last few months small isolated punctate lesions began to appear in the neighbourhood of the larger patches. The affected areas were slightly itchy.

The state of the leg was described as follows:—Below the knee on each leg there are large patches, 3 by 5 inches in area, of cayenne-pepper-like punctate deposits of pigment, so closely aggregated as to produce plaques of pigmentation, forming curiously angular shapes with sharply linear and sometimes serpiginous outlines. The general effect is that of buff-coloured tattooing of the skin. There is in addition a slight degree of scaling.

Dr. Douglas Heath remarked that the disease was probably more common than it was supposed to be, and that it might often be mistaken for varicose pigmentation.

Dr. J. J. Pringle thought the condition was essentially one of capillary dilatation with a very small amount of hæmorrhage. He had certainly seen a considerable number of cases, although seldom consulted expressly for it.
—WM. BARBOUR.

Pelade and Exophthalmic Goitre. By R. Sabouraud (*Ann. de Derm. et de Syph.*, 1913, No. 3, p. 140).—The author states that certain cases of alopecia areata and Basedow's disease appear to be directly connected; these cases are almost always chronic and severe, some of them being aggravated, while others are improved by the disease. In children of patients with Basedow's disease, who have symptoms of thyroid insufficiency, there may be present alopecia areata without vitiligo, or vitiligo without alopecia areata. He also refers to his previous observations on the relation of alopecia areata to ovarian troubles, and considers it worthy of note that these two ductless glands appear to play a part among the obscure causes of alopecia areata.

—WM. BARBOUR.

A Case of Folliclis or Papalo-necrotic Tuberculosis of the Skin Mistaken Clinically for Lichen Ruber Planus. Kaufmann-Wolf (*Archiv. f. Derm. u. Syph.*, May, 1914, cxx, No. 1).—This lesion in an otherwise healthy woman, aged 48 years, was apparently produced by an electrode which had been strapped on to the patient's left wrist by a dentist. After the application the wrist became very red and painful, and a fortnight later the spots appeared. Clinically, they presented the appearance of typical lichen ruber planus. They were situated on the dorsum of the left fore-arm in its lower third, and consisted of isolated pin-head size lesions, of firm consistence and light pink colour, and each presented a central depression.

Two papules were excised and examined by Prof. G. Arandt, who reported that histologically they bore no resemblance to lichen planus, but that the condition was one of papulo-necrotic tuberculide, or folliclis, the main features being groups of cellular infiltration with central necrosis. There were neither giant cells nor tubercular bacilli present. Two other cases of a similar diagnostic interest are cited.—WM. BARBOUR.

Books, Pamphlets, &c., Received.

The Intensive Treatment of Syphilis and Locomotor Ataxia by Aachen Methods, by Reginald Hayes, M.R.C.S. London: Baillière, Tindall & Cox. 1914. (3s. 6d. net.)

Cane Sugar and Heart Disease, by Arthur Goulston, M.A., M.D.Cantab. London: Baillière, Tindall & Cox. 1914. (5s. net.)

Essentials of Physiology, by F. A. Bainbridge, M.A., M.D.Cantab., D.Sc.Lond., F.R.C.P., and J. Acworth Menzies, M.D.Edin. With 134 illustrations. London: Longmans, Green & Co. 1914. (10s. 6d. net.)

A Manual of Physiology, with Practical Exercises, by G. N. Stewart, M.A., D.Sc., M.D.Edin., D.P.H.Camb. With coloured plate and 467 other illustrations. Seventh edition. University Series. London: Baillière, Tindall & Cox. 1914. (18s. net.)

Syphilology and Venereal Disease, by C. F. Marshall, M.D., M.Sc., F.R.C.S. Third edition. London: Baillière, Tindall & Cox. 1914. (10s. 6d. net.)

Lead Poisoning: From the Industrial, Medical, and Social Point of View. Lectures delivered at the Royal Institute of Public Health, by Sir Thomas Oliver, M.A., M.D., F.R.C.P. London: H. K. Lewis. 1914. (5s. net.)

Physiological Principles in Treatment, by W. Langdon Brown, M.A., M.D.Cantab., F.R.C.P. Third edition. London: Baillière, Tindall & Cox. 1914. (5s. net.)

A Clinical Study of the Serous and Purulent Diseases of the Labyrinth, by Dr. Erich Ruttin. With a foreword by Professor Dr. Victor Urbantschitsch. Authorised translation by Horace Newhart, A.B., M.D. With 25 textual figures. London: William Heinemann.

The Secrets of the German War Office, by Dr. Armgaard Karl Graves, late Spy of the German Government. Fiftieth thousand. London: T. Werner Laurie, Limited. (2s. net.)

The Infant Nutrition and Management, by Eric Pritchard, M.A., M.D.Oxon., M.R.C.P.Lond. London: Edward Arnold. 1914. (3s. 6d. net.)

Mentally Defective Children, by Alfred Binet and Th. Simon, M.D. Authorised translation by W. B. Drummond, M.B., C.M., F.R.C.P.Edin. With an Appendix containing the Binet-Simon Tests of Intelligence by Margaret Drummond, M.A., and an Introduction by Professor Alexander Darroch. London: Edward Arnold. 1914. (2s. 6d. net.)

A Short Handbook of Cosmetics, by Dr. Max Joseph, Berlin. Second English edition. Revised, with Appendix. London: William Heinemann. 1914. (2s. 6d. net.)

Our City Slums: The Experiences of a Medical Practitioner, by H. E. Jones. Glasgow: John Cossar. 1914. (6d.)

Obiter Scripta: Throat, Nose, and Ear, by A. R. Friel, M.A., M.D. Bristol: John Wright & Sons, Limited. 1914. (2s. 6d. net.)

Essentials of Human Physiology, by D. Noël Paton, M.D., B.Sc., F.R.C.P.Ed. F.R.S. Fourth edition, revised and enlarged. Edinburgh: Wm. Green & Sons. (12s. net.)

GLASGOW.—METEOROLOGICAL AND VITAL STATISTICS FOR THE FIVE WEEKS ENDED 24TH OCTOBER, 1914.

	WEEK ENDING				
	Sept. 26.	Oct. 3.	Oct. 10.	Oct. 17.	Oct. 24.
Mean temperature,	51·4°	51·3°	53·7°	49·3°	47·8°
Mean range of temperature between highest and lowest,	26·5°	19·3°	13·0°	21·8°	20·1°
Amount of rainfall, . ins.	0·06	0·25	0·06	0·18	0·01
Deaths (corrected),	356	312	309	308	303
Death-rates, .	17·7	15·5	15·4	15·3	15·1
Zymotic death-rates,	1·1	0·9	1·1	1·4	1·1
Pulmonary death-rates,	3·0	2·5	3·1	3·3	2·7
DEATHS—					
Under 1 year,	92	74	75	67	71
60 years and upwards,	83	80	75	61	71
DEATHS FROM—					
Small-pox, .	...	...	...	...	...
Measles, .	1	1	1	1	...
Scarlet fever,	5	3	6	9	8
Diphtheria,	2	2	3	5	4
Whooping-cough,	11	11	6	8	7
Enteric fever,	2	2	5	4	3
Cerebro-spinal fever, .	...	2	...	...	2
Diarrhœa (under 2 years of age),	54	28	26	13	16
Bronchitis, pneumonia, and pleurisy,	31	27	38	48	41
CASES REPORTED—					
Small-pox, .	...	...	...	...	...
Cerebro-spinal meningitis, .	1	...	...	1	2
Diphtheria and membranous croup,	42	32	35	40	32
Erysipelas,	44	43	34	34	47
Scarlet fever,	145	159	174	175	144
Typhus fever,	...	...	...	...	...
Enteric fever,	15	12	12	11	10
Phthisis, .	53	39	57	42	37
Puerperal fever,	2	3	10	6	5
Measles,*	8	10	21	17	18

* Measles not notifiable.

SANITARY CHAMBERS,
GLASGOW, 31st October, 1914.

THE

GLASGOW MEDICAL JOURNAL.

No. VI. DECEMBER, 1914.

ORIGINAL ARTICLES.

SOME MANIFESTATIONS OF CONGENITAL SYPHILIS.*

By LEONARD FINDLAY, M.D., D.Sc.,

Physician, Royal Hospital for Sick Children, Glasgow ;

AND

MADGE E. ROBERTSON, M.B.,

Assistant at the Dispensary, Royal Hospital for Sick Children, Glasgow.

(*From the Royal Hospital for Sick Children, and Pathological Department, the University, Glasgow.*)

(*Wassermann reactions were in part done by Dr. H. F. Watson.*)

OUR ideas regarding not only the prevalence but also the pleo-morphism of syphilis have within recent years undergone a marked change. For a definite diagnosis of this disease we no longer depend wholly on the clinical history, or on the evidence of active or healed characteristic clinical manifestations, but are relying more and more on the results of the complement deviation test originally devised by Wassermann. By means of this test our suspicions regarding the *rôle* played by syphilis in such pathological states as locomotor ataxia, general paralysis,

* Towards the expenses of this research a grant was made by the British Medical Association.

aneurysm, and chronic endocarditis have been confirmed. And, further, many conditions, *e.g.*, mental deficiency and epilepsy, in which syphilis was not supposed to be a predominant factor, have been shown, on the strength of this same reaction, to be due not infrequently to the ravages of the spirochæta pallida.

Now, since the truth, or otherwise, of these conceptions regarding the frequency of the disease itself, and the part which it plays in the etiology of many serious pathological changes, depends in great measure, if not entirely, on the specificity or reliability of the Wassermann test, it would seem not out of place here to consider in the first instance the *rationale* of the reaction and the evidence adduced as to its reliability. When many organic substances (*e.g.*, albumen, microbes, or their toxins) are injected into the body, anti-substances are developed, and it is the interaction of the "substance" and this "anti-substance" which gives rise to some of the manifestations of disease. For their interaction, however, another factor, viz., complement— always present in the blood plasma—has been found to be necessary, and it is the application of this knowledge which has led to the modification of the intrathecal treatment of disease of the nervous system. Cerebro-spinal fluid, as shown by Martin and M'Kenzie,[1] does not contain complement; hence, in cerebro- spinal fever, to allow of the antibodies in the antimeningococcic serum exerting their antimicrobic influence on the meningococci, it is necessary to inject at the same time fresh human serum.

This reaction, the combination of substance and anti- substance in the presence of complement, can take place not only *in vivo*, but also *in vitro*, and is specific, *i.e.*, the anti- substance and the particular substance (the so-called antigen) calling it forth alone combine with the absorption of complement. Thus, if complement is absorbed in the presence of a known antigen, it can only have occurred through the agency of its specific anti-substance. This is the *rationale* of the Bordet- Gengou reaction devised for the detection of an anti-substance, and it was for the purpose of discovering specific antibodies in the blood serum in syphilis that Wassermann introduced the test. As at that time spirochætes could not be cultivated, an extract of a congenital syphilitic liver, rich in spirochætes, was used as antigen; but soon afterwards it was shown that an extract of normal liver, of ox liver, or solutions of other chemical substances, *e.g.*, lipoids, acted as efficiently, or even more efficiently, and thus the reaction, or in other words the absorption of complement, could not depend, as was at first believed, on the combination of an antigen with its specific anti-substance. It was soon discovered, too, that normal serum acted to a certain extent in the same way, as did also the serum of patients suffering from leprosy, frambœsia, sleeping sickness, and also, at least according to some writers, malaria.* Nevertheless, it has been demonstrated that in this country at least it is the syphilitic serum which most actively deviates, or absorbs, complement. Thus the test is, as Professor Muir says, a quantitative and not a qualitative one, and the important point for us to decide is how much complement must be absorbed by a certain amount of the serum before we can look upon it with suspicion. We suppose everyone will admit that it is wiser to make the requirements so high that the tendency will be rather to under-estimate than to over-estimate the number of what we call positive reactions.

Many attempts have been made to intensify the power of the syphilitic serum to absorb or deviate complement, and make it more markedly divergent in its behaviour from that of normal serum. Browning, Cruickshank, and M'Kenzie,[2] after much labour, were successful in their endeavours in this line, and they have shown, on the grounds of very extensive and numerous examinations, that lecithin and cholesterin cause a syphilitic serum to become much stronger in deviating complement, while affecting not at all, or only very slightly, the behaviour or power of normal serum. These authors and their colleagues at the Pathological Institute of Glasgow University, working in very different fields of medicine, have accumulated during the past few years a vast amount of material, and this Browning[3] has recently brought together and published.

As we have throughout practised the Browning, Cruickshank, and M'Kenzie technique, often spoken of as the Glasgow method, we will take the liberty of quoting some of the figures published by Browning. He and his co-workers showed that a positive

---

* Fletcher has recently shown that with the Glasgow technique a positive Wassermann reaction is not obtained in malaria (*Lancet*, 13th June, 1914, p. 1677).

reaction was obtained in 95 per cent of cases of syphilis in the secondary stage, in 75 per cent of cases in the tertiary stage, in 50 per cent of cases in the latent stage, and in 95 per cent of cases of congenital syphilis with lesions. In a series of 364 children selected because there was nothing to suggest syphilis either on physical or historical grounds, a positive reaction was only obtained in 13, or 3·5 per cent. We ourselves have investigated a similar series of 22 apparently healthy children, and did not obtain a positive reaction in a single case. These figures show pretty conclusively that the test, although not specific, is practically only found in syphilis.

No one, it must be admitted, will have much experience of this biological test without encountering difficulties and disappointments. Sometimes a complement which is deviated too easily or only with great difficulty will be met with, and then no reliance can be placed on the results. The antigen, too, varies slightly in its behaviour, and therefore it is always advisable, indeed, according to Browning, imperative, to compare the conduct of any serum under question with that of a known syphilitic and non-syphilitic serum. Only a method in which all these factors are thoroughly controlled can be relied upon, and, in our opinion, the Glasgow technique fulfils such requirements. In any series of examinations so many cases can be pronounced as definitely positive, and so many as definitely negative, but there always remains a proportion of doubtful or borderland cases. In such it is advisable to repeat the examination, but not infrequently this is done with no happier result. In our tables we have classified our results under these three headings. This does not necessarily detract from the great value of the test, but simply impresses us with the fact that it is an aid to diagnosis which must be left in the hands of a recognised expert. If this be done, and especially if the laboratory worker has in addition an intimate knowledge of the clinical aspects of his cases, nothing but help of the highest order can accrue from its use. The Wassermann test is of value not only in the diagnosis of anomalous forms of the disease, but also in gauging the efficacy of our treatment. In the present paper we intend to demonstrate by its aid the great importance of syphilis as an etiological factor in some not infrequent conditions of hitherto unknown cause.

Eczema oris syphiliticum.—Last year H. F. Watson and one of us (L. F.)[4] described a variety of eczema in the neighbourhood of the mouth, met with chiefly in children, but also in adults, which in consequence of the results of the serological tests we named *eczema oris syphiliticum.* When we published an account of this disease we had met with twenty-one examples, in all of whom or in the members of their families the blood reacted positively. Since then some twelve more cases have come under our notice, and all again have reacted positively, thus supporting our previous statement that this variety of eczema was syphilitic in nature. The first case observed was treated with mercury and neo-salvarsan, and after several intramuscular injections of the latter drug the eczema disappeared without leaving any trace, and the blood test became negative. Ten months later, however, this same patient again came under observation with the condition as bad as ever, and examination of the blood revealed once more a positive reaction. Extended experience but confirms our published opinion as to the specificity of the lesion.

Dermatologists and others have doubted the correctness of our view, and some have even stated that what we were describing was merely the scarring from the rhagades occurring in the early stages of the disease. But in our opinion there is not the slightest resemblance between the cicatrices from these early or initial manifestations and the condition of *eczema oris syphiliticum.*

Eczema oris syphiliticum is a diffuse infiltration of the skin around the mouth, usually situated at one or both angles, and continuous with the mucous membrane of the lips. It may be dry and scaly, or moist with the discharge accumulating in the form of crusts, and when it heals, as we have seen it do under the influence of antispecific treatment, not the slightest vestige of its existence remains. (Plates illustrative of the lesion are published in *The Medical Annual*, 1914.)

Congenital heart disease.—Congenital heart disease is in most text-books ascribed either to some form of aplasia or to foetal endocarditis, but concerning the nature of the toxin which induces this latter condition the majority are silent. As long ago as 1875 Coupland[5] showed before the Pathological Society of London the organs of a child of three months, which presented, in addition to gummata of the liver, lung, and myocardium, a patent interventricular septum. Since then many writers, including Lancereaux, Warner, Eger, Virchow, Hutchinson, and Fournier[6] have recorded cases of morbus cæruleus, which on clinical grounds alone they ascribed to syphilis. With the introduction of the Wassermann test a fresh impetus has been given towards the solution of this question, but the findings of different workers have markedly varied. Browning[3] records the observations of Watson, who found the Wassermann reaction positive in seventeen out of twenty-five cases, and concluded that syphilis was responsible for much congenital cardiac disease. Holt,[7] more recently, investigated a large series of sick children, and in six cases of this malady did not obtain one positive reaction.

We have been able to collect in all eleven cases of congenital cardiac disease, and have subjected either the children themselves or their parents to the serological test. As will be seen from the accompanying abstract of cases (No. 1) the mischief was characterised by cyanosis, clubbing of the fingers, and a loud murmur in five of the patients. In two of them instead of cyanosis there was marked pallor. In not one child were specific stigmata noted, yet in seven of the patients themselves, and in one of the parents of other two of the cases, a positive Wassermann reaction was obtained, thus showing evidence of syphilis in nine of our cases, or 81 per cent.

I.—ABSTRACT OF CASES OF CONGENITAL HEART DISEASE.

M = male, F = female.

CASE 1.—M., 1½ years. Great cyanosis with clubbing of fingers and toes; heart enlarged to right and left. No cardiac murmur; second pulmonic sound audible. Saddle nose (?) Wassermann strongly + in mother and child.

CASE 2.—F., 11 months. Cyanosis. V.S. basal murmur with absence of second pulmonic sound. History of rash on body at age of 3 weeks. No specific stigmata. Wassermann strongly + in child.

CASE 3.—F., 15 months. Cyanosis when crying, but at other times unduly pale. Heart enlarged with apex 1 inch outside nipple line in sixth space. V.S. murmur loudest in pulmonic area, with absence of second pulmonic sound.   Previous child was stillborn.   Wassermann negative in child and both parents.

CASE 4.—M., 2 years.   Cyanosis of face, hands, and feet, with clubbing of fingers and toes.   Heart enlarged.   V.S. murmur over tricuspid area; second aortic and pulmonic sounds audible.   No specific stigmata.   Wassermann strongly +.

CASE 5.—M., 14 months.   Marked cyanosis with clubbing of fingers and toes.   Heart enlarged.   V.S. basal murmur with second pulmonic sound audible.   No specific stigmata.   Wassermann strongly +.

CASE 6.—F., 4 years.   Great cyanosis, clubbing of fingers and toes.   Heart enlarged to right.   V.S. murmur all over precordium with second pulmonic sound quite audible.   Child died; no *post-mortem.*   Wassermann strongly +.

CASE 7.—F., $1\frac{10}{12}$ years.   Slight cyanosis.   Loud V.S. murmur audible all over precordium and back of chest.   Second pulmonic sound loud.   Saddle nose with chronic rhinitis.   Died of broncho-pneumonia.   No *post-mortem.*   Wassermann weakly + in mother and definitely + in child.

CASE 8.—F., 2 months.   Pallor; no enlargement of heart.   V.S. basal murmur, with loud second pulmonic sound.   Wassermann + in father.

CASE 9.—M., $5\frac{4}{12}$ years.   Extreme degree of cyanosis, clubbing of fingers and toes.   Heart enlarged to right and left.   Loud V.S. murmur all over precordium.   Second pulmonic sound sharp.   Wassermann + in mother and child.

CASE 10.—F., 6 months.   Pallor; attacks of dyspnœa.   Heart very much enlarged to right and left.   No murmur; second pulmonic sound audible.   Died; no *post-mortem.*   Wassermann weakly + in mother; child not examined.

CASE 11.—F., 2 years.   Slight cyanosis; no clubbing of fingers or toes.   Great enlargement of heart.   Basal systolic thrill.   Loud V.S. murmur, with absent second pulmonic sound.   Wassermann negative in child and also in mother.

It is impossible to say whether the lesions in these cases were due to aplasia or endocarditis, because the majority of the patients are still alive, and in none of those that died was an opportunity for a *post-mortem* examination obtained. Theoretically there seems no reason why both types of the mischief could not be due to the spirochæte, since not improbably the same factor which would call forth an

inflammatory lesion in a more or less fully developed organ
would interfere with the normal growth of the developing
organ.   It is well known, too, that the myocardium of the
foetus is a favourite medium for the treponema pallida.
Warthin[8] has shown that in congenital syphilis the spirochæte
may be found only in the heart, and he describes a patchy
and disseminated myocarditis in such cases.   In twelve
examples of congenital syphilis in infants, children, and
adolescents presenting cardiac symptoms he discovered these
changes with the spirochæte in all, and concludes that syphilis
must always be reckoned with in congenital cardiac lesions,
and also in chronic heart disease of children and young adults.
Further research, however, on lines similar to the above is
required to solve this problem.

Spastic diplegia.—Spastic diplegia is another disease which
has of late years been ascribed to syphilis.   We refrain from
speaking of the malady as " Little's disease " because, although
undoubtedly injury at birth, as first pointed out by Little, can
induce meningeal hæmorrhage, with atrophy of the cortex and
secondary degeneration of the pyramidal tracts and consequent
spastic paralysis, many examples of spastic diplegia are met
with in which no history of injury at birth can be obtained.
One of us (L. F.) has observed (in association with Dr. Barclay
Ness) a typical case of spastic diplegia in which there was no
history of a difficult labour or of syphilis (this was before the
introduction of Wassermann's test), and in which minute
examination of the brain and spinal cord revealed aplasia of the
whole motor system from the cerebral cortex to the anterior
horns.
     Dean[9] was perhaps the first to suggest that syphilis might
account for some cases, yet in a series of 15 patients he only
obtained a positive Wassermann reaction in 1.   Holt[7] more
recently did not meet with 1 positive reaction in the course of
the investigation of 8 cases.   During the past two years we
have had opportunities of observing 33 examples of spastic
diplegia at the out-door department of the Glasgow Children's
Hospital, and in 13 a definite positive reaction was obtained,
while in other 2 the reaction was of the borderland type.   In
the following abstract of cases (No. II) is supplied information

regarding the question of injury at birth, the presence of specific stigmata, the evidence of syphilis in the family history, and the result of the serum test in our cases.

II.—Abstract of Cases of Spastic Diplegia.

M = male, F = female.

No. 1.—M., $2\frac{1}{2}$ years. No specific history in mother; no stillbirths or abortions; no injury at birth; no specific stigmata. Wassermann definitely +.

No. 2.—M., 11 years. No specific history in mother; no stillbirths or abortions; no injury at birth; no specific stigmata. Wassermann negative.

No. 3.—M., 2 years. No specific history in mother; no stillbirths or abortions; no injury at birth; no specific stigmata. Wassermann negative.

No. 4.—M., $4\frac{1}{2}$ years. No specific history in mother; no stillbirths or abortions; history of injury at birth; no specific stigmata. Wassermann definitely +.

No. 5.—M., 7 years. No specific history in mother; five miscarriages; no injury at birth; no specific stigmata. Wassermann negative.

No. 6.—F., $1\frac{8}{12}$ years. No specific history in mother; no stillbirths or abortions; no injury at birth; no specific stigmata. Wassermann definitely positive in mother and child.

No. 7.—F., $4\frac{1}{2}$ years. No specific history in mother; one miscarriage; no injury at birth; no specific stigmata. Wassermann negative.

No. 8.—F., 5 years. No specific history in mother; no stillbirths or abortions; history of injury at birth; no specific stigmata. Wassermann negative.

No. 9.*—F., 7 years. No specific history in mother; no stillbirths or abortions; history of injury at birth; no specific stigmata. Wassermann negative in mother and child.

No. 10.—F., $3\frac{1}{2}$ years. No specific history in mother; nine miscarriages; history of injury at birth; no specific stigmata. Wassermann negative.

No. 11.—F., $4\frac{3}{4}$ years. No specific history in mother; no stillbirths

---

* This child is a twin. The other child was born without difficulty, and is quite normal.

or abortions; injury at birth doubtful; No specific stigmata. Wassermann negative.

No. 12.—M., 10 years. No specific stigmata. Wassermann definitely positive.

No. 13.—F., 6 years. Left upper central incisors notched; eczema oris. Wassermann definitely positive.

No. 14.—M., 13 years. No specific history in mother; no stillbirths or abortions; no injury at birth; no specific stigmata. Wassermann negative.

No. 15.—M., 8 years. History of injury at birth; no specific stigmata. Wassermann negative.

No. 16.—F., 14 years. No specific stigmata. Wassermann negative.

No. 17.—M., 13 years. No specific stigmata. Wassermann negative.

No. 18.—M., $10\frac{1}{2}$ years. No specific stigmata. Wassermann negative.

No. 19.—M., $5\frac{1}{2}$ years. Hemiplegia; no specific stigmata. Wassermann definitely +.

No. 20.—M., 2 years. No specific history in mother; no stillbirths or abortions; history of injury at birth; no specific stigmata. Wassermann definitely +.

No. 21.—M., $1\frac{1}{2}$ years. No specific history in mother; no stillbirths or abortions; history of injury at birth; no specific stigmata. Wassermann negative.

No. 22.—M., 3 years. No specific history in mother; no stillbirths or abortions; no injury at birth; no specific stigmata. Wassermann strongly + in mother and child.

No. 23.—F., $2\frac{2}{12}$ years. No specific history in mother; no stillbirths or abortions; history of injury at birth; no specific stigmata. Wassermann negative.

No. 24.—F., $2\frac{1}{2}$ years. No specific history in mother; no stillbirths or abortions; history of injury at birth; no specific stigmata. Wassermann—borderland case.

No. 25.—F., 6 years. No specific history in mother; no stillbirths or abortions; history of injury at birth; no specific stigmata. Wassermann definitely +.

No. 26.—F., $1\frac{3}{12}$ years. No specific history in mother; no stillbirths or abortions; no injury at birth; no specific stigmata. Wassermann strongly + in mother and child.

No. 27.—F., $2\frac{2}{12}$ years. No specific history in mother; no stillbirths or abortions; history of injury at birth; no specific stigmata. Wassermann strongly + in mother and child.

No. 28.—M., $2\frac{4}{12}$ years. No specific history in mother; 1 miscarriage;

history of injury at birth; no specific stigmata. Wassermann—borderland case.

No. 29.—F., $1\frac{2}{12}$ years. No specific history in mother; no stillbirths or abortions; history of injury at birth; no specific stigmata. Wassermann negative in mother and child.

No. 30.—M., 9 years. No specific history in mother; no stillbirths or abortions; hemiplegia; history of injury at birth; no specific stigmata. Wassermann definitely + in mother, weak in child.

No. 31.—F., 7 years. Mother a prostitute, specific history doubtful; no stillbirths or abortions; no specific stigmata. Wassermann definitely +.

No. 32.—F., 4 years. No specific history in mother; no stillbirths or abortions; history of injury at birth; no specific stigmata. Wassermann negative.

No. 33.—F., 2 years. No specific history in mother; no stillbirths or abortions; no injury at birth; no specific stigmata. Wassermann negative in mother and child.

How are we to explain the influence, if any, of syphilis in the etiology of this condition? In many of these cases there is no history of injury at birth, and, as previously mentioned, in one example of the malady *post-mortem* examination lent no support to the idea that a hæmorrhage of the meninges had ever taken place. To the naked eye the cerebral convolutions in this case presented a normal conformation, but minute examination revealed that the motor cells in the Rolandic areas were deficient in number, that the pyramidal tracts were small, and the cells in the anterior cornua not so abundant as normally. In view of the absence of sensory phenomena in this case, and, as a matter of fact, in most examples of this malady, it would seem that the anterior Rolandic areas are the seat of the lesion, while the posterior or motor-sensory escape. It is as though some selective action had been at work. Such is quite possible, indeed not unlikely, when we remember how strictly the spirochæte limits itself to definite tracts in locomotor ataxia. Nevertheless, in congenital syphilis alterations have been described in the cerebral capillaries which would tend to extra-vasation of blood, and we know, too, that in general paralysis there is a change in the meninges characterised by hæmorrhage. Subrazès and Dupérié[10] have shown that the spirochætes in congenital syphilis attack the cerebral capillaries, causing a proliferation of the endothelium and connective tissue with colloid degeneration of the vessel wall. It may be that where there is every likelihood, or even definite proof, of a rupture of vessels being the determining cause, syphilis has been the prime factor in the case. Had the meninges been normal the injury would probably not have been sufficient to bring about extravasation of blood, but in the presence of syphilitic changes a rupture of vessels is very liable to occur. In 15 of our own cases there was definite history of injury at birth, and 5 of these reacted positively to the blood test, whereas in 10, 4 of which reacted positively, this factor could be eliminated, so that syphilis would seem to be almost equally important from an etiological point of view whether there is a history of injury or not. In this connection it is interesting to note that the statistics of Hannes [11] make it very doubtful if difficulty at birth with the production of asphyxia is specially prone to be followed by cerebral mischief. He found that of 150 children born asphyxiated, 3 per cent were mentally abnormal; of 150 children instrumentally delivered but not asphyxiated, 3 per cent were mentally abnormal; and of 150 children born spontaneously and without any accident, 3 per cent were also mentally affected.

Undoubtedly the percentage of positive results in our series is higher than any previously recorded, but this we are inclined to think is due, as was first suggested by Dean,[9] to the early age of most of our cases. The Wassermann reaction wanes as the child gets older, and he surmised that any series of young children would probably give a fairly high percentage of positive results.

Mental deficiency.—The part played by syphilis in idiocy and mental deficiency is a question that has always interested pediatrists and alienists. Before the Wassermann test was introduced, evidence was based on the family history, or on the presence of so-called stigmata, and from a comparatively limited experience of the subject we are not astonished that the majority of authors were inclined to lay little stress on this infection as an etiological factor. Various workers have estimated the frequency of syphilis in mental deficiency very differently—Shuttleworth [12] 1 per cent, and Ziehen [13] 17 per cent.

Although it is a truism that congenitally syphilitic children are unduly slow in developing, comparatively few of the cases of idiocy that one meets with at the out-door department of a children's hospital present specific stigmata. Nor can we expect to receive much help from the family history since it is, in our experience, the exception rather than the rule to obtain evidence of infection of the mother of undoubtedly syphilitic infants. Some writers would hold that stillbirths and miscarriages are strong evidence of the mother being syphilitic, but the truth of this teaching we very much doubt; at least, the statistics which we have been able to collect at the dispensary of the Glasgow Royal Hospital for Sick Children are decidedly against such a story being of any diagnostic value. In 97 syphilitic families 19 per cent of 427 pregnancies ended in abortions or stillbirths, and in 19 non-syphilitic families also 19 per cent of 123 pregnancies ended in a similar fashion. It might seem from these figures that syphilis was not a predominant cause of infantile mortality, but it must be remembered that this ante-natal loss only represents a tithe of the mortality from syphilis, since a great number of children born apparently healthy succumb during the early weeks of life. These figures are, of course, too small to enable us to draw definite conclusions of any kind except that the history of miscarriages is not proof of a syphilitic infection.

With the help of the Wassermann reaction the frequency of syphilis has been found to be greater than previously supposed. Lippmann[14] found 13 per cent of his cases of mental deficiency gave a positive reaction; Dean,[9] 15 per cent; Krober,[15] 21 per cent; Raviart, Breton, Petit, and Cannæ,[16] 30 per cent; Chislett,[17] 57 per cent; and Fraser and Watson[18] found evidence of syphilis in either the patients or their families in 60 per cent of 205 mentally defective and epileptic children. These cases were all of school age, so that the comparatively early age of the children, and the fact that in many instances the families were also investigated, account for the very high proportion of syphilis in the series.

At the Glasgow Sick Children's Dispensary we have taken the opportunity of examining the serum of some 22 mentally deficient and epileptic children, and have obtained a definitely positive Wassermann reaction in 13, *i.e.*, 59 per cent, and in 2 a reaction of the borderland type. (See Table III for details.)

III.—ABSTRACT OF CASES OF MENTAL DEFICIENCY.

M = male, F = female.

No. 1.—F., 4 years. No specific stigmata, no specific history in parents. Wassermann—borderland case.

No. 2.—M., $8\frac{1}{2}$ years. No specific stigmata, no specific history in parents. Wassermann definitely +.

No. 3.—M., $9\frac{1}{2}$ years. Interstitial keratitis and Hutchinson teeth; one stillbirth. Wassermann strongly +.

No. 4.—F., $8\frac{1}{2}$ years. No specific stigmata, no specific history in parents. Wassermann strongly +.

No. 5.—F., $1\frac{3}{4}$ years. No specific stigmata, no specific history in parents. Wassermann strongly +.

No. 6.—M., $7\frac{1}{2}$ years. No specific stigmata, no specific history in parents. Wassermann strongly +.

No. 7.—M., 11 years. No specific stigmata; miscarriages. Wassermann negative.

No. 8.—M., 3 years. No specific stigmata, no specific history in parents. Wassermann definitely +.

No. 9.—M., 5 years. No specific stigmata, no specific history in parents. Wassermann negative.

No. 10.—F., 10 years. No specific stigmata, no specific history in parents. Wassermann negative.

No. 11.—M., 8 years. No specific stigmata, no specific history in parents. Wassermann negative.

No. 12.—M., $2\frac{1}{2}$ years. Epilepsy; no specific history in parents. Wassermann negative.

No. 13.—M., 7 years. No specific history in parents. Wassermann strongly +.

No. 14.—M., $3\frac{3}{4}$ years. No specific history in parents. Wassermann negative.

No. 15.—F., 2 years. No specific stigmata, no specific history in parents. Wassermann strongly +.

No. 16.—F., 3 years. No specific stigmata; two miscarriages. Wassermann definitely +.

No. 17.—F., $1\frac{1}{4}$ years. No specific stigmata; illegitimate child. Wassermann definitely +.

No. 18.—F., $4\frac{3}{4}$ years. No specific stigmata; 1 miscarriage. Wassermann—borderland case.

No. 19.—M., 4 years. No specific stigmata, no specific history in parents. Wassermann strongly +.

No. 20.—F., 5 months. Snuffles? illegitimate child. Wassermann negative.

No. 21.—F., 9 months. No specific stigmata, no specific history in parents. Wassermann definitely +.

No. 22.—M., 1¾ years. No specific stigmata; 2 miscarriages. Wassermann definitely +.

In our series the percentage of positive results is undoubtedly high, and this may be in part explained by the fact that most of the children are, as in Fraser and Watson's series, young. It should be noted that Chislett's, Fraser and Watson's, and our own results are all based on the same Wassermann technique, and, if the method can be relied upon, are confirmatory of one another.

In conclusion, we must state that in spastic diplegia and mental deficiency we could discover no one symptom, or combination of symptoms, other than the Wassermann test, or any point in the history, at least in the vast majority of the cases, by which the syphilitic could be differentiated from the non-syphilitic.

Conclusions.—1. The Wassermann reaction, at least in this country, is practically only found in syphilis, and, if properly controlled, is a test of great diagnostic value.

2. A condition of chronic eczema situated at the angles of the mouth, and invading the mucous membrane of the lips, is often of a syphilitic nature.

3. Congenital heart disease is not infrequently found in patients suffering from congenital syphilis, as evidenced by a positive Wassermann reaction.

4. About 45 per cent of cases of spastic diplegia and 60 per cent of mental defectives also seem to be the subject of congenital syphilis, as evidenced by a positive Wassermann reaction.

LITERATURE.

[1] Martin and M'Kenzie, *Jour. Path. and Bacteriol.*, 1908, No. 12.
[2] Browning, Cruickshank and M'Kenzie, *Diagnosis and Treatment of Syphilis,* London, 1911.
[3] Browning, *Brit. Med. Jour.*, 10th January, 1914.
[4] Findlay and Watson, *Lancet*, 29th March, 1913.
[5] Coupland, *Brit. Med. Jour.*, 1875, vol. ii, p. 542.
[6] Fournier, *Stigmates Dystroph. de L'Hérédo-Syphilis*, Paris, 1898, p. 162 (gives numerous references, with clinical summaries).
[7] Holt, *Amer. Jour. Dis. Children*, September, 1913, p. 167.
[8] Warthin, *Amer. Jour. Med. Sc.*, 1911, vol. 141, p. 398.
[9] Dean, *Proc. Royal Soc. of Med.*, July, 1910·
[10] Subrazès and Dupérié, *Zeit. f. Kinderheilk. Ref.*, 1913, Bd. vii, p. 35.
[11] Hannes, *Zeit. f. Geburt. and Gynœ.*, 1911, Bd. 68, p. 689.
[12] Shuttleworth, *Amer. Jour. of Insanity*, 1888, vol. 64, p. 381.
[13] Ziehen, *Psychiatrie*, Leipzig, 1908, p. 613 (quoted by Fraser and Watson).
[14] Lippmann, *Münch. med. Woch.*, 1909, vol. 56, p. 2416.
[15] Krober, *Med. klin. Woch.*, 1911, vol. 7, p. 1239.
[16] Raviart, &c., *Rev. de Med. Paris*, 1909, No. 28, p. 840.
[17] Chislett, *Jour. Mental Science*, 1911, vol. 57, p. 499.
[18] Fraser and Watson, *Jour. Mental Science*, October, 1913.

THE EDUCATION OF THE SEMI-BLIND.

By W. B. INGLIS POLLOCK, M.D., F.R.F.P.S.,

Assistant Surgeon, Glasgow Eye Infirmary; Ophthalmic Surgeon, Govan Parish School Board.

Acts of Parliament make it necessary that every child should receive an education. Recognising that some children are mentally or physically incapable of receiving education by the ordinary methods, it has been laid down as necessary that these children should be sent to special schools or institutions. For a blind child any parent can demand that the local educational authority provide teachers for it, or send it to a school for the blind. But between the blind and the normal sighted there are many children with more or less defective vision. Ophthalmic surgeons have also pointed out for many years that myopia and the cases of blindness resulting from it are nearly all due to the methods of education.

The modern lighting of schoolrooms, the school desks, the size of the type in school books, and the institution of medical inspection and treatment of school children have all arisen from the efforts to prevent the development of myopia. These improvements have already lowered the percentage of myopes, and the amount of short sight among school children, but they are not sufficient. These subjects have been dealt with by me in previous papers.[1] It is now six years since the late London School Board opened an experimental class for the education of high myopes by methods devised by Mr. Bishop Harman, their chief oculist. The class was such a success that children suffering from other diseases were soon admitted to it, and other centres had to be opened. These special classes are now to be found in many of the larger towns in England, where the Chief Medical Officer to the Board of Education has warmly supported them from the first. In this paper it is hoped to show what kind of cases are suitable, and to give a short description of the methods of education employed in these special classes.

The children may be divided into two groups. The first group is composed of children suffering from various diseases of the eyes, in which the eyesight is so defective that they are unable to read ordinary print or even specially large type. A number of these children are affected with syphilis of the eyes. Syphilitic iritis and keratitis are not uncommon; but retinitis, choroiditis, and optic neuritis are more rarely found. These affections are generally late manifestations of congenital syphilis, and are more or less amenable to treatment, which, however, may take three years or longer before useful vision is obtained. The following is a typical case:—

J. L., aged 12 years, was brought to me in February, 1910, suffering from syphilitic corneo-iritis. The cornea of both eyes was more or less opaque. The pupils were irregular, and occupied with membrane. The vision of the right eye was equal to counting fingers at 6 feet, and the left to fingers at 4 feet. He was treated internally with mercury and potassio-tartrate of iron, and given yellow oxide of mercury and atropine sulphate for local application. In November, 1911, or almost two years later, he could read by the aid of glasses the three largest letters of the test types at the normal distance, and a moderate-sized type of print. He was very anxious to get back to school, and it was a pleasure to observe how keen he was to be able to read.

Children suffering from congenital cataract may have fairly good vision, *e.g.*, cases with $\frac{6}{18}$ or even $\frac{6}{24}$ and $\frac{6}{36}$ with Snellen's test types can usually read ordinary print. Many ophthalmic surgeons advise such children not to have the lens removed so long as the cataract remains stationary, because after the operation the power of accommodation is lost, and they are therefore entirely dependent upon glasses; one glass being required for distant vision and another for near work. Other surgeons advise the operation to be performed if the vision is below $\frac{6}{18}$ with the test types, at least in one eye. The removal of congenital cataract is undertaken in several stages, and if it is done entirely by discission, they may cover a period of six months or a year. Some cases take much longer, particularly when the operation has been followed by iritis or cyclitis. Children are also kept off near work when the cataract is in a doubtful stage, and the surgeon is uncertain whether to operate or not, the period of observation extending to a year or longer. After the removal of the cataract it is often some time before the child is able to read ordinary print.

Optic neuritis is rare in childhood. When the condition is due to brain disease, tumour, tuberculosis, meningitis, or to renal disease, the child must be excluded from school entirely. Some cases are associated with uncorrected errors of refraction. Others follow influenza and the various forms of the exanthemata. In other cases it may be very difficult to establish the etiology. Complete rest from all reading and writing is necessary in every case, and may extend to a period of two or more years.

Nystagmus is not uncommon in childhood; it is often associated with albinism, congenital cataract, corneal opacities, retinitis, choroiditis, optic atrophy, or high degrees of astigmatism. The vision is comparatively poor in most cases, rarely rising above $\frac{6}{60}$ with the test types. As the child grows older the eyesight may improve. But for several years or during his entire school life the vision is so defective that the child is unable for ordinary print.

Corneal nebulæ and leucomata are frequently present in childhood, but often decrease or even disappear as the child grows up to adult life. The absorption of opacities in the cornea may be hastened by massage accompanied by the use of dionin, fibrolysin, iodolysin, yellow oxide of mercury, and other drugs. In a number of cases the eyesight is too defective during the school age for the reading of ordinary books.

Many children suffer from phlyctenular or strumous ophthalmia, an affection which is specially prone to recur again and again. The relapses frequently occur when the children return to school, and they are therefore often absent from school for prolonged periods. If these cases could be kept from all book work, and spend a large proportion of their time in the open air, the relapses would become much rarer. Several educational authorities have established open-air classes, or classes in rooms which are entirely open to the air on one side.

The second group is composed of children suffering from excessively high degrees of myopia. They are able to read ordinary print by holding it close to the eyes, which increases their myopia, and thus a vicious circle is set up. If proper precautions are not taken in their education during school life, the condition tends to progress more or less rapidly, and leads ultimately in many cases to blindness. The following are cases of myopia :—

. J. M'A., aged 10 years, was seen by me first in January, 1913, with high myopia. He was kept on atropine for nine months, and was not allowed to read or attend school. By this means the myopia was reduced in amount, and his vision had improved. In September, 1913, in response to his urgent request, I allowed him to begin reading and to attend school, at the same time prescribing glasses. He was then able to see with the glasses, $\frac{6}{24}$. In March, 1914, or six months later, he returned for stronger glasses. On examination he was found to be almost blind. His vision was $\frac{1}{60}$. He is now again under similar treatment, and the eyesight is slowly recovering; but it will be three years or more before he can be allowed to look at an ordinary book. In other words, this means that he will not receive any education by ordinary school methods.

M. D., aged 5 years, was brought to the Govan School Clinic in February, 1914, with high myopia. In the right eye central vision was destroyed by a patch of retino-choroidal atrophy occupying the macula. In the left eye there was thinning of the choroid at the macula, with pigment in the retina. His vision was $\frac{0.5}{60}$. He is a most intelligent child, and it has been a matter of great difficulty to keep him away from books. He has been under atropine without intermission since that date, and excluded from school. It may be four or more years before he can safely be allowed to read or attempt to do fine work.

Present educational methods.—Children suffering from these diseases of the eyes are being treated by educational authorities in three different ways.

By the first method they are permitted to attend school, but are not allowed to do any near work. This means that they sit in the class and pick up all the information they can. In the higher standards, where writing occupies a great deal of the time, they are not able to keep pace with the other children. Many of the headmasters prefer that these cases should be excluded from school, since their presence interferes to some extent with the routine of the classes. Nevertheless, I believe that these children are better to be attending school than outside it altogether, as will be shown immediately.

By the second method children with serious defects of vision or diseases of the eye may be entirely excluded from school. This is very unsatisfactory, because it often means exclusion for prolonged periods, even up to three or more years in a number of cases. The children are apt to loaf about the streets or to become household-drudges. If they are at all studious, and many of them are, they read books or papers at home, probably under the worst conditions of lighting and print, and the very object of exclusion is defeated. There is also a real loss to the child in being deprived of the communal life of the school, as it has been called. The children are frequently most anxious to get back to their classes.

By the third method such cases may be sent to a school for the blind. This has been done by some school authorities; but it has very serious drawbacks. The children lead the life of the blind, and acquire their habits, while retaining a certain amount of vision, which might be augmented by appropriate treatment, and would become of great value to them in after life. They learn Braille, which is, in my opinion, a pure waste of time for them. Moreover, when the teacher's back is turned, these children look down and peer into the Braille impressions, which are much more difficult to see than ordinary print. At home they use the ordinary books. Finally, they are liable to be stigmatised as blind children. In these days of Employer's Liability Acts few employers can run the risk of taking a child from a blind school.

Classes for the semi-blind.—It was for these reasons that Mr. Bishop Harman[2] devised the classes for the semi-blind. He lays it down as an absolute essential for success that the class shall be placed in an ordinary school for normal children, and worked as an integral part of this school. The scheme of work is as follows:—

1. Oral teaching is given with the normal children for such subjects as can be taught orally. This keeps the children up to the normal standard in their work. They are placed in the front seats in these classes.

2. All literary work must be learned without books, paper, or slates. The special classroom has a band of blackboard placed all round the room, 3 to 6 feet above the floor level. It does not require to be adjustable, as the teachers and the scholars can each reach that height. Bishop Harman has designed an inexpensive desk, which acts as a table for working, on, and when it is raised forms a blackboard. The first batch were made by the pupils of one of the deaf schools. All letters and figures must be large, and made free-arm fashion, so that the child stands back from the board at full arm's length. To obtain more permanent records for the older children large sheets of black paper are employed, and chalk is used. The chalk should be practically dustless. The oldest children are allowed to print their lessons, employing 1 and 2 inch types. Two sets of printing are provided for each class.

3. A full use is made of every kind of handicraft that will develop attention, method, and skill, with the minimum use of the eyes. Girls are taught knitting by touch, but are not allowed to use their eyes. They soon learn to do it automatically. The junior children, both boys and girls, are taught paper folding, stick laying, and felt weaving in colours. Seniors and some juniors are taught modelling maps and rough wood work. Advanced boys are given advanced basket work, bent iron work, and the making of nets, and girls cooking, laundry, and housewifery. The boys may be taught to become small traders, collectors, agents, and visitors, occupations which do not strain the eyes.

4. Drill and games enter largely into the curriculum. Some games are made instructive by drawing large scale maps on canvas laid on the floor, and making the children move from place to place as if travelling.

Conclusions.—The establishment of such classes allows children with serious defects of vision to obtain a good education, with all the benefits of regular school work. The medical treatment they may be receiving does not interfere with their work, nor do these special methods of education harm their eyes. The children only require to attend their dispensary or school clinic once a month in many cases. Older children can easily find their way to a centre. Younger ones are brought by their parents or by older children, or by a guide.

Many of the parents welcome the classes, since by these means their children resume school attendance, and they help by watching the children at home. The intelligence of the children has already been mentioned, and they can be relied upon to take up their part enthusiastically. Those who have been so defective that they cannot see their books rush at work immediately their sight recovers, and it will be a great benefit if they have, by the establishment of such classes, managed to keep up with their playmates.

Each case should be watched carefully. Their myopia or disease will probably improve to such an extent that there will be little fear of its progressing. The worst cases will pass the critical period of 7 to 14 years, when the eyes are soft and tender, receiving an all-round education, but without books.

The establishment of such classes will undoubtedly act as a powerful preventive of many of the cases of separation of the retina and macular atrophy resulting from myopia, which end in blindness, and are commonly seen in our hospitals and in private practice.

I trust that everyone with an influence in scholastic matters will aid in the establishment of such special classes in every town and county in the country.

REFERENCES.

[1] "The Eyesight of School Children," *Trans. Roy. Glasg. Philos. Soc.*, 1906; "The Relationship of Myopia to School Work," *Glasg. Med. Journ.*, November, 1907; "Visual Acuity of School Children," *Brit. Med. Journ.*, 2nd October, 1909.

[2] Bishop Harman, *Trans. Roy. Soc. Med.* (Section of Ophthalmology), 1913-14.

ŒSOPHAGOTOMY FOR THE REMOVAL OF A TOOTH–PLATE.*

BY WALKER DOWNIE, M.B., F.R.F.P.S.,

Lecturer on Diseases of the Throat and Nose, Glasgow University
and Western Infirmary.

I SHOW you this evening a gentleman, aged 24 years, on whom I performed œsophagotomy for the removal of a tooth-plate, which had become firmly impacted in the gullet.

As the result of an accident he had lost a central incisor tooth, which he had had replaced by an artificial one attached to a vulcanite plate. The artificial tooth had in turn got lost, but he continued to wear the vulcanite plate.

On the evening of Friday, 25th August, he bought a syphon of lemonade, and on his way home he attempted to relieve his thirst by taking a drink direct from the syphon. The fluid entered his mouth with greater force than he anticipated, an attack of violent coughing followed, accompanied by a sense of suffocation, and he thought that the tooth-plate had gone down his throat. He went to an infirmary late that night, where examination with x-rays gave no indication of the presence of a foreign body, nor could the doctor who examined him discover it by the use of the instruments at hand. The patient left the infirmary next morning at his own request, although he still had considerable pain on swallowing. The pain on swallowing continued, but he thought it was probably due to injury caused by the passage downwards of the tooth-plate, and the subsequent attempts to reach and remove it, rather than to its continued presence. He therefore did not consult another doctor until ten days had gone past, when he called on Dr. James Stevenson, of Clydebank, who referred him to me.

* Read at a meeting of the Northern Medical Society held on 6th October, 1914.

By the gentle passage of a bougie, the presence of the tooth-plate was detected at a distance of 9 inches from the incisors. Bromide of potassium was prescribed until he could come into a home for œsophagoscopy and removal of the foreign body. He went into a home on 9th September, and on the same evening was examined with the œsophagoscope. When the plate was brought into view it was found that the rounded roughened anterior edge was uppermost, and that the free extremities of the plate expanded the gullet laterally, causing the former to be firmly fixed.

The plate was caught with tube forceps, by which attempts were made to remove it, by pulling upwards gently, by raising one edge and depressing the other; and other methods of manipulation were employed, but it could not be dislodged. Attempts were then made to break the plate with cutting forceps, but these attempts were also futile. I then determined to do an œsophagotomy for its removal, but postponed the operation until the gullet walls had recovered from the results of the attempts to remove the plate by the direct method.

On 15th September, with the patient under chloroform, and assisted by Dr. W. Walls Christie, I performed a left lateral œsophagotomy. Even when the plate was exposed it was found to be so firmly impacted that it could not be extracted, so I broke off one end with forceps, then tilted the plate round and removed it. A soft rubber stomach tube was then passed through the nose, and the skin at the upper end of the incision only was brought together with two sutures. The wound was otherwise left open, and lightly packed with iodoform gauze.

The tube was kept in position for six days, and through it the patient was given hot water, milk, and soups. The tube was withdrawn on 21st September, when he could swallow with ease, and no food escaped through the wound. Two days later—that is, on the ninth day after operation—the patient went home with the wound almost healed.

This is the fourth case of œsophagotomy which I have done for the removal of a dental plate fixed by hooklets, or otherwise firmly impacted in the gullet, and each patient has recovered completely, with no subsequent œsophageal discomfort. It is important in the performance of the operation to cause as little injury to the gullet as possible before and during the operation, and so to shape the wound in the neck as to prevent the retention of any discharge. It is also very important to treat the wound as an open wound.

The plate in this case measured $2\frac{1}{5}$ inches (5·5 cm.) from one extremity to another, and while there were no metallic bands or hooklets, each end terminated in a comparatively sharp point, which, by penetrating the walls of the gullet, enabled it to become so firmly fixed as to defeat the attempts made to remove it through the œsophagoscope.

Obituary.

WILLIAM DOUGLAS ERSKINE, M.B., C.M. Glasg., UDDINGSTON.

WE regret to announce the death of Major (retired) W. D. Erskine, Royal Army Medical Corps, which occurred on 24th October. Major Erskine, who studied at the University of Glasgow, took the degrees of M.B., C.M., in 1887, and afterwards became house surgeon, first in the Glasgow Royal Infirmary, and, later, in the Royal Infirmary, Dundee. Entering the Army Medical Service, he had attained the rank of Major at the time of his retirement, which, until recently, was spent in Bournemouth. He returned a short time ago to Scotland, and took up residence in Uddingston, where his death, the result of an accident upon the railway line, took place at the age of 50 years.

WILLIAM FENWICK, M.D. Glasg., ROME.

WE regret to announce the death of Dr. William Fenwick, which occurred on 26th October. A student of Glasgow University, Dr. Fenwick took the degree of M.D. in 1864, and in 1872 he became a Fellow of the Faculty of Physicians and Surgeons of Glasgow. He had for many years an extensive practice in Pollokshields and Strathbungo, but retired from it about fifteen years ago. Since his retirement he had lived in Rome, where he died after a brief illness at the age of 80 years.

CURRENT TOPICS.

UNIVERSITY OF GLASGOW: GRADUATION CEREMONY. — A graduation ceremony was held at the University on 14th November, when the following .medical degrees were conferred:—

DOCTORS OF MEDICINE (M.D.)

I. WITH HONOURS.

George Herbert Clark, M.B., Ch.B.
Wm. MacAdam, M.A., B.Sc., M.B., Ch.B.
John William M'Nee, M.B., Ch.B.
John Boyd Orr, M.A., B.Sc., M.B., Ch.B.
William David Henderson Stevenson, M.A., M.B., Ch.B.

II. WITH COMMENDATION.

David Rutherford Adams, M.B., Ch.B.
William Barrie Brownlie, M.B., Ch.B.
Albert William Gregorson, M.B., Ch.B.

III. ORDINARY DEGREES.

John Ewing Adam, M.B., C.M.
Gertrude Jane Campbell, M.B., Ch.B.
James Alphonsus Joseph Conway, M.B., Ch.B.
Robert Douglas, M.A., M.B., Ch.B.
Gilbert Garrey, M.B., Ch.B.
Alexander Gibson Henderson, M.B., Ch.B.
William Johnstone, M.B., Ch.B.
John Wilson Mathie, M.B., C.M.
Henry Joseph Milligan, M.B., Ch.B.
Frank Anderson Murray, M.B., Ch.B.
William Seaton Paterson, M.B., C.M.
William Wallace, M.A., M.B., C.M.

Edin., India; Cromwell Gamble, M.B., Ch.B.Edin., Ireland; James William Edington, M.B., Ch.B.Edin., Dowlan, Coldingham; Stephen Ramchandra Rao, F.R.C.S.Edin., &c., India; Lakshmi Prasad Chaliha, F.R.F.P. & S.G., &c., India; John Hamilton Boag, M.B., Ch.B.Edin., Edinburgh.

The quarterly examinations of the above Board, held in Edinburgh, were concluded on 20th October with the following results:—

Final examination.—The following candidates, having passed the final examination, were admitted L.R.C.P.E., L.R.C.S.E., L.R.F.P. & S.G.:—Allan Beresford Hawkins, British West Indies; Florence Winifred Heyworth, Liverpool; Norman Hamilton Brewster, British West Indies; William Henry O'Grady, Co. Mayo; John Ramsay Fleming, Airdrie; Gerald Christopher Stanley Perera, Ceylon; William Clarke Fraser, Dundee; Arthur Edwin James, Auckland, New Zealand; Leonard Owen Weinman, Colombo; Arthur Alexander Murison, Dumbarton; John Martin, Glasgow; Gwilym Llewelyn Pierce, Llangollen; William Smith O'Loughlin, Limerick; and Khusru Roostamji Mehta, Calcutta; and 4 passed in medicine, 10 in surgery, 12 in midwifery, and 11 in medical jurisprudence.

APPOINTMENTS.—The following appointments have recently been made:—

J. Fletcher, M.B., C.M., D.P.H.Glasg. (1890), to be District Medical Officer to the Cockermouth Union.

Alexander MacLennan, M.B., C.M.Glasg. (1894), to be Consulting Surgeon to the County Council of Lanarkshire.

M. Macnicol, M.D.Glasg. (M.B., 1893), to be Certifying Factory Surgeon for the Leven District, County of Fife.

H. J. Milligan, M.B., Ch.B.Glasg. (1905), D.P.H., to be Tuberculosis Officer and Deputy Medical Officer of Health to the Borough of Bootle.

Royal Navy (27th October): To be Surgeons for temporary service in His Majesty's Fleet—D. K. Adams, M.B., Ch.B.Glasg. (1914); H. G. Anderson, L.R.C.P. & S.E., L.R.F.P.S.G. (1907); R. A. Barlow, B.Sc., M.B., Ch.B.Glasg. (1913); W. G. Clark, M.B., Ch.B.Glasg. (1910); G. Cochran, M.B., Ch.B.Glasg. (1911); R. W. Brander, M.B., Ch.B.Glasg. (1914); W. W. Rorke, M.B., Ch.B.Glasg. (1909); T. L. G. Stewart, M.B., Ch.B.Glasg. (1911);

C. L. Sutherland, M.B., Ch.B.Glasg. (1910); G. D. Muir, M.B., Ch.B.Glasg. (1905); J. C. Watt, M.B., Ch.B.Glasg. (1913).

9th November: Staff Surgeons A. A. Forrester, M.B., Ch.B. Glasg. (1897), and W. W. Keir, M.B., Ch.B.Glasg. (1898), to be Fleet Surgeons, with seniority of 8th November.

18th November: Temporary Lieutenants T. L. Stewart, M.B., Ch.B.Glasg. (1911), to *Victory*, additional for Royal Naval Division, to date 17th November; G. M. Fraser, M.B., Ch.B. Glasg. (1908), to *Victory*, additional for disposal, to date 19th November.

20th November: Surgeon C. W. F. Greenhill, M.B., Ch.B. Glasg. (1912), to *Columbine*, additional for Queensferry Sick Quarters, to date 24th November.

Royal Army Medical Corps (20th October): Lieutenant R. W. Simpson, M.B., Ch.B.Glasg (1906), to be Captain.

26th October: To be temporary Lieutenants—J. W. M'Leod, M.B. Ch.B.Glasg. (1908); D. R. Mitchell, M.B., Ch.B.Glasg. (1904); J. H. M'Nicol, M.B., Ch.B.Glasg. (1909); D. W. Hunter, M.B., Ch.B.Glasg. (1901); J. S. Somerville, M.B., Ch.B.Glasg. (1909); W. B. Watson, M.B., Ch.B.Glasg. (1907); J. M. Forsyth, M.B., Ch.B.Glasg. (1912).

27th October: Scottish Horse Mounted Brigade Field Ambulance—S. M. Sloan, M.B., Ch.B.Glasg. (1897), to be Lieut.-Colonel; G. B. Buchanan, M.B., C.M.Glasg. (1893), F.R.F.P.S., to be Captain. Attached to Unit other than Medical Unit— Lieutenant J. M'Houl, M.B., Ch.B.Glasg. (1904), to be Captain.

28th October: 1st Lowland Field Ambulance—A. W. Sutherland, M.B., Ch.B.Glasg. (1903); G. B. Eadie, M.D.Glasg. (M.B., 1901); and P. J. Moir, M.B., Ch.B.Glasg. (1914), to be Lieutenants.

30th October: To be temporary Lieutenants—G. W. Milne, M.D.Glasg. (M.B., 1901); J. A. Smith, M.B., Ch.B.Glasg. (1913).

3rd November: Major J. S. M'Naught, M.D.Glasg. (M.B., 1890), to be Lieutenant-Colonel. Lowland Mounted Brigade Field Ambulance—A. M. Young, M.B., Ch.B.Glasg. (1913), to be Lieutenant.

5th November: To be temporary Lieutenants—M. J. Murray, M.B., Ch.B.Glasg. (1912); W. H. Brown, M.D.Glasg. (M.B. 1901); A. T. M'Whirter, M.B., Ch.B.Glasg. (1910); D. W. Reid, M.B.,

Ch.B.Glasg. (1912); T. T. Rankin, M.D.Glasg. (M.B., 1905); J. T. W. Stewart, M.B., Ch.B.Glasg. (1911).

14th November: To be temporary Lieutenants—D. N. Knox, M.B., Ch.B.Glasg. (1909); J. B. Orr, M.B., Ch.B.Glasg. (1912); J. G. Duncanson, M.B., C.M.Glasg. (1892).

Territorial Force: 2nd Lowland Field Ambulance—J. W. Burton, M.B., Ch.B.Glasg. (1912), to be Lieutenant. 4th Scottish General Hospital—J. R. Riddell, F.R.F.P.S., to be Captain. Attached to Unit other than Medical Unit—G. J. Wilson, M.B., Ch.B.Glasg. (1911), to be Lieutenant.

16th November: To be temporary Lieutenants—H. Y. Riddell, M.B., Ch.B.Glasg. (1911); P. Drummond, M.B., Ch.B.Glasg. (1910); W. A. Hislop, M.B., Ch.B.Glasg. (1909); A. G. Gilchrist, M.B., Ch.B. Glasg. (1909); T. B. Johnstone, L.R.C.P. & S.G., L.R.F.P.S.G. (1910); P. H. Robertson, M.B., Ch.B.Glasg. (1903).

18th November: To be temporary Lieutenants—A. R. Muir, M.B., Ch.B.Glasg. (1911); A. Hunter, M.B., Ch.B.Glasg. (1906).

NEW JUSTICES OF THE PEACE.—The following amongst other appointments to the Commission of the Peace for the County of the City of Glasgow have been made by His Majesty the King on the recommendation of Sir D. M. Stevenson, Bart., during his tenure of the office of Lord Provost and as Lord Lieutenant of the County of the City of Glasgow :—F. Stewart Campbell, M.D. Glasg. (M.B., 1888); David Coutts, M.B., C.M.Glasg. (1891); Ebenezer Duncan, M.D. Glasg., F.R.F.P.S.; J. P. Granger, F.R.C.S.E.; William Macfarlane, M.B., C.M.Glasg. (1881); John M'Kie, M.B., C.M. Glasg. (1890); Samuel M'Lean, M.B., C.M. Glasg. (1898); P. J. O'Hare, M.B., Ch.B. Glasg. (1906).

ROYAL FACULTY OF PHYSICIANS AND SURGEONS.—The annual meeting of the Fellows of the Royal Faculty of Physicians and Surgeons of Glasgow was held in their hall, St. Vincent Street, on 2nd November. Dr. John Barlow was re-elected President; Dr. Ebenezer Duncan, Visitor; Dr. W. G. Dun, Treasurer; and Dr. Alexander Napier, Honorary Librarian. The following new Councillors were elected:—Dr. James A. Adams, Dr. A. Freeland Fergus, and Dr. Robert Jardine. Dr. J. H. Macdonald and Dr. George M'Intyre were the new elections to the Board of Examiners for the Fellowship. Mr. George M'Intyre was appointed to the Finance Committee, and Dr. A. Maitland Ramsay to the Library Committee. Dr. Leonard Findlay and Dr. William H. Manson were appointed Inspectors of Drugs. Dr. J. Wallace Anderson and Mr. D. N. Knox were the new appointments as Managers of Glasgow Royal Infirmary, and Mr. A. G. Faulds was appointed Director of Glasgow Asylum for the Blind.

The Fellows unanimously agreed to subscribe 100 guineas to the Prince of Wales's Fund and 25 guineas to the Belgian Relief Fund.

GLASGOW NORTHERN MEDICAL SOCIETY.—The first meeting of this Society for session 1914-15 was held in the Royal Philosophical Rooms, 207 Bath Street, on 6th October, 1914, the President, Dr. Alex. Dickson, in the chair.

It was reported that the Hon. Treasurer, Dr. James H. Martin, had been called up with the Territorial Forces, and Dr. Stanley Richmond was unanimously elected Interim Hon. Treasurer.

To help to alleviate distress occasioned by the war it was unanimously agreed that the Society make the following donations:—The National Relief Fund, £5, 5s.; the Belgian Relief Fund, £5, 5s.; the Red Cross Society (Scottish Section), £5, 5s.

Dr. Walker Downie showed a patient from whose œsophagus he had removed an impacted tooth-plate by œsophagotomy. His remarks upon the case will be found as an original article upon another page.

Major Alex. MacLennan, R.A.M.C. (T.), described several interesting cases in the wards of the Glasgow Military General Hospital. He showed skiagraph plates illustrating the methods of localising bullets, and also specimens of extracted missiles. Major MacLennan's paper will appear as an original article in an early issue of the *Journal*.

CARE OF MENTAL DEFICIENTS.—The Glasgow District Board of Control met on 4th November under the presidency of Mr. James Cunningham. Twenty-two applications were submitted for the position of medical superintendent at Stoneyetts. On a vote Dr. Charles G. A. Chislett, at present deputy medical superintendent at Woodilee, was appointed.

Mr. Stephen J. Henry proposed that a committee be appointed to consider the question of additional accommodation for insane poor and mental deficients, and to report to the Board. He referred to the inadequacy of the accommodation in their different institutions, and said that for several years they had been running very close to the total amount available in Gartloch and Woodilee Asylums. The result was that they had been boarding out patients in other institutions, and that was not a condition of affairs that should be allowed to continue, as it meant that they had no control over those patients, for whom they were responsible. Owing to recent legislation the Board would have to deal with an increasing number of mental deficients, and they would not have the necessary accommodation to meet the demands that would be made upon them.

Mr. Low seconded, and the motion was adopted.

EDUCATION OF DEFECTIVE CHILDREN.—The second annual meeting of Phœnix Park Kindergarten Association was held at 600 Dobbie's Loan, Glasgow, on 14th November. Lady MacAlister presided. In the annual report, submitted by Miss M. A. Hannan Watson, it was stated that more than a year had passed since they started work in their proper surroundings, and they felt they had just cause for pride in their work. The work of the school was now fully developed. Two years ago they began with only a small number of children, and they thought it was best so, as it was important that the first pupils should be fully imbued with the spirit of the school, and serve as models to those who followed. Now there were 27 pupils on the roll, and the teachers felt that tradition had been established, and that work had become easier instead of heavier. The children were more capable, and in much better training.

Dr. Dyer, Chairman of Glasgow School Board, who moved the adoption of the report, complimented the Association on the pioneer work it had done. He emphasised the necessity for looking at the root problems involved, and said it was not sufficient to go on doing the work. They ought to consider why they were doing it, and why it was necessary. He wished to impress on the public of Glasgow and the teachers that, while it was their duty to do the best they could for the children, they had a much more difficult and important duty—to bring about conditions which would render such schools to a large extent unnecessary. If the parents were properly educated and did their duty, if the children had proper food, and if they lived under proper conditions, he was assured by all who knew anything about physiology and hygiene that in a very short time there would be very few defective children. The kindergarten, of course, only touched a very small part of a very large subject, and he hoped it would be used as the introduction to the study of larger problems.

CIVIL MEDICAL PRACTICE.—In view of the fact that further calls are now being made by the military authorities on the civilian medical practitioners for service with the Forces, the Scottish Medical Service Emergency Committee makes a fresh appeal to all retired medical men and other qualified persons who are willing to assist in the present crisis. The Committee has so far been successful in finding medical men to carry on the practices of their military colleagues during their absence, but in order to maintain an adequate supply of *locum tenens* additional names are required for registration. The Committee therefore invites all those who are able and willing to assist to send in their names without delay, giving at the same time full particulars as to qualifications, nature of practice preferred, &c. All communications should be addressed to the Convener, Medical Emergency Committee, Royal College of Physicians, Edinburgh.

Glasgow practitioners may at the same time be reminded of the appeal sent out in connection with the scheme of the Local Medical and Panel Committees for the Burgh of Glasgow, noticed in our November issue.

PROFESSIONAL CLASSES WAR RELIEF COUNCIL.—Directly the war broke out the distress expected to arise therefrom among the industrial population was anticipated and taken in hand by the establishment of the National Relief Fund. The response to the Prince of Wales' appeal was immediate and generous, with the result that there is little fear of irremediable upheaval of conditions among the industrial classes.

This fund, however, as everyone knows, makes grants only to the Local Distress Committees and the Soldiers' and Sailors'

Families Association. It does not, therefore, touch in any way the great distress already prevalent among the professional classes, for men and women of this class cannot appeal for help to the Local Distress Committees, who possess no adequate machinery for dealing with such cases. Yet these classes must necessarily suffer severely from the dislocation of business, and it is certain that the effects of the war upon the professions will continue to be felt for some time after the declaration of peace. In many instances distress has already arisen, and although the majority of the professions have their own benevolent funds, which must remain independent, and which are sure to be severely taxed, there is no centralised organisation or general fund to meet the conditions which already prevail. In view of this deficiency there has been formed during the last few weeks an organisation to be called the Professional Classes War Relief Council, with its headquarters in London. Representatives from the chief professional institutions, with representatives of the principal societies organising relief, have united in its formation, so that it is well acquainted with the circumstances and needs of each profession, and will be able to cover a wide ground. The intention is to assist by advice and indirect help rather than by monetary assistance. The benevolent funds of the institutions which represent the larger professions can give some financial help to their own members, and the Council does not intend to interfere in any way with the work of the committees controlling the various benevolent funds, but it thinks that considerable advantages will flow from bringing into close touch the professional institutions and the societies organising relief. The Council will also be in a position to organise certain special kinds of assistance in a way which will cause those funds to go further and do more ultimate good than would be possible without co-operation; while the risk of overlapping will be avoided. In the directions of education, training, maternity assistance, and the provision of temporary employment, it will be possible to deal with the family as a unit, and to help the dependents of professional men and women so as to promote their welfare in a more efficient and economical manner than would be possible by mere grants of money. The main object will be to bridge over the temporary difficulty caused by the war, and to pave the way to permanent profitable employment. The Council is under the provisional chairmanship of Major Leonard Darwin, and influential committees have been set up to deal with each of the departments of activity mentioned above. In connection with the department of maternity assistance, special mention may be made of the Maternity Nursing Home shortly to be opened at 13 and 14 Prince's Gate, London, kindly lent for the purpose by Mr. J. Pierpont Morgan. It is to be equipped with a voluntary medical and nursing staff of well-known medical men and women and of certificated nurses, and is to be open throughout the war to the wives of professional men for the sum of two guineas a week. · It is hoped in time to establish similar homes in the provinces, while to those for any reason unable to make use of the homes assistance will be given by the sending of free maternity nurses to their own homes, and also other help, such as layettes, &c., and arranging for free attendance by the local doctor. The secretaries for the scheme are Messrs. Theodore Chambers and Alexander Goddard and Mrs. A. C. Gotto, to any of whom subscriptions or donations may be sent at Kingsway House, Kingsway, London, W.C. The Maternity Nursing Home is also in need of articles of furniture, house and table linen, blankets, cutlery, plate, screens, bassinettes, and baby-cloths. Offers to provide these should be made to Mrs. Hills, 38 Prince's Gardens, London, S.W.

Co-operation of Trained Nurses.—The annual meeting of the Glasgow and West of Scotland Co-operation of Trained Nurses was held on 19th November in the Charing Cross Halls, Glasgow. Lady Stirling-Maxwell, president, occupied the chair. In their report for the past year the executive committee stated that the primary purpose of the association was to supply thoroughly trained and fully qualified nurses for those requiring their services, and at the same time to secure to nurses on the staff regular employment, adequate remuneration, and the advantages of a central home. At present there were 187 nurses on the roll. The number of cases attended during the year was 2,069, and the amount earned by the nurses £14,525. Since the outbreak of war, 62 nurses had volunteered for service in nursing the wounded. Some of these were now on the Continent, and a large number were engaged in the various district hospitals. Others were ready to give their services when required.

The approval of the report was moved by Sir Samuel Chisholm, Bart., who congratulated the Co-operation on the great progress it had made since its formation twenty-one years ago. Ex-Bailie J. W. Stewart seconded, and the report was adopted. On the motion of Colonel John A. Roxburgh, seconded by Dr. John Barlow, the office-bearers, including Mr. G. Wink Wight, C.A., as secretary, were re-elected, and Nurses Elizabeth Beaton, Farquhar, E. W. Miller, and Whincup were elected members of the executive committee in room of those who retired by rotation. Professor Glaister proposed a vote of thanks to the executive and medical committees, the honorary physicians and surgeons, the subscribers to the funds, and Miss Rough and her assistants. This was seconded by Dr. L. R. Oswald and agreed to. On the motion of Dr. W. L. Reid, chairman of the executive, Lady Stirling-Maxwell was thanked for presiding.

SANITARY SERVICES: CIVIL AND MILITARY CO-OPERATION.— The Local Government Board for Scotland has issued for the information of the local authorities a copy of instructions issued by the Army Council to Home Commands, directing that medical officers of health shall be informed of any proposed billeting in their districts, with a view to obtaining their expert advice and co-operation in billeting the incoming troops under the best sanitary conditions available. Medical officers of health are also to be consulted and their visits encouraged wherever camps are formed and maintained.

The object of these directions by the War Office, and of this circular, is to secure that the assistance which local authorities and their expert sanitary officers can give in connection with the sanitary condition of military quarters, the prevention of infectious disease, and other matters affecting the health of troops shall be fully utilised.

On 10th September the Board issued to all medical officers of health a circular letter, reproduced in our October issue, setting out the lines of action on which medical officers of health should co-operate with the military sanitary services.

The Board are confident that this work will be continued and extended, and in particular that local authorities will give every facility to the medical officer of health and the sanitary staff generally to carry out the close and continued oversight of the sanitary condition of billets and military camps.

Local authorities realise that at the present time it is essential that the civil and military authorities should work in the closest co-operation in preventing the spread of disease, and in removing all conditions which are favourable to the spread of disease. In some instances it may be necessary that the local authority should provide additional assistance for their officers in carrying out their duties.

After referring to the regulations adopted by the local authority for regulating the duties of the medical officer of health, the circular continues:—

The manner in which services can be rendered by the local authority and their officers necessarily varies with local conditions of military occupation, and with the arrangements already made for local co-operation with military authorities. There should be close co-operation between neighbouring authorities, so that no question of local boundaries may impair the assistance to be given to the troops.

The duties of the medical officer of health of a district or burgh in which troops are quartered should include—

1. Inquiring for, and bringing to the notice of the local authority, any conditions in which sanitary services can be rendered by them to the military population, *e.g.*, by extending water mains, opening or extending sewers, providing latrines or baths, providing hospital accommodation for cases of infectious disease, disinfecting clothing and blankets, destruction of refuse, making special arrangements for scavenging. Reports on these matters should be dealt with as urgent, and special meetings of the local authority should be called to consider them if necessary.

2. Inspecting systematically billets, and also camps or other places solely in military occupation, as regards the water supply, methods of disposal or removal of all solid and liquid refuse, general cleanliness, and for the prevention of exposure to infection.

3. Taking action by recommendations to the military authorities, by reports to the local authority, or otherwise,

with a view to the removal of any dangerous or objectionable conditions.

4. Giving information to the medical officer with the troops as to local cases of infectious disease as soon as they come to knowledge, and as to any localities, premises, bathing places, &c., which on health grounds should not be frequented by soldiers. In some districts troops will need to be cautioned against the consumption of sewage polluted shellfish.

5. Ascertaining what hospital provision is available for cases of infectious disease among troops in the district, and assisting in making arrangements for such provision. Existing civil resources should be made available to the greatest practicable extent for infectious cases among troops, care being taken not to diminish the accommodation for the civil population unduly.

The assistance desired by the War Office in the establishment of billets is of great importance.

When a medical officer of health of any local authority learns by an official intimation or otherwise that billeting is likely in his district he should at once communicate with the Chief Constable or Superintendent of Police, and obtain from him any further information of impending billeting which he may possess.

When the medical officer of health finds it necessary to make formal written recommendations, these should be addressed to the Deputy-Director of Medical Services, Scottish Command, Edinburgh. Usually these written communications should be restricted to matters of importance in which the medical officer of health, after local inquiry and conference, finds it necessary to put his advice on record. Copies of all formal written recommendations should be sent to the Board.

STATE INSURANCE: PANEL DOCTORS' PRESCRIPTIONS.—The Scottish Insurance Commissioners have issued a memorandum giving full particulars as to staff, salaries, and duties of a bureau for checking the prescriptions of Scottish panel doctors and the accounts of panel chemists, which it is proposed to establish in conformity with the recommendation of the conference of insurance committees held early in October. The bureau would be under the control of a joint committee representative of and appointed by the insurance committees.

Its staff would consist of a superintendent, assistant superintendent, 14 technical clerks as checkers, 10 ordinary clerks, 8 sorters, and a messenger, and its estimated cost, including office accommodation, printing, &c., is £2,800 a year. This expenditure would represent 1s. 10·4d. per 100 prescriptions (assuming 3,000,000), or 0·45d. per insured person (assuming 1,500,000).

From inquiries which the committee have made, both in England and Scotland, it is found that so far as the checking of prices is concerned a highly expert checker is able to dispose of about 10,000 prescriptions per week, and that a good average checker can dispose of about 6,000 within a similar period. To price as well as check the prescriptions would, of course, take longer, but it is thought that about 14 checkers would be sufficient for the pricing and carrying out of an analytical check of 3,000,000 prescriptions in Scotland. It is suggested that the most equitable method of distributing the cost of a central bureau would be to charge each insurance committee in proportion to the number of its prescriptions dealt with by the bureau. Each committee would thus contribute strictly in accordance with the amount of work performed on its behalf. Glasgow's contribution per year would be about £840 when the scheme was in proper working order, but for the first year £928.

A memorandum dealing with the scheme has been prepared for the Glasgow Burgh Insurance Committee by Mr. William Jones, its clerk. He explains that the proposal is to effect a combination of insurance committees, and to form a joint committee of control consisting of members of insurance committees. While nominally the proposed central bureau might be under the immediate direction of the joint committee, it might be anticipated that the Commissioners would retain to themselves such powers of approval as would make the joint committee more or less the instrument of the Commissioners. While nominally the combination would be one of insurance committees, it was proposed that doctors and chemists should make a proportionate contribution towards the cost of the bureau. Were they willing to do so they would naturally seek representation on the joint committee, and there would be created a new *ad hoc* body with a membership much in excess of the number suggested by the Insurance Commissioners. The volume of work which it is proposed that the staff should overtake suggested that the bureau would confine itself to the technicalities of correction, and chemists and committees alike would be asked to accept its results without question. The main feature of the new scheme was that it would be analytical as well as arithmetical. Under present conditions the burden falling upon the committee in connection with the check of the chemists' accounts represented less than 10 per cent of the funds available for the administration of medical benefit, as compared with 26 per cent on the basis of the new estimate. Whether the whole increase would fall to be borne by the committee was, of course, dependent upon the view of the doctors and chemists. Whatever the view of these bodies, the committee would not be relieved of the whole of its present charges, and its administration would be otherwise adversely affected. The committee should also keep in view that under the new financial arrangements their income for the administration of medical benefit was reduced by about £1,000 per annum. To incur additional expenditure in connection with the administration of that benefit was probably to involve them in financial difficulty.

The memorandum has been considered by the Sub-Committee on Medical Benefit, who disapproved of the scheme for the institution of a central bureau.

STATE INSURANCE: SANATORIUM BENEFIT IN ARGYLLSHIRE.— The National Health Insurance Committee for the county of Argyll met on 30th October in the Christian Institute, Glasgow. The Rev. M. M'Callum, Muckairn, chairman, presided. Reports of the sub-committees were submitted and approved. In the report of the Medical Benefit Sub-committee it was mentioned that the number of insured persons in the county was 18,122. The committee approved of a proposal to establish a sanitary bureau for the analysis and checking of chemists' accounts, on the understanding that the cost be chargeable in equal portions to the Insurance Committee, the Panel Committee, and the Pharmaceutical Committee, and that the funds of the committee for administration purposes be made sufficient to meet the increased charges upon it. It was reported that since the last meeting of the committee the applications of nine persons for sanatorium benefit had been referred to the County Council, and that the applicants were now receiving treatment at the cost of the County Council, the funds of the Insurance Committee for sanatorium benefit having been exhausted in September last. It was resolved, on the recommendation of the Sanatorium Benefit Committee, to enter into an agreement with the County Council, in terms of Section 64 of the National Health Insurance Act, whereby, in consideration of the committee paying over to the County Council the whole funds available to them for sanatorium benefit, the County Council should undertake to provide the treatment necessary for insured persons recommended by the Committee for Sanatorium Benefit, the arrangement to endure for a period of five years.

THE WELLCOME CHEMICAL RESEARCH LABORATORIES.—We are requested to intimate that Dr. Frederick B. Power will retire from the directorship of the Wellcome Chemical Research Laboratories on 1st December, in order to return to the United States of America, where, for family reasons, he will make his future home. His period of service dates from the foundation of these laboratories by Mr. Henry S. Wellcome in the spring of 1896.

The character of the research work carried out in these laboratories by Dr. Power and under his direction during these eighteen and a half years is so high that it has been truly said of him that he has, during the period of his administration, inaugurated a new era in his field of research in England.

Dr. Power will be succeeded by Dr. Frank L. Pyman, whose researches and contributions to chemical science are well known. The character and policy of the Wellcome Chemical Research Laboratories will continue as in the past.

CITY OF GLASGOW DOCTORS' AMBULANCE.—We are informed by Mr. J. Inglis Ker, secretary to the Scottish Motorists' Committee of the Red Cross Society, that the total amount subscribed to the City of Glasgow Doctors' Ambulance up to 18th November was £169, 15s. Should £300 be subscribed, the Transport Committee would undertake to provide an ambulance which could be depended upon to give every satisfaction, and Mr. Inglis Ker appeals to the profession to make up the deficit.

The medical profession of Glasgow has already contributed very generously to the various War Funds, and many of its younger members have given not only their money but themselves in aid of the cause for which we fight. But this is an appeal, the object of which has peculiar claims upon all those of the profession who cannot go to the front. An ambulance supplied and equipped by them, and representing them, is the nearest equivalent they can offer for personal service, and would bring them, at least in spirit, into closer touch with their colleagues and friends in the field. We trust that even before these lines appear in print the sum of £130 which is still lacking may be made up, and we are confident that the doctors of Glasgow will not suffer such a beneficent enterprise to perish for lack of support.

THE COLLEGE OF AMBULANCE.—There has recently been inaugurated at Nos. 3 and 4 Vere Street, London, a College of Ambulance, which has arisen out of the desire of those attending classes at the Polytechnic to present Mr. James Cantlie with a testimonial appropriate to the enormous labours he has devoted, and still devotes, to ambulance work. It is in accordance with Mr. Cantlie's own wishes that the testimonial has taken the shape of the establishment of this College, for which the buildings at Vere Street have been provided by Mr. James Boyton, M.P., free of rent for a period of twelve months. The object of the College is to form a centre for higher training in ambulance work, which shall comprise both a museum of ambulance, with models of appliances, waggons, field and other military hospitals, and also classes of instruction for medical men in ambulance work and drill. The College will hold examinations and give diplomas, the examinations being open to all who possess the necessary knowledge, wherever acquired. Those who hold certificates of existing ambulance associations will be granted from five to twenty per cent of the available marks necessary to obtain the diploma, according to the certificates they hold.

The College has an additional object, to be the headquarters of a "Humanitarian Corps," whose work shall be first aid in time of need. It is intended to meet sudden emergencies, and to act in advance of those bodies which are organised for the relief of destitution, but which, because their help must be preceded by enquiry, are unable to deal with an immediate necessity. Women and men will be eligible for the Corps, and a uniform and badge are issued by the central authority to those approved. It is hoped that representatives of the Corps may ultimately be found in every town and village, and the amount of good that could be done by the prompt assistance of such a body, not in money only, but in the distribution of food and in the provision of help and comforts for the sick in the remoter districts, must be at once apparent.

The constitution of the College has already been drawn up, and it is to be hoped that an institution for which there is so much room may shortly be in complete operation. Classes are now being held for first aid, home nursing, and hygiene, and also for bandaging, signalling, and drill, while special instruction is being given daily to those who intend going on active service. All communications are to be addressed to the secretary, Mrs. Colin MacDonald, 3 and 4 Vere Street, London, W.

ANÆSTHETICS IN WAR.—The following appeal, recently published in the *Glasgow Herald,* is of special interest to the medical profession:—"The fighting in the north of France and south-west of Belgium has been of such unprecedented severity, and the number of casualties so numerous, that an exceptional strain has been thrown upon surgical equipment, and this not the least upon the supply of anæsthetics. Hence there is a very real shortage in some of the hospitals across the Channel. Anæsthetics are essential not only to save the wounded from needless suffering, but also to diminish the shock of operation, and thereby increase the probability of recovery. The military hospitals under the direct control of the War Office are doubtless supplied adequately, but several other hospitals are already in urgent need. Information has been received through the French Red Cross, the Belgian Legation, and other official sources that some of the hospitals in Boulogne, St. Malo, Dunkirk, Havre, Calais, and other towns are running short of supplies, and should have their stocks replenished at once.

To these hospitals, and also to any in Great Britain and Ireland where need has come or may arise, we are desirous of sending chloroform, ether, and any other type of anæsthetic that they may be needing, together with apparatus for administration if wanted for use in the case of the wounded. It is desired to make a wide appeal to enable an emergency anæsthetic centre to be formed at once from which anæsthetics can be despatched at the shortest notice to hospitals in need. Donations should be sent to Mrs. William Sharp, hon. secretary, 49 Cambridge Street, Hyde Park, London, W., or to Mrs. D. M. Riddel, hon. treasurer, 15 Mount Street, Grosvenor Square, London, W.— (Signed) F. N. Maude, Colonel C.B. (late R.E.); D. M. Riddel, Vice-Admiral (retired); B. H. M. Riddel, Elizabeth A. Sharp."

FRENCH HONOURS TO THE ROYAL ARMY MEDICAL CORPS.— That the gallantry and devotion to duty of our medical officers in the field has been in accordance with the best traditions both of the army and of the medical profession is known to all of us through the unanimous testimony of war correspondents and of letters from the front. That they should have received signal recognition from our chivalrous allies is a source of deep gratitude to the profession as a whole, which feels that medicine is honoured in the persons of Major S. L. Cummins, M.D., who has been awarded the Cross of Officer of the Legion of Honour; of Captain G. E. Lewis, M.B.; J. T. M'Entire, M.B.; and H. S. Ranken, M.B., who have received the Cross of Knight of the Legion of Honour; and of the nine non-commissioned officers and men upon whom the Military Medal has been bestowed. The medical school of Glasgow has special cause to be proud of Captain H. S. Ranken, whose gallantry was such as to confer upon him not only the Cross of the Legion, but also the Victoria Cross. A medical correspondent of the *Times*, writing from Paris on 17th November, says of him :—" To-day the King has conferred the Victoria Cross upon an army doctor who, in a literal sense, gave his life for his friends. It was my good fortune to know Captain Harry Sherwood Ranken intimately during that period when we studied medicine together. The promise of these days has been fulfilled, for Ranken was of the very best type of British medical man, calm and fearless, and infinitely careful for those placed under his charge. During the supreme moments of his life, when he had been sorely wounded, that spirit of devotion made a hero of him; and laconic as is the official intimation—'for tending wounded in the·trenches under rifle and shrapnel fire at Hautvesnes on September 19 and on September 20, continuing to attend to wounded after his thigh and leg had been shattered'—it is enough." The heroism of Captain Ranken, though it reaped the sad reward of a noble death, will live as an inspiration to his comrades and successors.

RED CROSS SOCIETY.—The labours of the Scottish Branch of the Red Cross Society during the past month have been constant and strenuous, and it is good to know both that they have been productive of beneficent results and that they have been generously supported.

A report by Colonel M'Ewan at the end of October, relating to the goods despatched from St. Andrew's Hall, states that up to that date garments had been issued as follows:—To France, 27,592; to Belgium, 8,300; to Stobhill, 4,100; to the Navy, 2,800; and to various other outlets, 3,500—making a total of 46,292. In addition, there had been sent out 46 cases of books and magazines, 30,000 cigarettes, 60 lb. tobacco (a large proportion of these having gone to Stobhill), 10,000 bandages, and 2,000 splints, besides large quantities of foods, stationery, games, combs and brushes, razors, nail and tooth brushes, hot-water jars and hot-water rubber bottles, candles, soap, and many other gifts. For the Belgian wounded who had arrived at Stobhill it had been necessary to provide a very large quantity of clothing, the Red Cross Society supplying them with entire outfits, both in the hospital and for going out from it. Not less than £1,000 would be expended on this.

The Headquarters Organising Clothing Committee and the Countess of Eglinton and Winton's Committee for gifts in kind made an appeal for warm coats, ulsters, and dressing-gowns, also cardigan jackets, mufflers, helmets, gloves, mittens, body belts, and for surgeons' and nurses' operating gowns, at the same time thanking the public for their already generous response. Warm expressions of thanks to the Society for consignments of material were received from the French Ministry for Foreign Affairs and from the Belgian Government.

The Society also sent to Serbia a consignment of gifts in kind, which was much appreciated.

Early in November it was announced that the control of convalescent home and hospital accommodation in Scotland had been restored to the Scottish Branch of the British Red Cross Society, and that in the western district all offers of such accommodation should be made to Colonel R. D. M'Ewan, St. Andrew's Hall, Glasgow. It was proposed to establish an additional hospital of fifty beds at Carrick House, Ayr, and an appeal for funds was issued by Mrs. Oswald of Auchencruive, subscriptions to be sent to Mr. J. N. Robb, solicitor, Wellington Square, Ayr.

At a meeting of the Executive, held on 6th November, a report on the Scottish Hospital in France was submitted by Mr. N. P. Brown and Mr. Baird Smith, who had just returned from a visit to it. The personnel of the hospital had been quartered at Paris, while the equipment was at Rouen, an arrangement which was due to the fact that for some time there had been very few wounded at Rouen, and also, in the view of the deputation, to defective organisation of the Central Red Cross Committee in London. The negotiations of the deputation were ultimately successful in re-uniting at Rouen the personnel and the equipment of the hospital, which was to be employed as a unit at one of the military hospitals in the town, and before they left Rouen a large influx of wounded had given full employment to its staff. The motor unit, consisting of four ambulance and three motor lorries, had proved of much service in the transfer of wounded, and the deputation placed on record their sense of obligation to Mr. Anderson, of Paris, who had put the buildings and grounds of his linoleum factory at the disposal of the motor unit for the purpose of garage and housing the personnel. They expressed also their appreciation of the services of the Scottish Deputy Commissioner in France, Dr. C. E. Walker, to whom the directors of the Glasgow Cancer Hospital have given an extended leave of absence till the end of the year or longer if necessary.

An offer made by the directors of the North British Loco-motive Company of their administrative building at Springburn for use as a Red Cross Hospital has been accepted by the Executive. The building, which is well adapted for hospital purposes, is able to accommodate 150 patients, and will soon be in working order, being equipped and maintained by the Scottish Branch. It has been found impossible to make use of a number of the smaller private hospitals placed at the disposal of the Society, since each hospital train which comes north carries 100 wounded soldiers, and it is impracticable to deal with smaller units.

The hospital on Irvine Moor was in readiness for the reception of patients on 7th November.

Mrs. Brooman White, of Ardarroch, has issued an appeal to the county of Dumbarton for funds for a Dumbartonshire motor ambulance; and a movement, towards which over £400 have already been subscribed, has been set on foot in Coatbridge to provide a motor ambulance in the names of the Coatbridge Branches of the St. Andrew's Ambulance Association and Red Cross Society.

The Headquarters Organising Committee, in view of the colder weather, made in the middle of November a special appeal for knitted gloves and mittens, urging work parties to knit these instead of socks for the next few weeks.

On 16th November the members of the second detachment of personnel to staff the extension of the Scottish Red Cross Hospital at Rouen were received in the Municipal Buildings by the Lord Provost and Corporation, the Lord Provost conveying to them the best wishes of the Corporation and of the Red Cross Executive.

Sir George T. Beatson, chairman of the Scottish Branch, who addressed them at the request of the Lord Provost, said that the detachment was going out to a hospital already in working order. He had received a letter, dated 11th November, from Dr. Struthers, surgeon in charge of the Scottish Hospital at Rouen. Dr. Struthers wrote that on Saturday, 7th November, they took 42 patients into their three wards, which had been full since then. Each ward had 14 beds. There was plenty of room for the beds, and the general result was comfortable. The clinical work, Dr. Struthers added, was interesting, and mainly surgical. With regard to the Red Cross work, Sir George T. Beatson said that, taking everything into consideration, and looking to the very heavy demands made on the medical service of the Army, it was satisfactory to know that those demands had been very fully met, and to know that in no small measure that was due to the help given by the Red Cross Society. They were not a society that had been established to go and do work just where they liked. The principle of their Society was that it was supplementary to the medical service of the Army. The tendency, he knew, was for everybody to feel that they must rush. While that was natural, it led to confusion and overlapping and want of real efficiency. The great principle was that the Red Cross should only go forward to help when they were asked to do so by the military authorities. They asked them for that hospital and they gave it, and in those circumstances the Red Cross were welcome in France, and the military were doing everything they could to make them comfortable and give them a proper place. When he was over in France he had opportunities of seeing the means that were taken for the care of the wounded. He went through No. 8 General Hospital, Rouen, with General Woodhouse, Director of Medical Services for the Expeditionary Force, on a day when about 800 wounded had arrived, and he had no hesitation in saying, from what he witnessed there, that the British soldier was getting the best treatment that was going.

The party, who numbered twenty-two, and consisted of Dr. Charles M'Neill, eight nurses, and thirteen orderlies, left for France on the following morning.

On 20th November the headquarters of the Organising Committee issued a further appeal for sheets (sizes 96 in. by 60 in.), and pillow cases (25 in. by 16 in.), face and bath towels, games of all kinds, dressing gowns and warm coats, and all knitted garments, but especially for gloves and mittens, cuffs, lumbago belts, and mufflers. Large numbers of these garments were being despatched weekly from St. Andrew's Halls, Glasgow, to all the hospitals, both at home and in France, to re-equip the wounded soldiers and sailors when leaving, and also for use on the transport hospital ships. The committee asked that all requisitions for garments sent from the private hospitals and convalescent homes be made in tens instead of dozens in future.

The use of the rest stations has steadily increased from week to week. For the week ending on 14th November about 300 wounded soldiers were met on coming from the trains by the orderlies, their wounds were attended to, and they were conveyed by motor and other conveyances to their destination. Many comforts are supplied, and these have largely been received as gifts—biscuits from M'Vitie & Price, cocoa from Messrs. Cadbury, also Oxo and Camp Coffee. An interesting further use of the rest stations has developed. One lady has made her particular service that of conveying the wives of wounded soldiers to the hospitals to see their husbands, and the rest stations have proved a serviceable meeting place from which the wives are conveyed to the hospitals. Rest stations have also been used by convalescent soldiers visiting the city. Simple refreshments are supplied to them when required.

Donations for the "Scotch Lassie" motor ambulance are still wanted, and are being received by Miss Stewart Wright, 26 Lansdowne Crescent, Glasgow, and Miss J. Aitken, 53 Hamilton Drive, Hillhead, Glasgow.

Since the work began the following garments have been issued :—

To France, 52,500; to Belgium, 8,300; to Stobhill Hospital, 10,740; to the Navy, 4,200; to various other outlets, mainly local small hospitals and convalescent homes, 18,700; to Indian Hospital, 1,800; to Canadian Contingent Hospital, 310; and to Servia, 6,400—a total of 102,950.

In addition there have been sent out 60 cases books and magazines, 55,000 cigarettes, 95 lb. tobacco, 14,000 bandages, and 3,200 splints. Parcels which are not included in these figures continue to be sent to St. Andrew's Halls for "Stobhill." From notes in county branch reports it is indicated that they continue to send parcels direct to "Stobhill." It would be better that each of these were sent to St. Andrew's Halls, Glasgow; the record of garments would then be complete; every requisition which the hospitals send there is duly complied with. A large number of private hospitals and convalescent homes has been opened for the relief of the military hospitals, and to these considerable supplies of garments have been sent. The following is the list:—Mrs. Cunninghame, Craigends, Johnstone; Southwood, Stirling; Pollok House, Glasgow; Riding School, Hamilton; Royal Alexandra Infirmary, Paisley; Marchioness of Bute, Mount Stuart; Dalzell House, Motherwell; Hyndwood, Bridge of Allan; Drumpellier, Coatbridge; Falkirk Infirmary; Carrick

House, Ayr; Wallside, Falkirk; The Crescent, Ardrossan; Princess Louise, Roseneath; and Lady Eglinton's Hospital, Irvine.

Two motor ambulances for service at the front, which have been subscribed for by the Baptist churches in Scotland, were formally handed over to the British Red Cross Society (Scottish Section) at a meeting held in Adelaide Place Church, Glasgow. The Rev. T. W. Lister, Dennistoun, presided over a large gathering, which was representative of the Baptist denomination. The vehicles were received on behalf of the Red Cross Society by Major Fleming, who warmly thanked the donors in the name of the Society.

NEW PREPARATIONS, &c.

Maltona.—This is stated to be composed of Oporto wine with extract of malt. It is manufactured by a firm with its address in Glasgow, and is advanced for use in anæmia and debility. It is claimed to contain no drugs nor to be liable to create a habit. On sampling the wine it was found to have a pleasant aroma and taste, and to possess those characteristics that one associates with a good port wine.

Riedel's Mentor, 1914.—This is a well-bound book written in German. It is divided into four parts. Part I deals with technical and analytical work. Pharmaco-therapeutic work of the year 1913 is discussed in the succeeding part. The third part is arranged alphabetically, and gives the names and a short description of newer remedies and proprietary products. Finally, the special products of Riedel are described.

It is quite an interesting production, and exemplifies the enterprise of the German chemist.

From Messrs. James Spicer & Sons, Limited, London.

A sample of "Economic" antiseptic waterproof material, intended to take the place of oiled silk and mackintosh fabric for bandages and bed sheets. It is a khaki-coloured material, apparently consisting of thin cartridge paper, thoroughly waterproofed, tough, and difficult to tear, and at the same time very pliable. It can be supplied both in small sizes and in large-sized sheets, and would seem to be exceedingly useful for the purposes for which it is designed.

REVIEWS.

Quain's Elements of Anatomy. Eleventh Edition. Editors—
Sir EDWARD ALBERT SCHÄFER, LL.D., Sc.D., M.D., F.R.S.,
JOHNSON SYMINGTON, M.D., F.R.S., and THOMAS HASTIE
BRYCE, M.A., M.D. In Four Volumes. Vol. II, Part 2—
Splanchnology. By J. SYMINGTON. London: Longmans,
Green & Co. 1914.

QUAIN is so much a classic, and the editors of successive
editions men of such established reputation, that it seems
almost unnecessary to say what an excellent account of the
viscera this volume gives. One could wish, however, that in
many instances the account were more exhaustive. There
seems a tendency, for example, to ignore alternative views,
which in a book of this character might well be included, since
Quain is as much a book of reference as a text-book ; and while
there is some attempt to include a bibliography, it is so
hopelessly incomplete that one questions if it would not have
been wiser to omit it altogether. Unfortunately, too, as it
seems, it is just in those sections of the volume on the subject of
which much work is at present being done that the references
are most defective.

While one recognises the good qualities of this volume, the
descriptions of the various viscera are far from uniformly
excellent; and while, for example, the account of the
peritoneum, of its pouches, folds, and abnormalities, is splendid,
the section dealing with the ductless glands can only be
described as poor. Why, even from the meagre account given,
all description of the pituitary gland is omitted, and one is
referred for this to another volume, is quite incomprehensible.
Surely it matters little whether the body in question lies in the
skull or the abdominal cavity: if it is a ductless gland it should
be described with the other comparable structures. There is in
this section for some reason a lamentable incompleteness; why,
it is difficult to understand, since much of the work on ductless

glands is recent and therefore easily accessible. As an example of incompleteness, the description of the parathyroids is striking, almost no reference being made to the many variations in their position, some account of which, at least, is given in every student's text-book. Under spleen, too, one finds much to cavil at. The description of the renal surface as flat, the slumping of the pancreatic impression with the base, the cheerful assumption that arterial capillaries open into the pulp spaces directly, the complete absence of all mention of Wall's excellent account of the spleen lobules—all leave one with the impression that at least this section might have been improved by careful revision.

Here, too, while there is no mention of the so-called scapular body, the equally dubious cardiac glands are described as if they were old and tried friends.

One finds, however, with satisfaction that some attempt to bring the topography of the stomach into line with skiagraphic findings has been made. While this is the case, one cannot but regret that it has not been more thoroughly carried out, and that the geometrical factor in the apparently contradictory findings is not emphasised. It may be that in this, a subject to which one has given careful consideration, one is apt to be hypercritical, but it seems unfortunate that the difference between a solid and its projection is not mentioned. Among other defects might be mentioned the incompleteness of the description of the so-called ligaments of the uterus, the lack of colour in the illustrations, and in many of these, too, the unfortunately flat impression they give. One could wish also that some of the illustrations had been larger, and others smaller; for example, that the large and very diagrammatic sections of the lower abdominal cavity, which recur so frequently, were smaller, and that some of the really excellent reproductions of frozen sections were larger.

In the space at one's disposal it has been impossible, of course, to do more than record in a more or less impressionist manner one's opinion of this volume, and if this account of it seems to describe only the faults, it is because they are rendered the more obvious by contrast with the many excellencies of the work, and because Professor Symington has achieved so much that one cannot but wish he had achieved more.

Quain was so long a classic, so long the "best" text-book on anatomy, that it is with the utmost regret one comes to the conclusion that, even in the slightest degree, the idol is less stable on its pedestal.

The Dietetic Treatment of Diabetes. By B. D. BASU, Major, I.M.S. (retired). Fourth Edition. Allahabad: The Panini Office. 1913.

THE popularity of Major Basu's little volume is sufficiently attested by its having reached a fourth edition in the brief space of four years. It will be found by those who are unfamiliar with it to be a compendium not only of the practice but of the theory of the dietetic treatment of diabetes, and although for Occidental readers much that is said of the value of Indian food-stuffs is superfluous, there yet remains much that must prove of value to those embarrassed with the difficult problem of affording the diabetic an adequately varied diet.

Pain: Its Origin, Conduction, Perception, and Diagnostic Significance. By RICHARD J. BEHAN, M.D. New York and London: D. Appleton & Co. 1914.

THIS elaborate work is the result of Dr. Behan's conviction that the significance of pain is in a diagnostic sense very frequently misunderstood, and represents his endeavour to collect in one volume all that is known of the nature and significance of pain. With this end in view, he has laid under contribution the fruits of a very extensive acquaintance with the literature—how extensive may be seen from the bibliography with which his volume ends—and he has brought to the analysis of his great stores of material no small amount both of critical and constructive faculty.

The first part of the book deals with general considerations, and is divided into chapters devoted to sensation in general, the nature and distribution of pain, the perception of pain-sensation, the classification of pain, and the intensity of pain. The author then passes to the consideration of pain in connection with diseases of the nervous system, of the muscles, the bones, the circulatory system, and the glandular tissues. He next takes up the subject of regional pain, and this discussion is followed by chapters on pain in the organs of special sense written by representative members of the Vienna medical school. Pain in the abdominal wall and in the abdominal viscera next receives attention, and upon this follows a consideration of pain in the genito-urinary system, and, finally, of thoracic pain due to diseases of the heart or lungs. The treatment of every subject is very thorough, and in each section much is to be found which is of profit to the physician or surgeon.

The illustrations, whether diagrammatic or photographic, are numerous and technically excellent, but there would seem to be no good reason for the prevalent American custom of using photographic illustrations of the female nude figure for the purposes of a scientific work.

Diagnosis of the Malignant Tumours of the Abdominal Viscera. By Professor RUDOLF SCHMIDT. Translated by JOSEPH BURKE, M.D. London : William Heinemann (Rebman, Limited). 1913.

THIS book is much to be commended for the light it throws upon what is often an exceedingly difficult subject. The diagnosis of malignant abdominal tumours is too often allowed to rest upon mere probabilities, and many unnecessary laparotomies are the consequence. No doubt the diagnosis can always be certainly made as the result of operation, but it is too little remembered that laparotomy is in itself a shock, and if its only result is to discover an inoperable tumour, it can do nothing but harm to the individual patient. In order that an operation should be successful, accurate and early diagnosis is required; and it is no small achievement of Professor Schmidt's that he has produced a volume which is calculated to be exceedingly helpful in many a doubtful case. His book is divided into a general and a special part, the former dealing with abdominal examination and with the bacteriology, symptomatology, and etiology of malignant abdominal disease, while the latter discusses the special diagnosis of malignant affections of the several abdominal organs. Following these two parts there comes a series of illustrative case-histories, to which frequent reference is made in the text, and which constitutes a valuable feature of the book. The translator, though in other respects he has done his work well and accurately, has unfortunately adhered too closely to the German idiom for the achievement of an easy English style; but, in spite of this drawback, the volume may be commended to the careful study of the diagnostician.

Abel's Laboratory Handbook of Bacteriology. Second English Edition, Translated from the Fifteenth German Edition by M. H. GORDON, M.A., M.D., B.Sc. London: Henry Frowde and Hodder & Stoughton. 1912.

THIS is one of the Oxford Medical Publications. It can be carried in the pocket, and, considering its size, contains a great deal of information most useful to the laboratory worker. Incorporated with the translation is an account of some recent methods in use in this country.

After a chapter each on the microscope, sterilisation and disinfection, nutrient media, culture methods and staining methods, there is an account of the special media for, and the cultivation and staining of, a list of some twenty-nine organisms, including yeasts and moulds. The chapter on "Methods of obtaining material from the body" is revised and amplified by Dr. Horder, and that on "Methods of examining the blood in relation to immunity" is edited by the translator. "Inoculation and *post-mortem* examination of animals," and "Methods of preserving preparations, cultures, and organs" are each the subject of a chapter. The chapter on the examination of water, milk, sewage, &c., is revised and amplified by Dr. Houston, and, similarly, that on the examination of dust and air, by the translator.

Some of the translated English is rather laboured, and we would take exception to one or two of the abbreviations, *e.g.*, "B.i." for the influenza bacillus, "B.ty." for B. typhosus, "aq.

com." for—what? And so far as we have seen there is no explanation of the meaning of a *plus* and *minus* sign occurring together in some of the tables. On p. 117 it is stated that B.ty. does not change the colour of neutral-red glucose-agar; and lower down on the same page the fermentation of this sugar is cited as a means of differentiating it from the dysentery bacillus.

Transactions of the American Surgical Association. Vol. XXXI. Edited by ARCHIBALD MACLAREN, M.D. Philadelphia: Wm. J. Dornan. 1913.

THIS volume of *Transactions* for the year 1913 contains many interesting papers in different fields of surgery.

Fractures, congenital dislocation of the hip, amputations, blood-vessel surgery, surgery of the thyroid gland, and diseases of the sigmoid flexure are among the subjects considered.

It is to reports like these that the surgeon must turn when desirous of becoming acquainted with the best work of our American *confreres,* and we can assure him that he will find much profitable reading within the covers of the present volume.

Tuberculin in Diagnosis and Treatment: A Text-Book of the Specific Diagnosis and Therapy of Tuberculosis. By Dr. BANDELIER and Dr. ROEPKE. Second English Edition. Translated from the Seventh German Edition by W. B. CHRISTOPHERSON. London: John Bale, Sons and Danielsson. 1913.

"BANDELIER and Roepke" bids fair to become in its English dress as indispensable to the tuberculin therapist in this country as the speedy exhaustion of seven German editions shows it to have become in Germany. The second English edition, ably translated by Mr. Christopherson, puts in the hands of English workers a complete compendium of the diagnostic and therapeutic uses of tuberculin. Beginning with a discussion of the theoretical basis of the tuberculin reactions and of tuberculin therapy, the authors pass to a general consideration of the application of the tuberculin tests with their indications and contra-indications, and then treat of their particular application in diseases of the different organs of the body. The remainder of the book is occupied with the subject of tuberculin therapy, general principles being first discussed, and the merits of the various tuberculin preparations considered in detail. The authors give the preference to bacillary emulsion (tuberculin B.E.) for therapeutic use. The special section on the treatment of pulmonary and other forms of tuberculosis follows, and the volume ends with a bibliography useful for German literature, but containing very little reference to English publications. The illustrations showing the appearances of the cutaneous and percutaneous reactions, and the charts showing the courses of cases treated by tuberculin, form a valuable addition to the book, which may be warmly commended to all interested in tuberculin therapy.

Surgery of the Vascular System. By BERTRAM M. BERNHEIM, A.B., M.D. With 53 Illustrations in Text. London: J. B. Lippincott Company. 1913.

THIS book is intended to be a practical and suggestive aid to surgeons interested in the surgery of the vascular system, and the author has, by taking for granted a fundamental knowledge of the conditions to be treated, attempted to make the text as simple as possible.

In a historical note prefixed to the volume, the author points out that previous to the work of Carrel blood-vessel surgery comprised chiefly the treatment of aneurysms. Nowadays the subject has widened to include the repair of injured blood-vessels, transplantation of arterial or venous segments, anastomosis, and direct transfusion of blood.

The various chapters deal with these subjects, beginning with a consideration of general technique. Transfusion is then taken up. The methods of Crile and Elsberg are described, and are followed by the details of the author's method by a two-pieced tube. End-to-end suture, lateral anastomosis, transplantation of a segment of vein or artery, and reversal of the circulation by arterio-venous anastomosis come in for lucid and detailed description. We note the author's preference for lateral anastomosis, a procedure which he supports by good reasoning.

A chapter on varicose veins, which seems to be comparatively of minor importance, follows, and the concluding pages are devoted to aneurysms. Following on a description of treatment of aneurysms is a *revue* of the results of operation by different methods on aneurysms of the large arterial trunks. This chapter is freely furnished with statistical tables, and these with the comments thereon are of great interest and value.

The volume is most interesting, and it cannot fail to help those engaged in or about to take up blood-vessel surgery. The descriptions throughout are simple and easily comprehended. The illustrations are numerous and well executed.

Modern Problems in Psychiatry. By ERNESTO LUGARO. Translated by DAVID ORR, M.D., and R. G. ROWS, M.D. With a Foreword by Sir T. S. CLOUSTON, M.D., LL.D. Second Edition. Manchester: At the University Press. 1913.

THIS is in every way a most admirable translation of a remarkable work by "one of the master spirits of biological science, who, while knowing and using the details and facts of his subject, is not content with a narrow and technical view of it, but has pressed into its elucidation all the correlated sciences of anatomy, physiology, biology, and psychology. Lugaro seems to me," proceeds Sir T. S. Clouston in his highly instructive and eulogistic foreword, "to have been able to set the whole problem of psychiatry before his mind, to have realised its extraordinary difficulties, and to have pointed out future lines of research more clearly and fully than almost any of our modern authors. He combines caution with scientific enthusiasm. . . . He is reliable and practical, while retaining the subtle mental qualities of his race. . . . One cannot read the book without receiving an overpowering impression of the author's love of truth and of his intense craving to get nearer to solid ground in the abstruse questions with which psychiatry abounds."

" We Britons," concludes Sir Thomas, " needed such a clear, logical, and illuminating treatise. Even its abundant theorising will stimulate us to think. It is wider in its scope and more philosophical in its methods of treating the subject than any book of our own. In short, it exhibits more of the scientific spirit. All our alienists and most of our physicians will do well to peruse it."

Mental Diseases : A Text-book of Psychiatry for Medical Students and Practitioners. By R. H. COLE, M.D., M.R.C.P. London: Hodder & Stoughton. 1913.

IT has been the author's aim in this volume concisely to delineate the general features of psychiatry in such a manner that the subject may appeal to the student and general practitioner rather than to the specialist. He therefore prefixes to his account of abnormal mentation an analytic description of the normal processes of mind, from which he proceeds to discuss the general diagnosis and etiology of insanity, and afterwards describes its various clinical forms. Their relation to general diseases is then considered, and a chapter on the pathology of insanity follows. The next chapter is devoted to the subject of prognosis, then comes a chapter on the legal relations of insanity, and, lastly, a chapter on general treatment. The order in which the subjects are handled is thus a little promiscuous, and it is difficult to see the justification for interpolating a consideration of legal considerations between the subjects of prognosis and treatment. That part of the book which deals with the special forms of insanity is undoubtedly the best; the descriptions are clear and they are emphasised by excellent illustrations. The section devoted to normal mental processes borders, of course, upon the domain of philosophy, but is hardly sufficiently philosophical to help the student very far in his endeavour to comprehend the human mind. The remarks upon general diagnosis are too brief, and rather suggest notes for a chapter on the subject than the completed chapter. Taken as a whole, the book, while conveying in a limited compass a fair and temperate statement of the forms of insanity, yet fails to leave any very arresting picture of them upon the mind's eye.

ABSTRACTS FROM CURRENT MEDICAL LITERATURE.

———

EDITED BY ROY F. YOUNG, M.B., B.C.

———

MEDICINE.

The Treatment of Hæmoptysis in Pulmonary Tuberculosis.

By N. B. Burns, M.D. (*Boston Medical and Surgical Journal*, 17th September, 1914).—The author considers the following points of importance :—

1. Absolute rest.
2. Immediate lowering of the blood-pressure.
3. The determination of blood to other parts of the body, this calling for (*a*) application of cold to thorax ; (*b*) purgation.
4. Positive assurance to the patient that he is in no danger.

The patient is placed flat on his back unless the hæmorrhage is extreme, in which case he should be turned on his side, the diseased lung being uppermost and the head hanging over the edge of the bed. Nitro-glycerine ($\frac{1}{100}$ gr.) is given immediately, and an ice bag placed on the chest for not more than one hour at a time. Cracked ice should be given by the mouth until the initial excitement is past. Magnesium sulphate is then administered in full doses unless there are positive contra-indications. The author emphatically discourages the use of morphia as tending to increase the pulmonary congestion, and failing to diminish, if it does not increase, the blood-pressure. In the after-treatment diet should be non-stimulating, and the cough checked by suitable drugs.

—David MacDonald.

Syphilis of the Lungs.

By E. A. Burnham, M.D. (*Boston Medical and Surgical Journal*, 10th September, 1914).—The author considers that in the differential diagnosis of diseases of the lungs the possibility of a syphilitic basis has been too much neglected. In its early stages syphilis produces acute pulmonary conditions like bronchitis and broncho-pneumonia ; but its most frequent occurrence is in the tertiary stage, when its lesions produce physical signs which are identical with those of pulmonary tuberculosis. Certain of the objective signs are dissimilar ; hæmoptysis is more frequent in tuberculosis, the temperature curve in syphilis is not so variable, and the loss of flesh and strength are not so rapid and marked ; the patient with syphilis does not appear to be so ill as one with a tubercular infection of the same extent. In syphilis the majority of the author's cases have shown lesions in the lower lobes. The absence of bacilli in the sputum, together with the presence of any of the stigmata of syphilis, and especially with a positive Wassermann reaction, should make the diagnosis certain.—DAVID MACDONALD.

SURGERY.

Wounds and Their Treatment. By G. K. Dickinson (*American Journal of Surgery*, October, 1914).—The author points out in the course of a discussion on the histology of wound-healing that the destroyed tissues furnish products which act as auxetics for cell-division. Microbes kill devitalised tissues, putrefactive organisms then provide auxetics, and thus "through death we live." The profound attraction of white cells ends in an excess, and pus is produced.

Organisms entering a wound are to be eliminated and controlled, but they are not to be driven more deeply into the damaged part. Antiseptics may be as injurious to tissues as micro-organisms. Tincture of iodine and potassio-mercuric iodide, however, disturb cell-life very slightly, yet potently influence germs. The action of yeast is proteolytic, while it is also chemotactic. The author quotes a case in which an abdominal operation-wound on the third day began to show gangrene at the margins, and the patient's condition was becoming desperate. The part was irrigated with an emulsion of yeast-cake, and afterwards packed with some of the yeast plant which had been softened in water, and healing then went on rapidly.

The author refers also to the use of citrated saline solution in cases of slowly healing wounds, in order to dissolve out fibrin and unnecessary leucocytes, and to the stimulating effect of applying freshly-drawn blood to the seat of ununited fractures.—CHARLES BENNETT.

Two Acute Abdominal Cases which Necessitated Extensive Removal of Bowel. By H. J. Godwin (*The British Journal of Surgery*, October, 1914).—The first patient was a girl of 8 years who had been subject to attacks of abdominal pain, with vomiting, since she was 2 years old. Recently she was admitted to hospital, having had pain, vomiting, and constipation for three days. On admission the temperature was 99°, pulse 116, and respirations 24. Abdominal distension was present, there was tenderness in the right iliac region, and signs of free fluid were made out. A mass was felt in the pelvis on rectal examination. Laparotomy revealed a mass of almost gangrenous small intestine twisted on its mesentery, while attached to the mass was a mesenteric cyst with a cord of blood-vessels. Four feet of intestine was involved, and this having been removed, entero-cæcal anastomosis was performed. Recovery was uninterrupted.

The second was a man of 27 years of age, who became ill with abdominal pain and vomiting, but did not take to bed ; nor did he seek medical advice until the fourth day, and then he walked six miles to his doctor, who sent him to hospital next day. Despite the virile condition of this patient, sufficient signs of abdominal mischief were found to make operation necessary. The appendix was gangrenous, and the necrotic process was so extensive that appendix, cæcum, and 6 inches of ileum had to be removed. This was followed by ileo-colostomy. The patient made a good recovery.—CHARLES BENNETT.

DISEASES OF THE EYE.

Some Emergencies in Ocular Therapeutics. By A. Darier, Paris (*The Ophthalmoscope*, August, 1914).—This paper, read before the Oxford Ophthalmological Congress, in July of this year, contains the author's opinions on the latest work in ocular therapeutics. He considers radium of great value in various kinds of tumours, and of analgesic and neurasthenic power in neuralgias and paralyses.

Salvarsan is not an absolute specific for syphilis ; but this "does not any the less prevent it from being the best of the antisyphilitic remedies, complimenting most happily" treatment by mercury and iodides. It is also a cure for traumatic or post-operative infections and sympathetic ophthalmitis.

The new salt of quinine, introduced recently by Morgenroth, possessing a special tropism for the pneumococcus, he has found reliable in pneumococcal ulcers of the cornea. It is also of value in gonococcal conjunctivitis, and in dendritic keratitis, through an "obvious bacteriotropic action."

This author has frequently laid great stress on the collateral or para-specific action of medicaments. He considers that sera, in addition to their specific action, exercise a marked influence upon lymphocytosis, polynucleosis, phagocytosis, and possibly other actions not yet understood. It is the influence of these different factors which shows the importance of the para-specific or collateral action of therapeutic agents. Such stimulation of the general defences of the organism in different infective processes is obtained with antidiphtheritic serum, yeast serum (Deutschmann), mycolysine, staphylase (Doyen), cultures of lactic bacilli or of coli-bacilli (Massol, Taponnier), metallic ferments, nuclein, &c.

In all infective diseases early interference is of the greatest importance to secure if possible an *abortive action.* Invaluable time is lost by awaiting the results of a bacteriological report. In these cases para-specific sero-therapy should be employed, while awaiting to administer to the patient the specific antitoxins and bacteriolysins indicated by the subsequent bacteriological report. In some cases the truly specific agents may not be required; in any case the action of the "specific remedies is greatly enhanced, the ground having been well prepared by para-specific therapy."

A passing reference to the work of Sir Almroth Wright fails to show whether the author now employs the opsonic index or not.

In ocular tuberculosis he considers that tuberculins exert a favourable action in the majority of cases. A series of questions are suggested on the action of tuberculins for inquiry from every ophthalmic surgeon in the country.

Reference is also made to the work of Wassermann on eosin and colloidal selenium in cancer.—W. B. INGLIS POLLOCK.

An Improvement in Local Anæsthesia in Operations upon

the Eye. By G. H. Pooley, Sheffield (*The Ophthalmoscope*, August, 1914).—
In this paper, read before the Oxford Ophthalmological Congress in July of this
year, Pooley describes his method of obtaining complete anæsthesia by a retro-
bulbar injection of a 1 per cent solution of alypin. The procedure was first used
for the removal of prolapsed iris in traumatic cases; and in cases in which large
pieces of steel had to be removed with the magnet. Since then the author has
used the method in all intra-ocular operations.

The iris and ciliary body contain a large number of sensory nerves, which
leave the eyeball by the long and short ciliary nerves. The latter enter the ciliary
ganglion in two groups. It is situated to the outer side of the optic nerve. The
shortest route for reaching this region is also from the external side of the
eyeball.

The conjunctival sac should be prepared in the usual manner' for an intra-
ocular operation. If time is not of importance a 5 or 10 per cent solution of
cocaine should be instilled at intervals of thirty, twenty, and ten minutes before
operation. If time is of importance a crystal of solid cocaine may be placed on
the fold of conjunctiva which is to be injected first. A graduated hypodermic
syringe with a specially strong needle has been made by Messrs. Weiss.

The formula is as follows :—

Alypin, ...	gr.	$15\frac{1}{3}$
Sod. chlor., ...	,,	12
Sol. adren. chlor. (1-1,000), ...	minim	10
Aq., ... ad	℥	$3\frac{1}{2}$

Three or four minims are first injected halfway between the cornea and
the fornix. The needle is again introduced at the outer fornix above or below
the insertion of the external rectus muscle. A few minims are injected
before the needle is pushed in the direction of the posterior pole of the eyeball.
Fifteen to 60 minims are then injected.

In non-inflammatory cases 15 to 30 minims are quite sufficient, while 30 to
60 minims are required for inflammatory cases. In eviscerations more than 60
minims may be necessary. The author has employed the procedure in 47 cases.
Apart from pulling on the recti muscles patients were unaware of any sensation.
In one very nervous patient a light general anæsthetic had to be given
in addition.

As regards complications, vomiting has occurred in 1 case of glaucoma, in 3
cases of cataract extraction, and in 1 case of evisceration. The vomiting was not
so severe nor so prolonged as that after general anæsthesia. It occurred in very
nervous patients. One patient had vomited after extraction of her other lens
under cocaine alone. There were no ill effects on the eye, except in 1 case of an
old blind glaucomatous eye, in which there was some hæmorrhage into the lips
of the wound. No permanant damage was done.

There was no obvious proptosis in any of the cases, although a slight proptosis
occurred in a case in which 70 minims had been injected for evisceration. No
toxic effects have been noted.—W. B. INGLIS POLLOCK.

PUBLIC HEALTH AND INFECTIOUS DISEASES.

Chemo-Immunological Studies on Localised Infections (Fourth Paper): Experimental Pneumococcic Meningitis and its Specific Treatment. By Richard V. Lamar, M.D. (*Journal of Experimental Medicine*, Vol. XVI, No. 5, 1912).—The experimental pneumococcic meningitis is produced by the injection of virulent pneumococci into the cranial or spinal cavities of monkeys, and a method of treatment is indicated by which its almost invariably fatal termination may be prevented.

In the experimental disease 0·1 c.c. of a 24-hour broth culture of virulent pneumococci commonly produced an inflammation of the meninges, and particularly of the pia mater, attended by bacteræmia. The inflammation became quickly purulent and fibrinous in character, extended readily from the cerebral to the spinal meninges and *vice versa*, and was so regularly attended by certain definite general symptoms that the whole constituted a definite disease entity.

The influence of treatment with immune serum is considered. A large quantity of immune serum, many times that required to protect a rat against the same quantity of culture as the monkeys received, was used. The eleven experiments show that immune serum has a distinct, though only slight, restraining influence upon infection. When administered within two hours it prevented the occurrence of infection in two instances. When given later a first injection seemed usually to restrain infection, but the restraining action was of short duration, the disease quickly developing into its usual course and producing death. An even apparently beneficial action of subsequent injections was rare. Thus, the serum was utterly powerless to stop an infection once well begun, and to prevent the death of the animal.

The next experiments deal with the influence upon treatment of a mixture of sodium oleate, immune serum, and boric acid. Each cubic centimetre of this mixture contained 0·1 c.c. of a 1 per cent aqueous solution of Merck's or Kahlbaum's sodium oleate, 0·2 c.c. of immune anti-pneumococcic serum, and 0·7 c.c. of a 5 per cent aqueous solution of boric acid. As in the experiments with immune serum, usually 2 c.c. of the freshly prepared mixture was injected once a day during the life of the animal, or until the spinal fluid gave no, or very little, growth of pneumococcus. Of the nineteen cases treated it was usual to notice an improvement in the physical condition, a clearing of the spinal fluid, and a reduction in the number of diplococci. This was true particularly of the first injection, which was usually followed by a disappearance of the bacteria in the circulating blood, and not only in these instances where recovery occurred, but also often even in those which terminated fatally. The subsiding of the bacteræmia is probably due not only to the control of the local infection, but also to the action of immune principles which have diffused from the cerebro-spinal fluid into the general circulation. The mixture of sodium oleate, immune serum, and boric acid exerted regularly a more powerful action than immune serum alone, and not only prevented the occurrence of infection, but also, when administered repeatedly, arrested the progress of an actually established infection, and led often to the enduring and perfect recovery of the inoculated animal.

—J. P. KINLOCH.

A Contribution to the Epidemiology of Poliomyelitis. By Simon Flexner, M.D., Paul F. Clark, Ph.D., and Harold L. Amoss, M.D.

(Journal of Experimental Medicine, Vol. XIX, No. 2, 1914). A strain of the poliomyelitic virus was propagated in monkeys for four years, during which time it displayed three distinct phases of virulence. The several phases covered different periods of time. At the outset the virulence was low, but by animal passages it quickly rose to a maximum. This maximum was maintained for about three years, when, without known changes in the external conditions, a diminution set in, and increased, until at the expiration of a few months the degree of virulence about equalled that present at the beginning of the passage in monkeys. The cycle of changes in virulence is correlated with the wave-like fluctuation in epidemics of disease, which also consist of a rise, temporary maximum, and fall in the number of cases prevailing. And an explanation of epidemics of disease is inferred in variations or mutations among the micro-organismal causes of disease, affecting chiefly the quality of their virulence.

—J. P. KINLOCH.

A Contribution to the Pathology of Epidemic Poliomyelitis. By Simon Flexner, M.D., Paul F. Clark, Ph.D., and Harold L. Amoss, M.D.

(Journal of Experimental Medicine, Vol. XIX, No. 2, 1914).—Epidemic polio-myelitis is a general disease affecting mainly the nervous system. Apparently the virus is not stored in the peripheral nerves, but seeks the parenchymatous nervous organs in which to multiply. The virus has been demonstrated by inoculation tests, not only in the spinal cord, but in the brain and in the inter-vertebral, Gasserian, and abdominal sympathetic ganglia.

All the ganglia show histological lesions, more or less severe, similar to those of the spinal cord and brain. The severest occur in the intervertebral ganglia, those next in severity in the Gasserian, while the mildest appear in the abdominal sympathetic ganglia. The interstitial lesions predominate over the parenchy-matous, and in pre-paralytic stages the intervertebral ganglia show interstitial lesions, especially pronounced at the pial covering.

The virus of poliomyelitis is highly resistant to glycerin, in which it survives for more than two years; to 0·5 per cent phenol, in which it survives for more than one year; while it succumbs after having been kept frozen constantly for several months.

It is unsafe to employ phenol to modify the virus of poliomyelitis for the purpose of active immunisation.

The cerebro-spinal fluids of convalescents tend to be devoid of the neutralising principles for the virus of poliomyelitis, although they may exceptionally be present within this fluid.—J. P. KINLOCH.

A Note on the Etiology of Epidemic Poliomyelitis. By Harold L. Amoss, M.D.

(Journal of Experimental Medicine, Vol. XIX, No. 2, 1914).—The globoid bodies or minute micro-organisms cultivated by Flexner and Noguchi from the central nervous organs of human beings and monkeys that have succumbed to epidemic poliomyelitis may be detected in the incubated brain tissues of infected monkeys in forms indicating *post-mortem* multiplication. Incubating the poliomyelitic tissues in kidney-ascitic fluid culture medium, and then crushing them, is a more certain method of obtaining cultures of the organism.

Identical bodies have been detected in blood films prepared on the twelfth day of the acute attack from a paralysed poliomyelitic monkey inoculated intraspinously.

The same organism has been cultivated from the blood of a monkey that had received intravenously a large dose of Berkefeld filtrate of poliomyelitic virus. No other micro-organisms were detected either in the sections of the brain or in film preparations of the blood. These observations tend to confirm the etiological relationship between the minute micro-organism and epidemic poliomyelitis, suggested by the successful cultivation and inoculation experiments of Flexner and Noguchi.—J. P. KINLOCH.

Intraspinous Infection in Experimental Poliomyelitis. By Paul F. Clark, Ph.D., and Harold L. Amoss, M.D. (*Journal of Experimental Medicine*, Vol. XIX, No. 2, 1914).—The routes by which the virus of polio-myelitis may be conveyed to the central nervous organs of monkeys, so as to produce infection and paralysis, are various, but not of equal certainty. The direct intracerebral injection yields the most constant results, next to which the intrasciatic and intranasal have been placed. Infection by way of the peritoneal cavity, subcutaneous tissues, and blood is obtained with far less certainty.

By intraspinous injections of specimens of poliomyelitic virus of suitable virulence infection can be caused regularly in Macacus rhesus monkeys.

The virus passes from the subarachnoid spaces into the nervous tissues, in which it multiplies, and into the blood.

The constant involvement of the pia-arachnoid membranes in this infection, even when no paralysis occurs, and the fact that infection can readily be produced by intraspinous inoculation, suggest anew that in the pathogenesis of poliomyelitis and interstitial tissue changes within the meninges, blood-vessels, and ground substance play a determining part.

While the virus injected into the subarachnoid spaces can be demonstrated there by inoculation tests forty-eight hours after the injection, it can no longer be detected on the sixth day, at a time when the first symptoms of infection make their appearance. The failure of the cerebro-spinal fluid from human and experimental cases of poliomyelitis to produce the disease when inoculated into monkeys is due to the fact that the virus is either fixed by the nervous tissues or passes into the blood.—J. P. KINLOCH.

The Relation to the Blood of the Virus of Epidemic Polio-myelitis. By Paul F. Clark, Ph.D., Francis R. Fraser, M.B., and Harold L. Amoss, M.D. (*Journal of Experimental Medicine*, Vol. XIX, No. 3, 1914).—The subject of the relation to the blood of the virus of poliomyelitis is of more than theoretical interest, as it may have a bearing on the manner of transmission of the disease.

Specimens of human blood taken during the paralytic stage of the disease and *post-mortem* have proved incapable of infecting Macacus monkeys.

Specimens of monkey blood taken at various stages of experimental polio-myelitis have not proved, as a rule, to be capable of infecting monkeys. In a single instance among ten tests, infection was secured with a specimen of blood removed at the beginning of the paralysis on the seventh day following an intracerebral inoculation.

When specimens of the spinal cord of a paralysed monkey have been injected into the brain, or simultaneously into the brain and spinal canal, the blood removed from one to forty-eight hours later fails to cause paralysis after intra-cerebral injection.

When large volumes of active filtrate are injected into the circulation the blood remains infective for seventy-two hours at least, but may not be infective when paralytic symptoms appear after ten days. When, however, the filtrate is injected in smaller amount, or when a filtrate of a less active virus is employed in large quantity, the blood either fails to convey the infection or conveys it irregularly.

It is only when overwhelming quantities of an active virus are injected into the blood that paralysis results. The injection of moderate doses is not followed by paralysis, although the virus may still be detected in a blood sample twenty-four hours after the injection. The existence of a mechanism capable of excluding the virus within the blood from the central nervous organs is therefore inferred.

Infection is accomplished far less readily through the circulation than by means of the more direct lymphatic and nervous channels of communication with the central nervous system.

Several series of feeding experiments conducted with the biting stable fly (*Stomoxys calcitrans*) resulted negatively.—J. P. KINLOCH.

Books, Pamphlets, &c., Received.

Urgent Surgery, by Félix Lejars. Translated from the seventh French edition, by William S. Dickie, F.R.C.S. (Third English impression.) With 20 full-page plates and 1,086 illustrations, of which 729 are drawn by Dr. E. Dalune and A. Leuba, and 198 from original photographs. Vol. I: Introductory — Head — Neck — Chest—Spine — Abdomen. Bristol: John Wright & Sons, Limited. 1914. (25s. net.)

The Practical Medicine Series. Under the general editorial charge of Charles L. Mix, A.M., M.D., and Rodger T. Vaughan. Series 1914. Chicago: The Year Book Publishers. (Price of ten vols., $10·00.)

Vol. IV—Gynecology, edited by Emilius C. Dudley, A.M., M.D., and Herbert M. Stowe, M.D. ($1·35.)

Vol. V—Pediatrics, edited by John Ridlow, A.M., M.D., with the collaboration of Charles A. Parker, M.D. ($1·35.)

Vol. VI—General Medicine, edited by Frank Billings, M.S., M.D., and J. H. Salisbury, A.M., M.D.

Indispensable Orthopædics: A Handbook for Practitioners, by F. Calot. Translated from the sixth French edition, by A. H. Robinson and Louis Nicole. With 1,252 original figures and 8 coloured plates. London: Baillière, Tindall & Cox. 1914. (21s. net.)

Life: Its Origin and Energy Mechanism, by Jadroo. London: Henry Kimpton. 1914. (1s. net.)

Quain's Elements of Anatomy. Eleventh edition. Editors, Sir Edward Albert Schäfer, LL.D., Sc.D., M.D., F.R.S., Johnson Symington, M.D., F.R.S., and Thomas Hastie Bryce, M.A., M.D. In four volumes. Vol. II., part II—Splanchnology, by J. Symington. With 349 illustrations. London: Longmans, Green & Co. 1914. (10s. 6d. net.)

Oxford Medical Publications. The Heart in Early Life, by G. A. Sutherland, M.D., F.R.C.P. London: Henry Frowde and Hodder & Stoughton. 1914. (6s. net.)

A System of Clinical Medicine dealing with the Diagnosis, Prognosis, and Treatment of Disease, for Students and Practitioners, by Thomas Dixon Savill, M.D.Lond. Fourth edition, thoroughly revised. London: Edward Arnold. 1914. (25s. net.)

The Blood: A Guide to its Examination and to the Diagnosis and Treatment of its Diseases, by G. Lovell Gulland, M.A., B.Sc., M.D., F.R.C.P.E., and Alexander Goodall, M.D., F.R.C.P.E. With twenty-eight text illustrations and sixteen coloured plates. Second edition. Edinburgh: Wm. Green & Son. 1914. (15s. net.)

Human Derelicts: Medico-Sociological Studies for Teachers of Religion and Social Workers, edited by T. N. Kelynack, M.D. London: Charles H. Kelly. 1914. (5s. net.)

Rose and Carless's Manual of Surgery for Students and Practitioners. Ninth edition. Revised by Albert Carless, M.B., M.S.Lond., F.R.C.S. University series. London: Baillière, Tindall & Cox. 1914. (21s. net.)

Hospital of the Protestant Episcopal Church in Philadelphia: Medical and Surgical Reports of Episcopal Hospital. Vol. II. Philadelphia: Wm. J. Dornan. 1914.

Cunningham's Manual of Practical Anatomy. Revised and edited by Arthur Robinson. Sixth edition. Vol. II—Thorax, Head, and Neck. With 267 illustrations in the text, and 11 plates. London: Henry Frowde and Hodder & Stoughton. 1914. (10s. 6d. net.)

Forensic Medicine and Toxicology, by J. Dixon Mann, M.D., F.R.C.P. Fifth edition. Revised and enlarged by William A. Brend, M.A., M.B., B.Sc. With frontispiece, plates, and 25 text illustrations. London: Charles Griffin & Co., Limited. 1914. (18s. net.)

Medical Nursing, by A. S. Woodwark, M.D., B.S. Lond., M.R.C.P. Lond. London: Edward Arnold. 1914. (4s. 6d. net.)

The Soldier's English and French Conversation Book, containing hundreds of useful sentences and words, enabling the British soldier to converse with the French and Belgian Allies, with the correct pronunciation of each word, an indispensable aid to the British soldier. Compiled by Walter M. Gallichan. London: T. Werner Laurie, Limited. (9d. net.)

A Text-Book for Midwives, by John S. Fairbairn, M.A., M.B., B.Ch.Oxon., F.R.C.P.Lond., F.R.C.S.Eng. With 3 plates and 104 Illustrations, 5 in colour. London: Henry Frowde and Hodder & Stoughton. 1914. (10s. 6d. net.)

GLASGOW.—METEOROLOGICAL AND VITAL STATISTICS FOR THE FOUR WEEKS ENDED 21st NOVEMBER, 1914.

	WEEK ENDING			
	Oct. 31.	Nov. 7.	Nov. 14.	Nov. 21.
Mean temperature, . .	47·2°	49·9°	47·0°	34·7°
Mean range of temperature between highest and lowest,	12·4°	8·8°	8·7°	7·5°
Number of days on which rain fell, ...	6	6	7	1
Amount of rainfall, . ins.	0·85	0·54	1·27	0·06
Deaths (corrected), . .	332	327	308	334
Death-rates, ...	16·5	16·3	15·3	16·6
Zymotic death-rates, . .	1·1	1·5	0·9	1·4
Pulmonary death-rates, .	4·0	3·4	4·6	3·6
DEATHS—				
Under 1 year, . . .	87	65	63	75
60 years and upwards, .	75	84	78	72
DEATHS FROM—				
Small-pox, ...	...	...	...	...
Measles, ...	2	5	2	1
Scarlet fever, . . .	7	7	5	8
Diphtheria, ...	4	4	3	9
Whooping-cough, . .	9	9	6	9
Enteric fever, . . .	3	...	1	2
Cerebro-spinal fever, . .	...	1	...	1
Diarrhœa (under 2 years of age),	14	13	7	6
Bronchitis, pneumonia, and pleurisy, . . .	56	53	72	53
CASES REPORTED—				
Small-pox, ...	...	...	...	...
Cerebro-spinal meningitis, .	1	1	2	1
Diphtheria and membranous croup, ...	46	42	44	50
Erysipelas, . . .	49	34	44	40
Scarlet fever, . . .	145	162	245	185
Typhus fever, . . .	...	...	...	...
Enteric fever, . . .	5	6	5	13
Phthisis, ...	41	51	33	29
Puerperal fever, . .	4	2	5	3
Measles,* . . .	24	27	30	20

* Measles not notifiable.

SANITARY CHAMBERS,
GLASGOW, 26th November 1914.

INDEX.

———o———

GLASGOW: PRINTED BY ALEX. MACDOUGALL.

The
Glasgow Medical Journal

EDITED BY

G. H. EDINGTON and W. R. JACK

WITH THE ASSISTANCE OF

R. F. YOUNG (Sub-Editor of "Abstracts")

A. J. BALLANTYNE
J. BROWNLEE
R. M. BUCHANAN
E. P. CATHCART
F. J. CHARTERIS

L. FINDLAY
A. A. GRAY
R. MUIR
E. H. L. OLIPHANT
J. R. RIDDELL

GLASGOW: ALEX. MACDOUGALL, 70 MITCHELL STREET
LONDON: H. K. LEWIS, 136 GOWER STREET, W.C.

All communications regarding Advertisements for this Journal are to be addressed to Mr. W. COWAN, 136 Buchanan Street, Glasgow

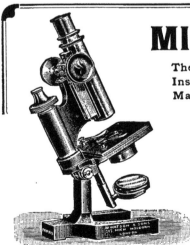

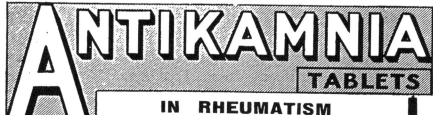

IN RHEUMATISM
AND NEURALGIA

In the administration of remedies to relieve **Pain**, the element of exhilaration should be considered, as many produce such delightful sensations as to make them dangerous to use.

Such is not the case with **Antikamnia Tablets.**

They are simply pain relievers—not stimulants—not intoxicants. Their use is not followed by depression of the heart.

In cases of **Acute Neuralgia**, tested with a view of determining the analgesic properties of Antikamnia, it has been found to exceed any of its predecessors in rapidity and certainty of the relief given. **Neuralgia, Myalgia, Hemi-crania,** and all forms of **Headache, Menstrual Pain,** &c., yield to its influence in a remarkably short time, and in no instance has any evil after-effect developed. Strongly recommended in Rheumatism. The adult dose is one or two tablets every one, two, or three hours. To be repeated as indicated. All genuine tablets bear the *AK* monogram.

TO TREAT A COUGH. Antikamnia & Codeine **Tablets** are most useful. It matters not whether it be a deep-seated cough, tickling cough, hacking cough, nervous cough, or whatever its character, it can be brought under proper control by these tablets. To administer **Antikamnia & Codeine Tablets** most satisfactorily for coughs, advise patients to allow one or two tablets to dissolve slowly upon the tongue and swallow the saliva. For night coughs, take one on retiring.

ANALGESIC.   ANTIPYRETIC.   ANODYNE.

Antikamnia Tablets, 5-gr.
Antikamnia & Codeine Tablets.

Supplied in 1-oz. packages to the Medical
Profession.

THE ANTIKAMNIA CHEMICAL COMPANY,
46 Holborn Viaduct, LONDON.

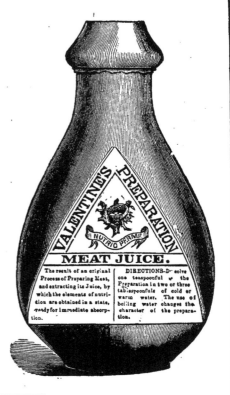

Lightning Source UK Ltd.
Milton Keynes UK
UKHW012200210219
337686UK00016B/1338/P